Betty B. Alford
Texas Woman's University

Margaret L. Bogle
Arkansas Children's Hospital

with a contribution
by Claire Zane

NUTRITION DURING THE LIFE CYCLE

Prentice-Hall, Inc., Englewood Cliffs, New Jersey 07632

Library of Congress Cataloging in Publication Data

ALFORD, BETTY B.
Nutrition during the life cycle.

Includes bibliographical references and index.
1. Nutrition. I. Bogle, Margaret L.
II. Title.
QP141.A613 613.2 81-19927
ISBN 0-13-627810-8 AACR2

Interior designed by F. Hubert
Cover by Wanda Lubelska Design
Manufacturing Buyer: Harry P. Baisley

Printed in the United States of America

10 9 8 7 6 5 4 3 2

ISBN 0-13-627810-8

PRENTICE-HALL INTERNATIONAL, INC., *London*
PRENTICE-HALL OF AUSTRALIA PTY. LIMITED, *Sydney*
PRENTICE-HALL OF CANADA, LTD., *Toronto*
PRENTICE-HALL OF INDIA PRIVATE LIMITED, *New Delhi*
PRENTICE-HALL OF JAPAN, INC., *Tokyo*
PRENTICE-HALL OF SOUTHEAST ASIA PTE. LTD., *Singapore*
WHITEHALL BOOKS LIMITED, WELLINGTON, *New Zealand*

contents

preface

ONCE WE ACQUIRE BASIC NUTRITIONAL KNOWLEDGE, the next step is to apply that information to individuals. This book has been written to increase understanding of the physiological, biochemical, and sociological factors that affect nutrient requirements and recommendations over the life cycle. It emphasizes practical applications, and includes appropriate food selections to meet nutrient needs. The text is designed to assist the student in acquiring the skills and knowledge necessary to translate the science of nutrition into the improvement of the nutritional status of individuals and groups. Although the book is intended for a course in life cycle nutrition as a part of the preparation of nutrition professionals, other health care professionals with basic nutrition knowledge should find it useful in working with clients.

Many texts provide information on the role of specific nutrients. Our intention is not to duplicate them, but rather to emphasize practical applications relating to food choices and selections to meet nutrient needs. Because of the current interest in nutrition research, the student is urged to keep up with the literature to augment the text.

The interrelationships of social, psychological, physiological, and biochemical factors and their impact on nutrient requirements and recommendations for food intake during specific stages of the life cycle are presented in each chapter to alert the reader to the influence of the total environment on an individual. The appendix includes the most up to date standards and recommendations of experts in the area of nutrition, as well as learning aids for the reader. Significant information from various authorities is charted or included in boxes for ease in comparing data.

The life cycle approach was chosen because of the relationship of nutrient needs to growth and development. Section I includes five chapters on specific stages of the life cycle—infancy, childhood, adolescence, the adult years and the later years. Considerations for adequate nutrition during each period are discussed. Implications for meeting the needs of each age are presented. Chapter summaries help the reader review the material and suggest areas in which further study and research are needed. The references at the end of each chapter include basic and clinical research, with both recent and classical work.

Section II, Chapters 7 through 12, discusses nutritional concerns common to all ages. In order to apply nutrition knowledge to the counseling of individuals and groups, a health professional must make an assessment of nutritional status.

Chapter 7 presents assessment methods for communities, groups, and individuals, giving specific techniques for practical as well as research activities in this area. Chapter 8, "Physical Fitness, Athletics, and Nutritional Needs," discusses a popular area of nutrition that has been dominated by much faddism and misinformation. The material in this chapter is presented in a manner calculated to help the reader distinguish fact from fiction. Weight control probably receives more attention than any other area of nutrition at all stages of the life cycle. Chapter 9 discusses weight reduction, fat theories, anorexia nervosa and regimens for gaining weight. The consumption of alcohol and the use of drugs have known influences on nutritional status from the fetus through the later years. Chapter 10 discusses alcohol and some of the more common drugs in relation to food intake and changes in nutritional status. The reader is directed to references giving extensive coverage to other drugs. Chapter 11, "Nutrition and Dental Health," discusses the relationship of nutrition to the development of good teeth and the influence of poor dental health on nutritional status. The prevention of dental caries is highlighted.

The final chapter is devoted to nutrition education, which is the element necessary to achieve and maintain good nutrition throughout the life cycle. Specific suggestions for methods, techniques, and the information needed at various ages include consideration of the total environment of the learner.

Acknowledgments

The support of co-workers, friends, and family was vitally important to the completion of the book. Special thanks go to Ms. Carmen Roman-Lopez, who used an initial draft of the text in a class she was teaching, Nutrition in the Life Cycle, at the Texas Woman's University. She made excellent suggestions for improvement that we incorporated into the final draft.

Mrs. Eloise Jackson was more than a typist. She assisted in proofing and organizing all the details related to the preparation of a book. Her patience and the attention to detail surely made the process easier.

Ms. Ann Blankenship, an Allsup-Lane Scholar at the Texas Woman's University, assisted with the obesity section of the weight control chapter.

Because writing a book took so much time, our families gave the most. My husband, Joe Alford, and my sons, Mark and Matthew Alford, endured having every holiday and vacation taken up with my writing.

My husband, Bill Bogle, my sons, Mark and Mike Bogle, and my daughter, Laurie Bogle, not only endured my writing at home, but the endless trips to Denton for manuscript preparation, review, and revision. A note of special appreciation to my former co-worker, Irma Shepherd, who encouraged us to write this book and provided lodging and personal support.

Betty B. Alford
Margaret L. Bogle

CHAPTER 1

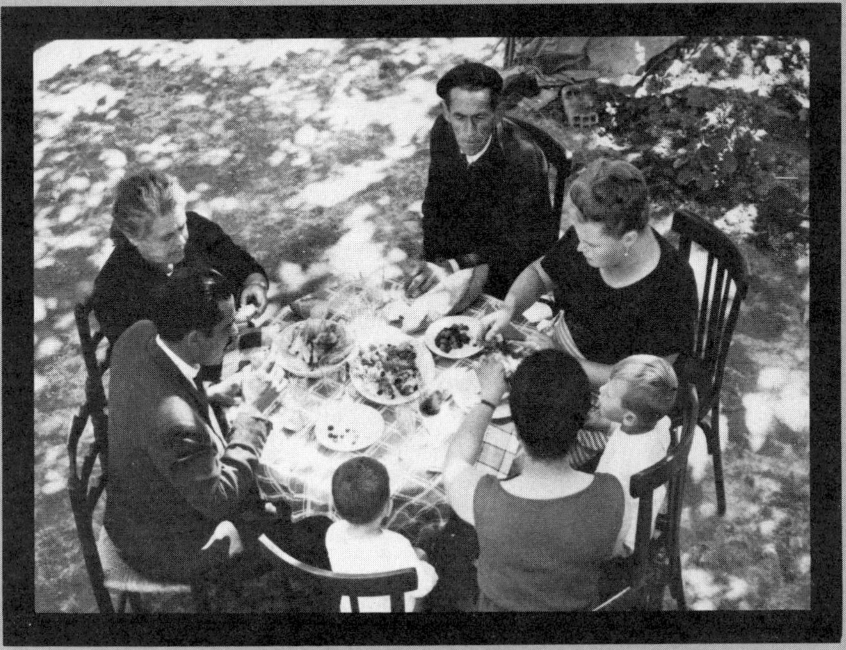

WHO photo by P. Almasy

introduction

NUTRITION HAS AN IMPACT AT EVERY STAGE OF THE LIFE CYCLE. This impact can be marked or subtle, but it is always present. Most of us are aware of the marked effects—we have all seen photographs of children in developing countries suffering from the effects of malnutrition and of diseases related to inadequate diet. But there are more subtle effects as well, effects that do not appear for many years and that we are beginning to know about now as better health care, immunization, and improved sanitation allow more people to live far longer than they did even less than a century ago.

Since 1900, the death rate has declined from 17 per 1000 people to less than 9. Mortality from many diseases such as tuberculosis, diphtheria, and poliomyelitis has been sharply reduced (see Table 1–1). Life expectancy in the developed countries is now 74 years, compared to 47 in 1900. Much of the increase in longevity is due to the reduction in the death rate, and especially to the sharp reduction in infant mortality in this century. But for us to make further progress, we will need to pay more attention to improving our health habits, including nutrition, and to following life styles that promote health and well-being (1).

In America today, thanks to the popular media, we are becoming more aware that what we eat makes a difference, and that we should devote as much attention to the quality of our food as we do to other aspects of our lives. But often, because of all the information we have at our disposal, and because of the promotion of fads and cure-alls, it is hard to make intelligent choices from the vast array of foods we have available to us. Millions of dollars are wasted each year on "health foods" and nutrient supplements; millions of people go from one kind of diet to another, each time hoping or believing that they have found the secret of health and long life.

SOURCES OF INFORMATION

In fact, we do have most of the basic information we need for sound nutrition. The two most useful tools for applying the science of nutrition are the Basic Food Groups and the Recommended Dietary Allowances (RDA). These were developed from data acquired through nutrition research. Both are based on the fact that nutrient and energy needs vary among individuals according to genetic makeup, the stage of the life cycle, and the state of health.

TABLE 1-1. Causes of Death by Life Stages, 1977

problem	INFANTS (UNDER 1) rank	INFANTS (UNDER 1) rate[a]	CHILDREN (1–14) rank	CHILDREN (1–14) rate[b]	ADOLESCENTS/YOUNG ADULTS (15–24) rank	ADOLESCENTS/YOUNG ADULTS (15–24) rate[b]	ADULTS (25–44) rank	ADULTS (25–44) rate[b]	ADULTS (45–64) rank	ADULTS (45–64) rate[b]	OLDER ADULTS (OVER 65) rank	OLDER ADULTS (OVER 65) rate[b]	TOTAL POPULATION (ALL AGES) rank	TOTAL POPULATION (ALL AGES) rate[b]
age groups														
Chronic Diseases														
Heart disease			7	1.1	6	2.5	2	25.5	1	351.0	1	2334.1	1	332.3
Stroke			8	.6	9	1.2	8	6.1	3	52.4	3	658.2	3	84.1
Arteriosclerosis											5	116.5	9	13.3
Bronchitis, emphysema, and asthma									10	12.2	8	69.3		
Cancer			3	4.9	5	6.5	1	29.7	2	302.7	2	988.5	2	178.7
Diabetes mellitus					10	.4	10	2.4	8	17.8	6	100.5	7	15.2
Cirrhosis of the liver							7	8.6	4	39.2	9	36.7	8	14.3
Infectious Diseases														
Influenza and pneumonia	5	50.6	6	1.5	8	1.3	9	3.0	9	15.3	4	169.7	5	23.7
Meningitis			8	.6										
Septicemia	6	32.7												
Trauma														
Accidents														
Motor vehicle			2	9.0	1	44.1	3	23.1	7	18.3	10	24.5	6	22.9
All other	7	27.7	1	10.8	2	18.4	4	18.5	5	25.5	7	78.1	4	24.8
Suicide			10	.4	3	13.6	5	17.3	6	19.1			9	13.3
Homicide			5	1.6	4	12.7	6	15.6						
Developmental Problems														
Immaturity associated	1	407.7												
Birth associated	2	294.4												
Congenital birth defect	3	253.1	4	3.6	7	1.6								
Sudden infant death	4	142.8												
All causes		1412.1		43.1		117.1		182.5		1,000.0		5288.1		878.1

[a] Rate per 100,000 live births.
[b] Rate per 100,000 population in specified group.

SOURCE: *Healthy People, The Surgeon General's Report on Health Promotion and Disease Prevention, 1979.* U.S. Dept. of Health, Education and Welfare, Public Health Service, No. 79–55071.

The food groups emphasize a variety of foods in the diet. No one food has all the essential nutrients in appropriate amounts or combinations for total nutrient needs. No single food is good or bad, but must be related to the contribution it makes to the total nutrient needs.

The RDA's provide a means of identifying specific nutrient needs of populations. Although the allowances are for a day, the average daily nutrient intake may be obtained over several days. The allowances are revised at five-year intervals based on knowledge obtained through research.

The USRDA are an adaptation of the RDA's for use in nutrition labeling based on the adult male allowances. The nutritional quality of a food is defined in a number of ways as seen in Table 1–2.

Of course, because our knowledge is not yet complete and because we need much more applied and developmental research (2), there is still controversy among scientists working in the nutrition field. Human nutrition involves not only the foods we eat, but the way in which the foods are grown and processed, the social environment in which we live, and our own individual metabolic systems. Changes in any one of these systems can have an effect on health. Since all nutrients and processes are not of equal importance in the health equation, it is often difficult to distinguish between cause and effect. In this book, we will attempt to provide factual information about nutrition in each phase of the life cycle so that informed applications of the research can be made to individual needs. The role of nutrition in the maintenance of good health will be stressed. It will provide information to enable individuals to make better food choices based on fact, not fiction.

The nutritionist must help others distinguish among sound nutrition concepts, hypotheses, and new areas of research, as well as undocumented statements (3). Some qualified nutrition scientists feel the public should be made aware of desirable changes in food intake even when we do not have proof that there will be a real benefit (4); others feel we should wait until all the evidence is in before suggesting that people change their habits. The most recent controversies involve polyunsaturated fats and cholesterol, sugar, and sodium. The differences are best illustrated by comparing the statements made in the Dietary Guidelines (USDA) and in *Toward Healthful Diets* (National Academy of Sciences). Many of the major themes are similar including eating a variety of foods and control of obesity. The differences arise from the emphasis on reduced cholesterol, sodium, and sugar intake for the entire population. Few experts disagree that these elements should be reduced for individuals at risk of specific diseases. General statements are not appropriate when linking nutrition factors with disease.

Nutrition, as we have said, is important to health—but it cannot solve all health problems. Some diseases, such as scurvy, pellagra, and beri-beri, are directly related to nutrition. Many diseases, however, are not caused or cured by changes in nutrition, although nutrition may be a factor in susceptibility or control.

TABLE 1-2. Defining the Nutritional Quality of Food

source	bases and/or purpose of deriving definition	definition
Federal Trade Commission	Nutrient Density Concept/1974 proposed Trade Regulation Rule on Food Advertising—nourishment claims	"An advertisement shall not represent food to be "nourishing," "wholesome," or "nutritious," or use any other term of similar import which in any way states, suggests, or implies that such food is a valuable or significant source of nutrition, unless a serving of the food contains at least four nutrients, including protein each of which is present in an amount of at least 10 percent of the U.S. RDA per 100 calories, and unless at least one of such nutrients is present in a serving of such food in an amount of at least 10 percent of the U.S. RDA."
Department of Agriculture		
Agriculture Research Service	1976 House Agriculture Hearings	Any food that has the potential for nourishing the body is considered nutritious.
Food and Nutrition Service	1978 proposed rule to define foods not to be sold in competition with lunches served under the National School Lunch Program	Foods of low nutritional value are those that do not make a positive nutritional contribution in terms of their overall impact on children's diets, dietary habits and appetites. These foods include soda water, frozen desserts, candy and chewing gum.
	Nutrient Density Concept/1979 proposed rule to define foods not to be sold in competition with lunches served under the National School Lunch Program	Limit the sale of any food which does not have at least five percent of the U.S. RDA for one or more of eight basic nutrients. The excluded foods are certain candies, chewing gum, soda water, and water ices.
Food and Drug Administration	RDAs/1973 nutritional labeling standards to aid consumers in making food selection.	Nutritional quality not specifically defined, except to provide for nutritional information on food labels when the food has been fortified by one or more nutrients that were not present or were present in small amounts in the food before processing and/or when nutritional claims are made.
Society for Nutrition Education	Nutrient Density Concept. Recommendations on the 1974 FTC's proposed Trade Regulation on Food Advertising—nourishment claims.	For a food to be called "nutritious" it should contain either (1) at least four nutrients in equal proportion to its energy (calories) or (2) at least two nutrients in double proportion to its energy contribution.

TABLE 1-2. (Continued)

source	bases and/or purpose of deriving definition	definition
Guarth Hansen, Professor of Nutrition, Utah State University	Nutrient Density Concept	A food is nutritious if it has at least four nutrients in equal proportion to calories for the leader nutrients intrinsically present. Leader nutrients are the nutrients commonly listed on the food label. Intrinsically present would be nutrients present in the foods when they are picked or grown.
Center for Science in the Public Interest		A nutritious food is one that contains no more than 10 percent of total calories from added sugar, 20 percent from added fat and oil, less than 0.5 percent added salt, and no artificial coloring or sodium nitrate; products containing any grain should be made from whole grain (not refined flour).

SOURCE: United States Government Accounting Office Report, 1980.

Nutrition during the Life Cycle: A Preview

Another factor in good nutrition is that humans have different nutritional needs at different points during the life cycle and in different life situations. Growth and atrophy or decay occur at the same time throughout life for everyone, but growth predominates in the early years and atrophy in the later years, and change is constant. Systematic change **(development)** occurs with age; it begins with conception and ends with death. We usually think of development as growth, as an increase in overall size. But body proportions can change without development: the accumulation of fat and water retention, for example, can contribute to weight gain without any growth.

The three major aspects of development are growth, differentiation, and morphogenesis (5). **Differentiation** is the change in a cell from a simple to a more specialized or complex cell. Differentiation is most rapid in the early months of fetal life, although it continues throughout life. **Morphogenesis** is the process by which the adult body and organs are formed. This process is controlled by genetic potential as well as environmental factors, so that rate of growth as well as final adult size vary from individual to individual.

Humans develop biochemically as well as structurally; chemical components of the body change in amount and in relative concentration. At any point in the life cycle, both structural and biochemical changes can be affected by nutrition, as we will see in the chapters of this book.

Section I of this book includes a brief discussion of social, psychological and physiological needs at various stages of the life cycle: infancy, childhood, adolescence, adult years, and the later years. Each chapter presents the interrelationships among physiological, biochemical, and sociological factors and their impact on nutrient requirements and recommendations. The role of nutrition in the maintenance of health is stressed.

Section II includes chapters on important nutritional concerns and problems common to all stages of the life cycle. Chapter 7 discusses techniques for measuring and evaluating nutritional status at all ages. Once status has been determined, the concepts of normal nutrition can be applied. Physical fitness and nutritional needs for athletic performance are currently receiving much publicity and interest. Chapter 8 discusses many of the fad ideas that have developed in this area and gives research support for a more realistic approach. Chapter 9 presents current knowledge and controversies surrounding obesity and weight control. In addition, problems of undernutrition and anorexia nervosa are discussed. Although anorexia nervosa is primarily a condition found in teenage girls, it can occur in males and at other times in the life cycle, like obesity. Consumption of alcohol and other drugs may have definite deleterious effects on the nutritional status throughout life through deprivation of food, toxic effects, or interactions with nutrients that render them useless. Chapter 10 covers these topics and presents concepts the student should be able to use in understanding the relationship of nutrition to drugs and alcohol.

Chapter 11 discusses the relationship between nutrition and the formation of strong teeth and healthy gums. In addition, it presents current information on dental caries as they relate to poor food habits and nutrition. Nutrition education, as discussed in Chapter 12, is a means of bringing the concepts of nutritional science to persons of all ages. Application of sound nutritional practices is the major thrust of this text. Chapter 12 presents the techniques to make this happen for individuals and groups.

references

1. *Healthy People,* The Surgeon General's Report on Health Promotion and Disease Prevention. DHEW (PHS) 79-55071, Washington, D.C., 1979.

2. HABICHT, J. "Translation of Scientific and Nutrition Findings to Social Policy." *Federation Proceedings* 38 (1979): 2551.

3. HARPER, A. E. "Dietary Goals—A Skeptical Review." *American Journal of Clinical Nutrition* 31 (1978): 310.

4. HEGSTED, D. M. "Dietary Goals—A Progressive View. *American Journal of Clinical Nutrition* 31 (1978): 1504.

5. HURLEY, L. S. *Developmental Nutrition*. Englewood Cliffs, N.J.: Prentice-Hall, 1979.

SECTION 1

LIFE CYCLE NUTRIENT NEEDS

CHAPTER 2

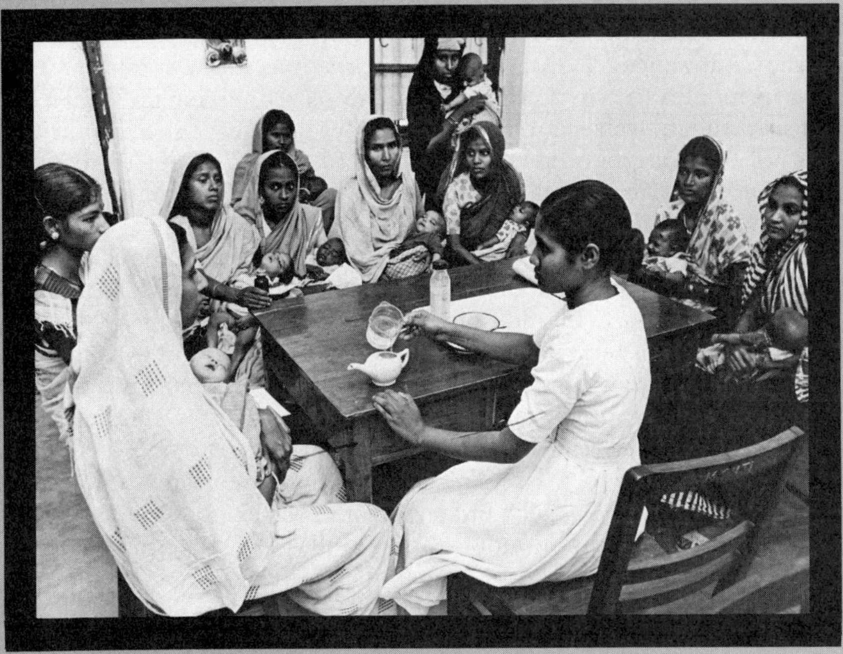

Photo by the United Nations

nutrition during infancy (birth to one year)

INFANCY IS THE PERIOD FROM BIRTH TO ONE YEAR OF AGE. In the current Recommended Dietary Allowances (RDA), the recommendations for nutrients are made for the first six months (0.0–0.5), when most infants are doubling their birth weight, and for six through twelve months (0.5–1.0). Because of the special nutritional problems of the preterm or low birth weight (LBW) infant, our discussion here will focus on full-term, normal weight infants. Birth length and weight are the basic reference points for evaluating the growth rate of the infant. The most rapid rate of postnatal growth for any period of the life cycle occurs from birth through four months (1); only during adolescence do individuals come close to matching this initial growth spurt. In addition to doubling birth weight by the end of four months, most full-term infants will triple their birth weight by the end of the first year. The average weight gain during the first four months is 20–25 g/day (5–6 g/kg/day), and approximately 15 g/day (2–3 g/kg/day) during the last eight months of the first year. By age 1, length increases by 50 percent of the birth length (from 20 cm to 30 cm). Proper nutrition is important for this growth spurt to be completed successfully. But an infant's social and psychological needs must also be met for healthy development. We will look first at these needs and at the sequence of physiological development before turning to the infant's nutritional requirements and how best to meet them.

SOCIAL AND PSYCHOLOGICAL NEEDS

Babies acquire a sense of self from how others treat them. Through contacts with parents and caregivers, they develop a sense of trust and well-being. Social isolation has a marked adverse impact on growth and development. The quality of care influences an infant's response to people and the way others react to the infant. A clean, sweet-smelling baby will be readily held and cuddled by adults and children; a dirty, foul-smelling baby will be ignored or rejected. Physical attractiveness enhances acceptance by others.

Infants are dependent on adults for feeding, care, and stimulation. The early attachment between mother and child is based on tactile stimulation, cuddling, and other forms of care, as well as feeding. Nurturance is more than physical care. Propping a bottle during feeding provides only for physical needs; holding, stroking, talking, and smiling during feeding are equally important.

In the early months, attachments are indiscriminate; after six months, primary attachments are formed to the parenting figure. These deeper attachments develop about the time of mobility, and their quality is important for the development of basic trust. An infant whose social and physiological needs are met promptly and lovingly is believed to develop a greater sense of trust than one who is physically abused, ignored, or starved.

The environment can also stimulate an infant's development. The infant needs to be exposed to a few safe, stimulating objects (2). In addition, playing with and talking to the infant, singing or reading to him or her, and paying attention to the infant's actions are vital for healthy development.

If all these conditions have been met, by the end of the first year the infant has a sense of self and others, acts with clear indication of intent, is skillful in imitating models, and can do some problem-solving in new situations (3).

Physiological Development and Function

The body composition of the infant is different at birth and at one year, and also different from that of the adult human (4). Table 2–1 shows some of these differences. For example, a greater amount of body water is found in the extracellular fluid of the infant than in the adult.

The protein content of the body increases progressively from birth to adult life in the fat-free body mass and the entire body. Nitrogen content is 2 percent in the infant body and 3 percent in the adult body. The fat in the body increases in adult life. The fatty acids consumed in the diet have some effect on the serum fatty acids and the adipose tissue fatty acids of the infant. A high intake of lino-

TABLE 2–1. Body Composition between Birth and One Year (Reference Male)

age	body weight (kg)	fat-free body mass (g/100 g)			whole body (g/100 g)			
		WATER	PROTEIN	OTHER	WATER	PROTEIN	LIPID	OTHER
Birth	3.5	84.3	12.8	2.9	75.1	11.4	11.0	2.5
4 months	7.0	81.7	15.4	2.9	60.2	11.4	26.3	2.1
12 months	10.5	77.5	19.2	3.3	59.0	14.6	23.9	2.5
Adult		72.4	20.5	7.1	62.6	16.4	15.3	5.7
range					(56–68)	(14–19)	(12–19)	(4–6)

SOURCE: Adapted from S. J. Fomon, *Infant Nutrition*, 2nd ed. (Philadelphia: Saunders, 1974); and F. Grande and A. Keys, "Body Weight, Body Composition, and Calorie Status." In *Modern Nutrition in Health and Disease*, 6th ed. Eds. R. S. Goodhart and M. E. Shils (Philadelphia: Lea & Febiger, 1980).

leic acid by an infant is reflected in the linoleic acid content of the adipose tissue.

The other part of body development includes the mineralization of the body. Mineralization of the skeleton is small, resulting in the soft, flexible bones characteristic of the infant. At this stage the crown and ends of the long bones are mostly cartilage (assessment of skeletal maturity is discussed in Chapter 7).

These measurements are difficult to obtain. Some are based on analyses of infants during autopsy, but most data are from indirect analyses based on indicators of body mass, such as total body potassium or creatinine. Measurements should be performed on well-nourished infants, for the malnourished child has reduced muscle mass, skin, tendons, cartilage, blood vessels, connective tissue, organ capsules, and bone matrix. This may amount to a reduction of 48 percent of total body protein in the malnourished infant.

The cell number and size of a tissue is based on the measurement of deoxyribonucleic acid (DNA) and the tissue weight. Deoxyribonucleic acid (DNA) is found primarily in the cell nucleus. The amount of DNA per diploid nucleus is 6.0 pg for the human and remains constant. By measuring the DNA in an organ or tissue and dividing by the DNA in the nucleus, the number of cells is determined. Once the cell number is determined, the weight of a cell, and its protein or lipid content, can be calculated.

Dietary fatty acids, serum fatty acids, and adipose tissue fatty acids demonstrate some resemblance. A high intake of linoleic acid has been reflected in the linoleic acid content of adipose tissue of infants.

the gastrointestinal system

Some aspects of gastrointestinal function are less well developed in early infancy than in later infancy and in the adult (5). The gastric acidity of the stomach is low in the newborn, but increases over the next few hours. Acidity appears lower in premature infants than in full-term infants, and secretion of hydrochloric acid and pepsin per unit of body weight is less for the infant than for the adult. Gastric digestion of protein appears to be relatively unimportant during infancy, although the lipolytic properties of gastric juice appear to be the same in infants and in adults.

In infants, the rate of gastric emptying depends on the size and composition of the meal and occurs in small amounts over several hours. Some absorption of protein, fat and glucose occurs in the duodenum; however, the greater amount of absorption takes place in the upper jejunum and the distal portion of the small intestine.

PROTEIN DIGESTION. The digestive activity related to protein is less for infants than in older children. Protein is digested less efficiently, and there is greater dependence on high-quality protein in the young infant. Digestion of protein by the infant depends primarily upon the presence of enzymes such as trypsin, chymotrypsin, elastase, and carboxypeptidases, which split the proteins into amino acids and small peptides for absorption. These enzymes are synthesized by the pancreas and secreted into the proximal portion of the duodenal lumen. In addition, there are enzymes that hydrolyze the small peptides in the brush border of the small intestine and facilitate approximately 20 percent of the peptide digestion. When conditions alter the brush border or intestinal flora, such as diarrhea or some antibiotic therapies, dilute protein feedings must be given until the proper level of protein-splitting enzymes has been reestablished. Most of the research regarding protein digestion and absorption has been conducted in the very young infant (less than 3 months) and the results extrapolated to the older infant.

FAT DIGESTION. Fat digestion depends on the fatty acid content of the fat and the age of the infant. For example, fatty acids from human milk are better absorbed than those from cow's milk. Fat of human milk is well absorbed by the infant, with 85 to 90 percent of fat intake absorbed. The most important determinants of fat absorption by the infant are these: 1) triglyceride structure, 2) fatty-acid chain length, and 3) degree of saturation of fatty acids. Pancreatic lipase hydrolyzes fatty acids from the 1 and 3 positions. Therefore, fats with palmitic or other long-chain saturated fatty acids located mainly in the 2 position are more efficiently absorbed. These fats are found in human milk.

Fatty-acid chain length affects fat digestion and absorption since short and medium chain length triglycerides increase fat absorption. The degree of saturation affects absorption in that *unsaturated* long-chain fatty acids, such as linoleic and oleic, are absorbed better than saturated fatty acids of the same length, such as stearic acid. These aspects of fat metabolism have given rise to the use of vegetable oils containing long-chain, unsaturated fatty acids in most infant formulas.

Studies have indicated that infants under 3 months of age absorbed vegetable oil in prepared formulas as efficiently as they absorbed human milk fat (6). These infants absorbed more fat and therefore excreted less in their stools than did infants fed cow's milk fat (butter fat). It is not until the infant is 4 to 6 months old that he or she begins to digest and absorb saturated fat equivalent to that absorbed in adulthood.

Lipase output per unit of body weight is independent of age during infancy and childhood. Neonates show a lower concentration of bile acids than older infants and adults. Differences in the composition of bile salts rather than in the quantity may be reflected in the decreased ability of infants to absorb fat when compared to adult capability. Long-chain saturated fatty acids are less well absorbed by infants than by older individuals.

CARBOHYDRATE DIGESTION. Infants have a smaller capacity to hydrolyze starch than children and adults. Feeding starch may increase the capacity. Lactase activity is high in full-term infants, and remains high throughout infancy. The rate of glucose absorption may be less in infants than in adults (4). The digestion of carbohydrate in the infant centers around the disaccharides; lactose, sucrose, and maltose and polysaccharides such as starch. Lactose (milk sugar) is well digested and absorbed by the infant whereas the ability of the infant to digest starch has been questioned. Lactose and other disaccharides are digested into monosaccharides by enzymes (lactase) found in the brush border of the intestinal tract. Concentration of lactase is sufficient for the digestion of milk sugar and reaches its peak soon after birth. Levels of this enzyme decline as the infant enters childhood and adolescence.

Disaccharides that are not digested pass into the colon, exerting an osmotic effect that can produce frequent loose bowel movements. The ability of the infant to split disaccharides is related to enzyme activity per unit of small intestinal mucosa and to the length of the small intestine. Considerably more research is needed for a complete understanding of the relationship between the amount of disaccharides eaten and the ability of the infant to digest it.

The digestion of starch (polysaccharides) in the newborn is questionable because of the low levels of pancreatic amylase in the small intestine. These levels do increase with age, but studies on starch digestion have been restricted to infants in the first few weeks of life and need to be conducted for older infants.

the kidney

From birth until adulthood, the human kidney goes through progressive stages of development. At birth, the infant kidney can handle only a small renal solute load and concentrate its urinary output. The functioning of the infant kidney is dependent upon sufficient intake of fluid. This ability to concentrate the urinary output increases with continuing development. The kidney of the normal infant can excrete a high solute load and produce an acceptable urine concentration of about 400 milliosmoles a liter if sufficient fluid is consumed (5).

the nervous system

The growth of the head indicates changes in the nervous tissue and fluid content of the cranium (4). The first months of life is the period of most rapid brain growth, and a too rapid or too slow rate during this time is cause for concern. The most common measurement of growth is head circumference (see appendix table).

Environmental stimulation and nutrition influence the physiological maturation of the central nervous system and the infant's behavior. As the interneuronal connections increase, so does nervous activity. As the fibers become larger and the myelin sheath develops, conduction times become more rapid. These changes affect patterns of sleeping and eating. At birth, the infant sleeps less than four hours, eats, and returns to sleep within the hour. There is little variation between day and night. By four months, most infants sleep for eight hours at night, with wakeful periods during the day. The duration of wakefulness increases from 2.5 hours at 1 week to 3.5 hours at 16 weeks, only one hour. But responsiveness and quality of behavior while awake increases greatly. The maturation of the central nervous system also affects ability to tolerate and consume a changing variety of food. Table 2-2 shows the sequence of these developments for the first year of life.

basal metabolism

"Basal" metabolic measurements for infants are made while sleeping after feeding (7); older children and adults are measured awake and 12 hours after eating. Table 2-3 shows the predicted heat production of full term infants in the normal weight-for-height classification. Heat production is related to the amount of active protoplasmic tissue. For overweight and obese infants, heat production is lower for a given weight. For the very slender, heat production may be somewhat higher than for the normal infant. No sex difference is evident before 10 months of age, but after 10 months heat production per given weight is higher for boys than for girls. Sleep depresses heat production to a greater extent (15 percent) than ingestion of food (8 percent) increases it.

Nutritional Requirements and Allowances

The requirement for individual nutrients has been defined as the amount that prevents deficiency symptoms. But many of the requirement values have been extrapolated from studies involving recuperating malnourished infants or animal models. The limitations of these methods are obvious (2). They are, however, the best we can do, since we cannot do experiments on healthy human infants.

Many of the stated "requirements" are based on the amounts of specific nutrients in human milk, for the assumption is that human milk is the perfect food for infants. The NRC-RDA adds a margin of safety of 50 to 100 percent to account for individual differences (8). Fomon uses the term "advisable intakes." He takes the fiftieth percentile of energy intake for breast-fed infants to estimate the intake of specific other nutrients from that amount of human milk. To these figures he has added a margin of safety depending upon the confidence that may be placed in the original estimate. The advisable intake is set to allow for maximum protection with minimal risk of overloading (4). The World Health Organization has also established recommended amounts of nutrients for infants (9).

Tables A–1 and A–2 in the appendix list the estimated requirements and/or recommended amounts of most nutrients for infants. These amounts should not be considered as absolute, nor should they be considered therapeutic for any given infant. They are a guide to determining adequacy of food intake with relation to nutritional status, with the caution that what may be marginal for one infant may be excessive for another. The overall needs of the infant may be

TABLE 2-2. Progressive Development of Infants and Relation to Feeding

age	activity	related food behavior
Birth	Sleep—onset at the end of nursing. Waking—crying continues until fed.	Up to 6 to 10 feeding periods. Upon waking, crying continues until fed.
1 month	Sleep—falls asleep with satiety. Interest in social stimulation.	Merging of two adjacent feedings.
3–4 months	Grasping—thumb in opposition to index finger.	
4 months	Sleep—soon after 6 P.M. feeding. Waking time varies (5–8 A.M.) usually without crying. Nap—after feeding; near 10 A.M. and 2 P.M. (two to four naps in 24 hr). Tongue projection. Inadequate approximation of lip to cup.	Able to wait for food and some adaptation to demands of the environment. Refusal of some feedings. Decrease in appetite for milk to 4 to 5 feedings. May not spontaneously wake for 10 to 11 P.M.. feeding. Spoon feeding difficult; must be placed on back of tongue. Much spilling of water or juice from a drinking cup.
4–6 months	Head erect when held in a sitting position.	Feeding while holding easier.
5 months	Sits with support.	Placement in a supporting chair for brief periods.
6–7 months	Reaches for objects	May reach for cup, spoon, or dish; needs to be secured.
7 months	Sleep—soon after 6 P.M. feeding; asleep 11 to 13 hours. Awake about 6 A.M.; half hour or longer before demanding feeding. Decrease in sucking demands. Positions mouth for spoon feeding; sucks food from a spoon. Awareness of cup.	Few 10 P.M. feedings; 3 to 4 feedings. Self-regulation or demand for food at first morning feeding. Follows a schedule for other feedings. Shows preference for solid foods, and milk intake may decline; large daily fluctuation. Early morning and 6 P.M. are best meals. Eagerness to eat; grasps spoon. Better approximation of lips to rim of cup. Can only take one or two swallows. Prefers water or juice to milk from a cup.
8 months	Can hold bottle after nipple is placed in mouth.	Some self-feeding.
8–10 months	Thumb opposition in picking up objects.	Can pick up chunk of food.
9 months	Sits without support for 10 minutes.	More variety of positions when fed.
10 months	Sleeps 6 P.M. to 5 to 7 A.M. Nap, morning and afternoon; or one long morning and brief afternoon. Preferences indicated. Likes to hold cup alone. Head tilts backward. Pulls to a standing position.	As much interest in morning company as in food; breakfast at 7 or 8 A.M. Solid foods well taken; some foods refused, usually because of temperature or texture. Juice, water taken well from cup; some milk.

TABLE 2-2. (Continued)

age	activity	related food behaviors
10 months (continued)	Patience developing.	Will wait for feedings; vocalizes anticipation rather than crying. Three meals a day, juice in afternoon; night bottles rare.
	Ability to sit erect.	High chair feeding (some may still need to be held for feeding).
	Lateral chewing movements.	Tolerance for a greater variety of food.
	Sense of satiety.	May refuse extra food beyond satiety.
	Interest in play.	Plays with food and dish.
	Good lip approximation.	Cup feeding more possible; blows bubbles.
	Hand coordination developing.	Finger feeds with bits from tray.
11 months	Stands with support.	None.
11–12 months	Walks with support.	None.
1 year	Sleep—similar to 10 months	Meal pattern similar to 10 months.
	Strong gross motor drive.	May prefer to eat in a standing position; needs toys while being fed; turns over dish if within reach. May refuse bottle and may still have difficulty with cup. Lower food intake.
	Holds cup with both hands and drinks.	
	Coordination improving.	Likes finger foods; finger feeds part of meal.
	Reaches for and picks up small objects without random movements.	
1–2 years	Develops ability to use fork and spoon.	Will still require assistance when tired.
	Runs.	

SOURCES: E. Hurlock, *Developmental Psychology*, 5th ed. (New York: McGraw-Hill, 1980); A. Gesell and F. L. Ilg, *Child Development* (New York: Harper & Row, 1949).

summarized as follows: energy, growth and replacement of body cells, and regulation of body processes.

energy

During infancy, energy needs are great. The amount of energy required by an infant depends upon basal metabolic rate, rate of growth, specific dynamic action of the food consumed, physical activity, and energy lost through bowel movements. Approximately 50 percent of calories needed are used for basal metabolism (see Figure 2-1). The largest variation is found in physical activity.

TABLE 2-3. Predicted Basal[a] Heat Production of Full-Term Infants, 1 Week of Age and Older and Within the Normal Weight-For-Height Classification[b]

weight in kilograms	1 week to 10 months[c] BOYS OR GIRLS	weight in kilograms	11 to 38 months[d] BOYS	GIRLS
	kcal./hr.		kcal./hr.	kcal./hr.
3.5	8.4	9.0	22.0	21.2
4.0	9.5	9.5	22.8	22.0
4.5	10.5	10.0	23.6	22.8
5.0	11.6	10.5	24.4	23.6
5.5	12.7	11.0	25.2	24.4
6.0	13.8	11.5	26.0	25.2
6.5	14.9	12.0	26.8	26.0
7.0	16.0	12.5	27.6	26.9
7.5	17.1	13.0	28.4	27.7
8.0	18.2	13.5	29.2	28.5
8.5	19.3	14.0	30.0	29.3
9.0	20.4	14.5	30.8	30.1
9.5	21.4	15.0	31.6	30.9
10.0	22.5	15.5	32.4	31.7
10.5	23.6	16.0	33.2	32.6
11.0	24.7			

[a]"Basal" heat production for infants includes the specific dynamic action of food and the measurements are made while the infant is sleeping quietly.

[b]For infants within the Slender weight-for-height classification, the heat production would be about 1 Calorie per hour higher than for Normal infants; for Underweight infants, the estimated heat production would fall outside the limit of plus 2 standard errors of estimate from the regression line for Normal infants; for Overweight infants, outside the limits of minus 2 standard errors of estimate.

[c]Computed from equation: kcal./hr. = 2.18 (weight, kg.) + 0.737; standard error of estimate = 1.6 kcal./hr.

[d]Computed from equations: For boys, kcal./hr. = 1.59 (weight, kg.) + 7.74; standard error of estimate = 2.2 kcal./hr.; for girls, kcal./hr. = 1.63 (weight, kg.) + 6.48; standard error of estimate = 1.9 kcal./hr.

SOURCE: D. Sargent, "An Evaluation of Basal Metabolic Data," *Home Economics Research Report* 8. Washington, D.C.: USDA, 1962.

Some infants sleep and are mostly inactive; others are awake, crying and kicking vigorously, which increases energy needs. The best method for calculating the energy needs of an infant is based on surface area of the body rather than other criteria such as weight and/or age in months; however, body weight is frequently used as a practical method for estimating total needs. In addition,

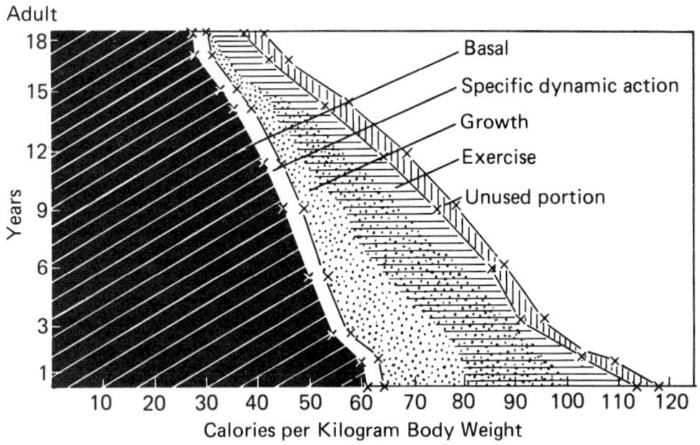

FIG. 2–1. Total daily expenditure of calories with approximate distribution among individual factors in relation to age and weight (calorie = large calorie = 1 kcal = 1 Cal). *Source:* V. C. Vaughan and R. J. McKay, *Nelson's Textbook of Pediatrics,* 10th ed. (Philadelphia: Saunders, 1975).

several other factors must be considered: the environment; temperature; interactions with mother or feeder, which may alter the amount an infant will ingest; and availability of food. In general, if energy intake is adequate during the first year of life protein needs will also be met, except when the traditional food for infants (milk of some sort) is not used. In some cultures, beans, gruel, or root starches are often given to infants at an early age. This decreases protein intake and may or may not alter energy intake. It may also result in protein calorie malnutrition.

In determining reasonable energy levels, Fomon expresses the amounts in growth and nongrowth percentages. He uses 32.8 percent of intake for growth from birth to 4 months, and 7.4 percent for growth from 4 to 12 months (10). These figures relate to the amount of energy believed necessary to build 1 gram of protein (0.5 kcal) and 1 gram of fat tissue (11.6 kcal). WHO has estimated that 5.0 kcal is needed for each gram of body weight gained (11). In recent studies with total parenteral nutrition (TPN) and elemental diets, the cost of tissue synthesis or weight gain was found to be 6.0 kcal per gram of weight gain (12). Animal studies have shown the energy cost of protein synthesis to be 7.5 kcal/g and 11.6 kcal/g for fat synthesis (13). Studies by Payne and Waterlow and Ashworth tend to substantiate these figures for infants (14, 15).

The energy requirement will be met by calories supplied by proteins, fats, and carbohydrates. There is some debate over the optimum ratios of these nutrients in infant formulas (16); Table 2–4 indicates the most commonly suggested ones.

proteins and amino acids

Proteins and amino acids are necessary for growth, synthesis of body tissue, and for nonprotein physiological compounds. Protein and amino acid requirements for infancy have been calculated from nitrogen balance studies and growth increments. In assessing protein needs energy intake from fats and/or carbohydrates

TABLE 2–4. Energy Distribution of Common Infant Formulas

nutrient	percentage of total calories HUMAN MILK	COW'S MILK	COMMERCIAL FORMULAS	FOMON'S FORMULA
Protein	7%	20%	9 to 15%	7 to 16%
Fat	55	50	45 to 50	30 to 55
Carbohydrate	38	30	35 to 45	35 to 65

SOURCE: S. J. Fomon, *Infant Nutrition*, 2nd ed. (Philadelphia: Saunders, 1974), p. 376.

must be adequate, or the estimates will be high. Protein will be used for energy rather than synthesis of tissue.

Nine amino acids necessary for tissue synthesis are not manufactured by the body and therefore are considered **essential amino acids.** They are listed in Table 2–5, and the amounts estimated by FAO-WHO, Holt and Snyderman, and Fomon are compared. These figures have been established using pure amino acids and proteins of high biological value (HBV). If proteins of lesser quality are used, the requirements are higher. Holt and Snyderman based their estimates on studies with infants where pure amino acids were fed and/or incorporated into basal formulas without the addition of whole proteins (17). Fomon used levels of amino acids that supported good growth in all infants studied. Individual amino acids were not manipulated and whole, intact proteins were used (18, 19). Some investigators have suggested that tyrosine and cystine may also be essential for small and/or immature infants (20). Interestingly, the amount of cystine in human milk is considerably greater than that in cow's milk. In addition, the ratio of methionine to cystine is approximately 1.0, which is unusual for animal protein.

Body protein content increases from 11.0 to 14.6 percent of total body weight during the first year. This tremendous growth and increase in other physiological compounds requiring nitrogen, such as enzymes, hormones, blood, and other fluids, make the protein requirement higher during this period than any other part of the life cycle. Apparently the need for essential amino acids is much greater for growth of new tissue than for repair of tissues. Table 2–6 shows estimates of protein needs during this period by various authorities.

Based on the estimates of protein needs in Table 2–6 and the protein in breast milk, the Committee on Nutrition of the American Academy of Pediatrics has set standards for infant formulas so that they provide a minimum of 1.8 g protein per 100 kcal, using protein with a protein efficiency ratio (PER) at least equal to casein. If the PER is less than that of casein, more protein must be provided in the formulas (21).

TABLE 2-5. Infant Requirements for Essential Amino Acids

AMINO ACID	FOMON MG/100 KCAL	WHO MG/KG/DAY	HOLT ET AL. MG/KG/DAY	FOMON, FILER MG/KG/DAY
Isoleucine	66	70	119	70
Leucine	132	161	229	161
Lysine	101	103	103	161
Methionine/cystine	24, 23	58	45 + cys	58[b]
Phenylalanine/ tyrosine	57[a]	125	90 + tyr	125[b]
Threonine	59	87	87	116
Tryptophan	16	17	22	17
Valine	83	93	105	93
Histidine	26	28	34	28

[a] No value given for tyrosine.

[b] Based on values of methionine:cystine and phenylalanine:tyrosine ratios in human milk.

SOURCES: FAO/WHO, *Handbook on Human Nutritional Requirements.* FAO Nutritional Studies No. 28, WHO Monograph Series No. 61, Rome, 1974. S. J. Fomon, *Infant Nutrition*, 2nd ed. (Philadelphia: Saunders 1974). S. J. Fomon and L. J. Filer, Jr., "Amino Acid Requirements for Normal Growth." In *Amino Acid Metabolism and Genetic Variation*, ed. W. L. Nyhan (New York: McGraw-Hill, 1971). L. E. Holt, Jr., and S. E. Snyderman, "The Amino Acid Requirements of Infants," *Journal of the American Medical Association*, 175 (1961), 100.

TABLE 2-6. Estimates of Infant Protein Needs

AGE (MONTHS)	FAO/WHO G/KG	NRC/RDA G/KG	FOMON'S ADVISABLE INTAKES G/100 KCAL
0 to 3	2.40	2.2	1.9
3 to 6	1.85	2.2	
6 to 9	1.62	2.0	1.7
9 to 11	1.44	2.0	

SOURCES: FAO/WHO, *Handbook on Human Nutritional Requirements.* Food and Agriculture Organization of the United Nations Nutritional Studies No. 28, WHO Monograph Series No. 61, Rome, 1974. S. J. Fomon, *Infant Nutrition*, 2nd ed. (Philadelphia: Saunders, 1974). Food and Nutrition Board, *Recommended Dietary Allowances*, 9th ed. (Washington, D.C.: Academy of Sciences, 1980). Reproduced by the permission of the National Academy of Sciences, Washington, D.C.

fats

Fat is a concentrated energy source important for the infant. In addition, lipids are carriers of the fat-soluble vitamins and a source of the essential fatty acids (22). Essential fatty acid deficiency results in a variety of metabolic disturbances, such as skin lesions and failure to grow (23). Fatty acids are also necessary for optimal development of the brain and myelinization of the central nervous system (24). Essential fatty acid deficiency has been described with the use of total parenteral nutrition and chemically defined (elemental) formulas. The essential fatty acid, linoleic acid, is higher in human milk than in cow's milk; it comprises 8 to 10 percent of the total fat. Cow's milk contains greater concentrations of saturated fatty acids, whereas long-chain, unsaturated fatty acids are in greater concentration in human milk. Fats in human milk are more completely absorbed than fats in cow's milk, a circumstance apparently related to the triglyceride arrangement of fatty acids, as well as the degree of saturation (25, 26). Lipids containing short and medium-chain fatty acids are more readily digested and absorbed than are the triglycerides of long-chain fatty acids. Absorption occurs without micelle formation, which eliminates the need for bile. These medium-chain fatty acids are bound to albumin and transported from the mucosal cell directly into the portal blood system. Consequently, commercial formulas containing MCT Oil for LBW and sick infants, particularly those with pancreatic or hepatic disorders, are now available (trademark of Mead Johnson) (27).

The American Academy of Pediatrics, Committee on Nutrition, recommends a minimum of 3.3 g fat per 100 kcal (30 percent of total calories) with 300 mg linoleic acid per 100 kcal (2.7 percent of total calories) in infant formulas. Skim milk is not recommended for infant formulas because of its low energy value, low satiety value, high protein and electrolyte content, and lack of sufficient linoleic acid (28).

major vitamins and minerals

The NRC-RDA for vitamins and minerals are listed for the 0 to 6 months group and for the 6 months to 1 year group. Just as individual variation is important with regard to calories and protein, so it is with needs for vitamins and minerals. To evaluate the vitamin and mineral intake of groups of infants, the values in Tables A–1 and A–2 of the appendix may be useful. In assessing the vitamin and mineral needs of specific infants, other factors must be taken into consideration, including heredity, particularly with regard to body size and/or certain chronic disease states; family history; dietary history; certain clinical laboratory studies; rate of growth; type of physical activity; and environment (29).

Primary vitamin deficiency diseases are unusual in the United States. With current levels of fortification of infant formulas, juices, cereals, and other basic foods, cases of primary deficiency diseases are rare. Some infants may exhibit vitamin deficiencies secondary to disease states or malabsorption syndromes. For example, deficiencies of the fat-soluble vitamins may be seen in infants with cystic fibrosis. Vitamin K deficiency is relatively common in the newborn and may occur in older infants with steatorrhea, as may deficiencies of other fat-soluble vitamins. In addition, LBW infants have been shown to have low serum levels of vitamin E, resulting in hemolytic anemia.

Determining the need for vitamins depends in part on the composition of the child's diet. As amounts of polyunsaturated fats increase in the diet, the need for vitamin E increases, just as the need for thiamin is proportional to carbohydrate intake and is often expressed as per kilocalories ingested. Vitamin B_6 (pyridoxine) requirements may be increased when protein intake is increased. Another example is the amino acid tryptophan, which may be converted to niacin, thereby reducing total amount of niacin needed.

Fortification of formulas and other foods commonly eaten by infants, as well as the availability of vitamin supplements, has given rise to the possibility of **vitamin intoxication (hypervitaminosis),** particularly with the fat-soluble vitamins, which accumulate in the body. Additional supplementation of vitamins is not necessary with commercially available formulas, which are fortified according to the listing given in Table 2–7.

The major minerals are those which occur in the body in the largest amounts —sodium, chloride, potassium, calcium, phosphorous, magnesium, and sulfur. The **trace minerals** are iron, fluoride, zinc, copper, chromium, cobalt, manganese, iodine, and molybdenum. Recommended amounts and estimated safe intakes are indicated in Tables A–1, A–2, and A–3 of the appendix.

The factors that must be taken into account in determining need for minerals are these:

1. *Amounts of other minerals in the diet*
2. *Chemical form of the mineral*
3. *Presence or absence of antagonists*
4. *Mineral status of the infant (biochemical indices)*
5. *Conditions within the gastrointestinal tract*

Iron deficiency anemia is the major nutritional deficiency seen in infants in the United States (30, 31). All the criteria above must be utilized in assessing an infant's iron stores. Adequate iron intake is a considerable problem for all infants, and particularly for preterm and LBW babies.

water and fluids

Water is a critical element for the infant. It is needed for growth and, more important, to replace losses from skin, urine, lungs, and feces. For practical purposes, the requirement for water is the amount needed to replace evaporative, fecal, and urinary losses (32). Evaporative losses account for the majority of the

TABLE 2-7. Minimum Levels of Vitamins and Minerals in Infant Formulas

nutrient	minimum amount per 100 kcal
Vitamins	
Vitamin A (μg RE)	75
Vitamin D (IU Units)	40
Vitamin K (μg)	4
Vitamin E (IU)	3 (with 0.7 IU/gm linoleic acid)
Ascorbic Acid (mg)	8
Thiamin (μg)	40
Riboflavin (μg)	60
Niacin (μg)	250
Vitamin B_6 (μg)	35 (with 15 μg/gm of protein)
Folic Acid (μg)	4
Pantothenic acid (μg)	300
Vitamin B_{12} (μg)	0.15
Biotin (μg)	1.5
Choline (mg)	7
Inositol (mg)	4
Minerals	
Calcium (mg)	50[a]
Phosphorus (mg)	25[a]
Magnesium (mg)	6
Iron (mg)	0.15
Zinc (mg)	0.5
Iodine (μg)	5
Copper (μg)	60
Manganese (μg)	5
Sodium (mg)	20 (6 meq)[b]
Potassium (mg)	80 (14 meq)[b]
Chloride (mg)	55 (11 meq)[b]

[a] Ca:P ratio no less than 1.1 nor more than 2.0.

[b] Milliequivalent for 670 kcal/liter of formula.

SOURCE: Reprinted with permission from Committee on Nutrition, American Academy of Pediatrics, "Commentary on Breast Feeding and Infant Formulas, including Proposed Standards for Formulas," *Pediatrics*, 57 (1976), 279. Copyright American Academy of Pediatrics 1976 and 1978.

infant's replacement needs. Conditions that increase evaporative losses, such as high environmental temperatures or fever, will therefore increase the requirement for additional water.

Fecal water losses normally account for a small percentage of total water losses. Diarrhea may increase fecal water loss and promote dehydration. An abnormally high water loss occurs with vomiting, and the lost fluids must be replaced to prevent dehydration. For an infant, vomiting and diarrhea episodes occuring frequently in a 12-hour period require medical treatment.

The amount of water lost through the urinary tract depends on the concentrating ability of the kidneys and the renal solute load. Maximum concentrating ability is not present at birth, so most infants excrete dilute urine (5). Under normal circumstances infants ingest more water than is required, but water intake must be carefully and frequently monitored under these conditions:

1. *Elevated body temperature*
2. *Decreased intake of formula and/or food*
3. *Diarrhea*
4. *Vomiting*
5. *Concentrated formula (or an error in formula dilution)*
6. *Use of high-protein formula*

Infants are dependent on others for water and cannot be expected to regulate intake by thirst mechanisms, as older children do. Careful sanitary precautions must be taken with water. Since water purity varies from place to place, sterilized water is recommended for the very young infant. The RDA lists 1.5 ml/kcal or 150 ml/100 kcal formula as being a reasonable water intake for most infants (7). Haycock gives an estimate of water needs, shown in Table 2–8. The requirement or maintenance values are based on bed rest (33). As body weight

TABLE 2–8. Fluid Requirements of Infants

body weight (kg)	amount of fluid (ml/kg/day)
Less than 10	100
10 to 20	50
20 and above	20

SOURCE: George B. Haycock, "Water and Electrolytes." In *Textbook of Paediatric Nutrition*, eds. D. S. Mc Laren, and D. Burman (London: Churchill Livingstone, 1976), p. 207.

increases, fluid requirements based on kg of body weight decrease. Fluid needs are met by the young infant from human milk or modified cow's milk or other correctly diluted proprietary formulas (.67 kcal/ml) (34).

MEETING THE NUTRITIONAL NEEDS OF INFANTS

During the first six months, the infant's nutritional needs are most adequately met with human milk, particularly if the mother is well nourished and producing adequate amounts. Breast milk need only be supplemented with a source of vitamin D, 10 μg (400 IU), and fluoride, 0.1–1.0 mg (7). Recent reports continue to emphasize the inadequacy of vitamin D in breast milk (35). In addition to meeting nutritional needs, there are other advantages of breast feeding (36, 37, 38):

1. *The warm psychological and emotional relationship between mother and infant.*
2. *The presence in human milk of helpful antibodies such as immunoglobins, especially IGA, which binds viruses and bacteria and prevents them from invading the mucosa of the gastrointestinal tract, and lactoferrin, which inhibits several pathogens under certain conditions.*
3. *There is less exposure to environmental contaminants.*
4. *It is convenient and always at the appropriate temperature.*
5. *The presence in human milk of lysozyme, which has an indirect effect on bacteria by stimulating the activity of antibodies.*
6. *There are no containers to wash and sterilize.*
7. *There is less chance of overfeeding.*
8. *The mother's hormonal mechanism delays the onset of ovulation.*
9. *It may, in some instances, be more economical.*

Human milk is relatively low in phenylalamine and tyrosine, another factor which suggests that it is best suited to the metabolic abilities of the young infant (39). The reduced incidence of infection is a significant factor in this and other countries where infant mortality rates remain high (40). Infection and diarrheal disease are major factors causing malnutrition in infants. Disease increases nutrient requirements, and diarrhea results in loss of nutrients and body fluid.

In breast feeding the supply (volume) of milk is dependent upon sucking (41). As the infant increases sucking time, more milk is formed and "let down" for subsequent feedings. For small infants a rigid schedule may be necessary, as these infants tend to sleep excessively without "demanding" feedings frequently enough to meet their growth needs. Most mothers compromise with rigid schedule and demand by allowing the infant to establish his or her own schedule. Initially, feedings are offered to the infant every two to three hours. There is great variation in appetite and capacity from infant to infant and in the same infant from feeding to feeding and day to day. This may make considerable difference in advising mothers as to number of feedings per 24 hours, amount per feeding, and total volume (42). A possible feeding schedule is given in Table 2–9, but it should be regarded as a guide only.

lactation

Meeting the nutritional needs of the infant always requires a discussion of lactation and breast feeding. The advantages for the infant have been noted, but it is necessary to point out the nutrition implications for the mother as well. (The physiological changes and nutritional needs of pregnancy are discussed in Chapter 5.) **Lactation,** or the process of milk production and breast feeding, is apparently increasing among all socioeconomic groups in the United States. Prior to the development of formula, breast feeding was the only method of nourishing the human infant. With formulas came advertising and the decline of breast feeding not only in this country, but also in developing countries, where other sources of infant foods and adequate sanitation practices were nonexistent. The result in these countries has been an increase in malnutrition for many infants.

Although most authorities agree that human milk is best for human infants, circumstances can prevent breast feeding—maternal mortality or disease, mental illness, drug addiction. In those instances it is better to have a well-fed infant on formula than a malnourished infant on breast feedings. The majority of women who desire to breast feed can be successful. Many find the support of other women who have breast fed or the La Leche League (an international group of mothers interested in promoting breast feeding) of great psychological and practical help in maintaining successful breast feeding.

In a recent review of lactation, Jelliffe and Jelliffe (38) note that success is the result of numerous interacting factors, including the vigor and maturity of the infant, as well as the health and nutritional status of the mother. Good maternal

TABLE 2–9. Suggested Feeding Schedule[a]

age of infant	number of feedings	volume per feeding	total volume
0 to 2 weeks	6–10	60–90 ml (2–3 oz)	600–700 ml
2 weeks–1 month	6–8	90–120 ml (3–4 oz)	700–750 ml
1–3 months	5–6	150–180 ml (5–6 oz)	750–850 ml
3–7 months	4–5	180–210 ml (6–7 oz)	900–1000 ml
7–12 months	3–4	210–240 ml (7–8 oz)	950–1000 ml

[a]This schedule may apply to both breast- and formula-fed infants.

nutrition increases birth weight and, therefore, the vigor and viability of the newborn. The stronger sucking ability of the vigorous infant directly influences the success of lactation. In addition, optimum nutrition during pregnancy allows for adequate maternal stores, protecting the mother who wishes to breast feed.

Physiologically, lactation is under the control of the endocrine glands, particularly the pituitary hormones, prolactin and oxytocin, which are influenced by the sucking process and maternal emotions. Only in recent years has human lactation begun to be studied scientifically, although it has been studied in animals whose milk products are important to the economy of a country.

The four stages of lactation as described by Jelliffe and Jelliffe are lactogenesis (milk initiation), galactopoiesis (milk secretion or the maintenance of lactation), milk ejection, and milk ingestion. These stages are dependent on the interaction of mother and newborn—both must actively participate. Milk initiation begins when colostrum secretion occurs after being triggered by decreases in placenta steroids and increases in the hormone prolactin, and continues because of the sucking of the newborn. Milk ejection is an active process within the breast controlled by the let-down reflex (Figure 2–2). Milk ingestion is then dependent on the rooting, sucking, and swallowing reflexes of the newborn. It may also be controlled psychologically in the mother by conditioned reflexes (sight or thought of the newborn, hearing a cry), or by stress, which can prevent the let-down. Figure 2–3 shows the complex interrelationships among the hormonal, nutritional, reflexive, and psychological controls on lactation. Failure of breast feeding in a healthy woman may also occur because of lack of knowledge of techniques, available foods, social pressures, competing professional pursuits, and attitudes of mother and father toward breast feeding.

maternal nutrient needs

Lactation increases the nutrient needs of the mother even above those of pregnancy (see RDAs in the appendix). Energy intake must be adequate to provide for the production of milk. The average healthy woman produces 850 ml of milk per day, the equivalent of 570 kcal. Production of milk is about 80 percent efficient, which means that the total energy requirement is 700 to 750 kcal per day (38). Maternal fat stores can be used for approximately 200 to 300 kcal per day for the first three months. An additional 500 kcal must be taken in food daily, or 200 kcal more than during pregnancy. If more than one infant is suckled or if lactation continues longer than three and one-half to four months, the energy requirement is even greater. The RDA for protein is 20 g above that of the nonlactating woman, or a total of 76 g daily. This amount of protein is necessary for the synthesis of milk protein. The protein content of human milk is relatively constant even from malnourished mothers, which would indicate that the amino acids necessary for milk protein are taken from the maternal stores when intakes are inadequate. Most women will consume adequate protein if their energy in-

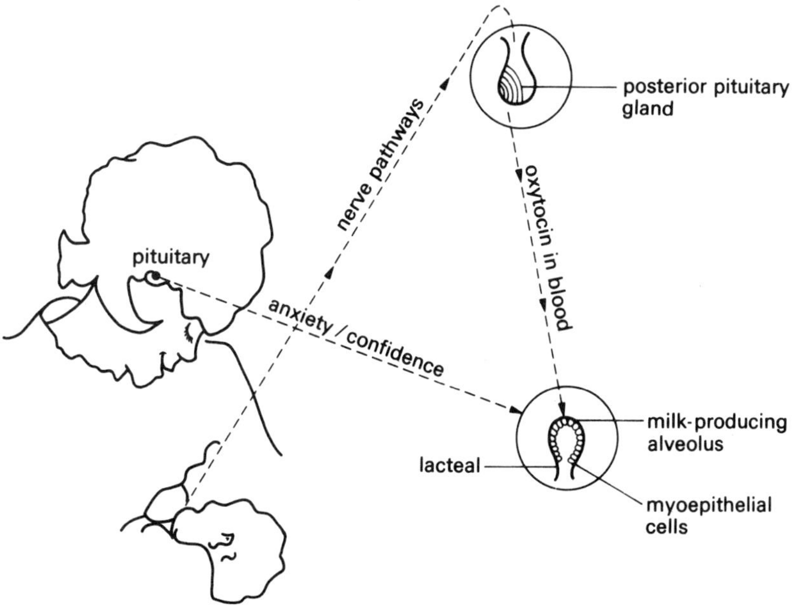

FIG. 2–2. The let-down reflex, simplified. *Source:* Derrick B. Jelliffee and E. F. Patrice Jelliffe, *Human Milk in the Modern World* (Oxford: Oxford University Press, 1978).

takes are adequate. However, because of the cultural demand of returning to thinness or because of low intakes in low socioeconomic groups, protein in the mother's diet must be carefully evaluated.

Breast milk will average 250 to 350 mg daily of calcium, although maternal intake may be less than that amount. Recent reports have confirmed that significant amounts of the mother's skeletal calcium is mobilized to meet these needs (43). This is equivalent to the calcium in one quart of milk and is difficult, if not impossible, to meet through food sources if milk is not consumed. The RDA for calcium is 1200 mg daily.

Other nutrients that need to be increased during lactation are vitamins A, D, E, and most water-soluble vitamins. There is some disagreement as to the most appropriate way to meet these needs, and considerable variation in the suggestions made by professionals. Fluid intake is important; two to three quarts of fluid should be consumed daily. Supplements of vitamins, minerals, or protein are not necessary if food intake is adequate.

Table 2–10 lists the foods and serving sizes necessary to meet increased nutrient needs during lactation. It should be used as a guide, with evaluation and planning of appropriate food intakes being done on an individual basis. There are many different ways to meet these needs, and there are no particular foods

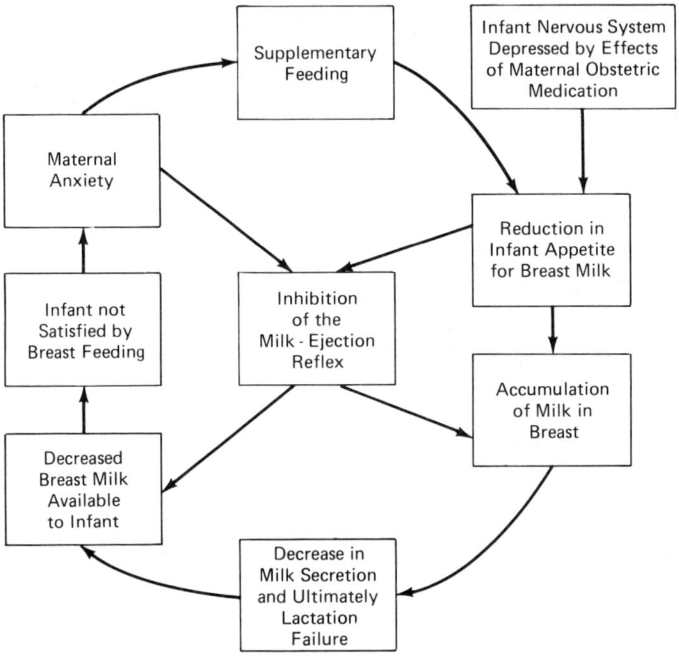

FIG. 2–3. Factors in the failure of lactation. Reprinted by permission of Alan Beer, M.D., Chairman, Department of Obstetrics and Gynecology, University of Michigan, Ann Arbor, Michigan.

that must be consumed or avoided. Monitoring of mother's and infant's weight is one means of evaluating adequacy of amounts of food. The mother who maintains good nutrition can minimize losses from maternal stores. Later in this chapter we will discuss the potential hazards of alcohol and drug use for breast feeding. Either may also play a role in significantly decreasing the amounts of food eaten, which can compromise the mother's nutritional status.

the composition of breast milk

The energy in human milk is provided by carbohydrates, fats and proteins. Lactose is the only carbohydrate in milk and is synthesized only by the cells of the lactating mammary gland. Lactose is a disaccharide composed of the monosaccharides galactose and glucose. It is synthesized in the mammary gland beginning late in pregnancy because of the influence of specific hormones and the protein alpha-lactalbumin. Alpha-lactalbumin is manufactured only in the presence of certain hormones, such as insulin, cortisone, estrogen, and prolactin.

The synthesis of lactose by the mammary gland locks up the glucose drawn from the blood that might go elsewhere in the body. Lactose provides a means

TABLE 2-10. Daily Food Guide for Lactation

food group	amount
PROTEIN FOODS	
Animal protein (eggs, beef, pork, chicken, fish). In addition to protein, supplies iron, riboflavin, niacin, B_6, B_{12}, phosphorus, zinc, and iodine.	Two 3-oz servings.
Vegetable protein (meat alternates, legumes, nuts). In addition to protein, supplies iron, thiamin, folacin, B_6, E, phosphorus, magnesium, and zinc.	Serving size varies; plan based on the protein composition of the food. Usually 2 4-8 oz servings.
MILK AND MILK PRODUCTS[a]	
Supply calcium, phosphorus, vitamin D, riboflavin, A, E, B_6, B_{12}, magnesium, zinc, and protein.	Four servings; one serving equals 8 oz of milk or its equivalent.
GRAIN PRODUCTS	
Supply thiamin, niacin, riboflavin, iron, phosphorus, zinc, magnesium (whole grains provide more magnesium and zinc), and fiber.	Three servings; one serving equals 1 slice of bread or ½ cup of macaroni, rice, or hot cereal.
VITAMIN C-RICH FRUITS AND VEGETABLES	
Supply ascorbic acid; when fresh, supply fiber.	One serving; approximately ½ cup fruit or ¾ cup of vegetables.
LEAFY GREEN VEGETABLES	
Supply folacin, A, E, B_6, riboflavin, iron, magnesium, and fiber.	Two servings; serving equals approximately 1 cup raw or ¾ cup cooked.
OTHER FRUITS AND VEGETABLES	
Include yellow fruits and vegetables, which supply large amounts of vitamin A as well as B complex, E, magnesium, phosphorus, zinc, and fiber.	One serving; serving equals approximately ½ cup.

[a]Vitamin D is necessary for the utilization of calcium. Milk is fortified with vitamin D; most other sources of calcium are not. A supplement to ensure an adequate vitamin D intake may be necessary if milk is not consumed.

SOURCE: Adapted from Maternal and Child Health Unit, California Department of Health, *Nutrition during Pregnancy and Lactation*, 1975, pp. 34–40.

of ensuring that glucose remains in the lactating cell and becomes part of the milk. The lactose content of the milk is approximately 7.5 g percent and is independent of maternal nutrition.

Fat supplies about half of the energy in breast milk. Although total fat content is relatively constant, the fatty acid composition of milk does resemble dietary intake. If more saturated fat is eaten by the mother, the milk will have increased amounts of saturated fatty acids (44). If maternal energy intake is inadequate, the fat content of the milk will be similar to that of subcutaneous fat, which the mother is mobilizing for energy.

Human milk contains more unsaturated fatty acids, with palmitic acid primarily in the 2 position of the glycerol molecule, a configuration which has been shown to favor absorption of fat (45). Commercial formulas are now being prepared by removing the butterfat and substituting vegetable oils. This has increased the absorption of fat from these formulas and decreased their saturated fatty acid and cholesterol content. The last milk suckled in a given feeding is higher in fat and the satiety value of the increased fat may serve as a natural regulator of appetite (46).

The protein content of human milk varies, being higher in colostrum and the milk of mothers who deliver prematurely and decreasing slightly in more mature milk (47). Estimates of protein content vary from 0.8 g to 1.6 g per 100 ml. In addition, human milk has been shown to have 20 percent more nonprotein nitrogen than cow's milk (48). The protein content of human milk is not dependent upon maternal food intake, but the volume of milk may be decreased in malnourished mothers.

Few data are available on the interaction between calcium intake and calcium in breast milk, although some lactating women have been found to be in negative calcium balance. It seems prudent to recommend increased amounts of calcium for the mother. Calcium levels have been reported to be comparable in milk from poorly nourished and adequately nourished women, so calcium content of breast milk may be at the expense of maternal stores.

The iron content of breast milk is less than in cow's milk, but is not influenced by the dietary intake of the mother. As noted previously, iron from breast milk is better absorbed than that of cow's milk and is a significant source for the breast-fed infant (49, 50).

The level of water-soluble vitamins in breast milk varies according to maternal dietary intake up to a point (51). Evidence shows that supplementation of an already adequate maternal diet does not significantly alter water-soluble vitamins in milk (52). For instance, riboflavin occurs naturally in large amounts, but only if the maternal diet is adequate in riboflavin. Deficiencies of vitamin B_{12} have been detected in infants breast fed by strict vegetarian mothers (53). Vitamin A concentration in milk is influenced by adequacy of the maternal diet during pregnancy and lactation. Decreased amounts have been observed in low socioeconomic status mothers whose dietary intakes were poor and in seasons when availability of carotene-containing vegetables and fruits was low. Fortification of the maternal diet with vitamin A has been shown to increase the amounts in breast milk.

Human milk is adequate to sustain growth and good nutritional status in the first six months of life in most babies of well-nourished mothers. Supplementation with fluoride may be necessary in areas where the water supply is not fluoridated, and with vitamin D if the infant does not get exposed to the sun. The duration of production and the volume of milk produced may be decreased in poorly nourished mothers, so that the infant's nutritional needs may not be met after four to six months lactation. Even though the nutritional quality of the breast milk of malnourished mothers is surprisingly good except for vitamin A and the water-soluble vitamins, the decreased volume produced means decreased energy available for the infant. When energy needs are not met, the infant's utilization of protein is impaired and growth may be compromised. In addition, the malnourished mother who continues to breast feed does so at the expense of maternal stores.

The relationship of oral contraceptives to lactation is now receiving some attention from researchers. The large-dose mixed oral contraceptive agents containing both estrogens and progestogens do decrease the production of milk, especially if they are started soon after delivery. The effects of OCA on milk composition have not been adequately studied in humans, but it is known that some hormones cross into the milk. The long-term physiological and behavioral effects of these hormones on the infant are unknown. Oral contraceptives promote metabolic changes typical of pregnancy, so serum levels of some nutrients are decreased while others are increased. More study is needed particularly in women who become pregnant and lactate after taking oral contraceptives, for long periods of time, as they could have inadequate stores of nutrients important to breast feeding (54).

Alcohol distributes in body fluids and is secreted in breast milk (55). The level of alcohol in human milk reaches almost the same concentration as in the mother's blood (56). Therefore, alcohol should not be consumed immediately before nursing an infant. Drugs such as anticoagulants, anticonvulsants, some antibiotics, thyroid suppressants, radioactive compounds, cathartics, and large amounts of aspirin appear in the breast milk and may be harmful to the infant (57, 58). More research is needed on the effects of other drugs and contaminants in breast milk, but indiscriminate use of drugs is not advised for the nursing mother.

FEEDING

formula feeding

Proprietary formulas made from cow's milk contain all the essential amino acids, and amino acids are added to formulas using soybean isolates in order to have them contain appropriate ratios of essential amino acids. The latter formulas thus have more total nitrogen, which may place greater demands on the young, immature kidney. In recent years, formulas that contain predigested protein with amino acids in recommended proportions have been introduced for infants with special physiological conditions. The ingredients of each commercially prepared formula should be monitored closely, as formulations change frequently to meet current research and demands.

The vitamin and mineral needs of the infant up to six months of age are adequately met with supplemented breast milk and/or commercial formulas which are fortified (59). Supplementation with vitamin D and/or fluoride is recommended for breast-fed infants where exposure to sunlight is inadequate and water supplies are not fluoridated (60). Because intestinal flora may not be well established in the newborn, the American Academy of Pediatrics, Committee on Nutrition, recommends intramuscular administration of vitamin K immediately after birth. Concentrations of prothrombin and clotting factors have been shown to be low until the intestinal flora begin to synthesize vitamin K—usually about one week after birth.

Iron must be carefully evaluated in individual infants. Full-term infants can maintain adequate iron with an intake of 1 mg/kg/day at 3 months of age. Low birth weight infants or infants born to mothers who had poor prenatal diets may not have sufficient iron stores to carry them for three months. These infants need an iron supplement of 2 mg/kg/day starting soon after birth. Supplemental iron may be in form of drops, iron-fortified formula, or foods rich in iron (meats and iron-fortified cereals).

Under most circumstances, if energy needs are met, other nutrient needs of the infant will be met; this is the basis for the use of "per 100 kcal" standards for supplementation (21). The infant who does not feed well and takes insufficient volume to meet energy needs must therefore be evaluated for other nutrient deficiencies as well.

feeding techniques

The infant should be held for all breast or bottle feedings (see Figure 2–4 for the appropriate technique and position for bottle feeding). Under no circumstances should bottles be propped or kept in bed with infants. Not only does this deprive the infant of positive security and a nurturing relationship, but it increases the possibility of strangulation, aspiration, and overeating (61). Another possible consequence is bottle-mouth syndrome, or decay of deciduous teeth from constant contact with sugar in formula and other liquids (62).

If bottle feeding is used, care must be taken in formula preparation and sanitation. The young infant has limited protection against infection. As the infant grows older, his or her immune production increases. Diarrhea can develop quickly in an infant from organisms introduced through food and water, and milk is an excellent medium for bacterial growth.

solid food

The early addition of foods other than breast milk or formula (usually referred to as **semi-solid food**) is often controversial (63). Some possible problems are overfeeding, allergic reactions, poor digestion of foods, and development of poor

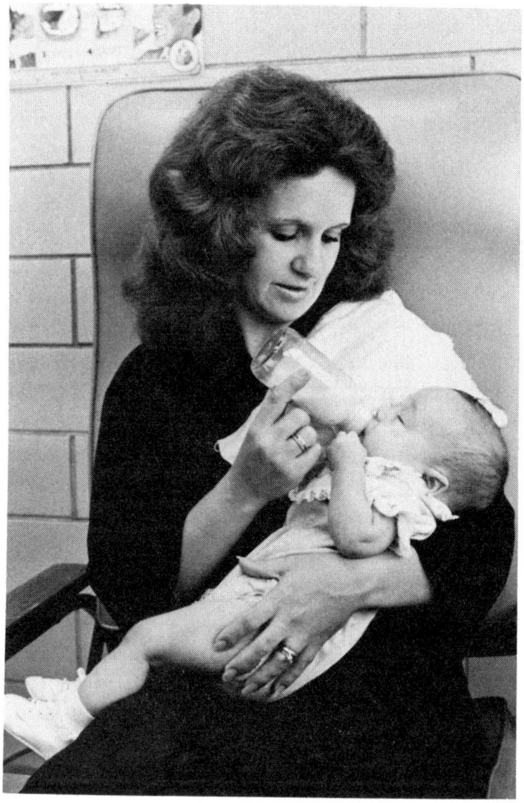

FIG. 2–4. Correct position for bottle feeding. Photo from Arkansas Children's Hospital.

food habits. There are no advantages to giving semi-solid foods before 4 to 6 months of age, but current social trends promote early introduction of solids as a sign of developmental achievement. Mothers are continuously comparing notes on what new foods have been accepted. Even though physiologically the infant does not need other food to meet nutrient needs, it may be necessary to offer some food from a spoon or glass by 4 to 6 months to keep up with developmental skills (64). As the infant develops improved swallowing techniques, small amounts of semi-solid food can be offered from a spoon. Infant feeders and plungers cause overfeeding, do not allow for self-regulation, and may cause choking. They are not recommended.

If semi-solid feedings are begun at approximately 4 months of age, by 6 months the infant should be taking amounts adequate to contribute to iron needs, particularly if iron-fortified cereals are used. Hypo-allergenic foods such as rice cereal should be introduced first. Each new food item should be offered in a small quantity two or three times daily, using the same food for at least three days before introducing another food. A possible schedule for introducing semi-solids is as follows:

Months	*Food*
3½–4	Iron fortified cereal
4½–5	Strained vegetables
5½–6	Strained fruit
6½–7	Strained meats
7½–9	Strained or mashed eggs

As the infant moves from one developmental stage to another, feeding should be altered to take advantage of new skills. Spoon feeding should not be attempted before good head control is achieved. As the infant begins to sit alone, he or she should be offered liquids from a cup or glass to prepare for eventual weaning from the bottle or breast. As sitting skills develop and hand to mouth movements are refined, the infant should be offered foods appropriate for finger feeding and requiring some chewing motions. This usually occurs at 9 to 12 months of age. At this time the child can also be expected to hold a small glass and drink small amounts from it unassisted. Until the infant is skilled at self feeding and the use of a spoon, the mother should be prepared for some playing in the food and untidiness. Not until after the period of infancy will the child be proficient at self feeding.

As foods other than formula are taken in significant amounts, the volume of formula should be reduced so that excessive calories are not consumed. Overfeeding at this age may begin lifelong habits of overeating. Solid foods given to infants, whether commercially prepared or prepared at home, will have less nutrient density than formula, with the possible exception of meats (65, 66). For this reason, the amount of formula and baby food eaten should be carefully monitored. For the poor feeder or slow gainer, formula is preferred over baby food because it has more nutrients in less volume. Also, for some infants the consumption of solid foods is frustrating and tiring.

SUMMARY

The nutrient needs change with the growth and physical development from birth to one year. Social and psychological factors are very important in these early months, for an infant needs attention and social contact.

The systems of the body develop rapidly, allowing for greater complexity in the diet. The nutritional needs of the infant can be met adequately during the first six months by breast feeding and supplementation with vitamin D and fluoride. If that is not possible, there are adequate commercial formulas available. Formulas made from protein of soy isolate are available for infants allergic to cow's milk proteins. Formulas without lactose are available for those who demonstrate lactose intolerance. Homogenized or skim milk is not recommended for the infant under one year. At 4 to 6 months foods other than milk may be introduced, beginning with strained or mashed foods and then those requiring real chewing.

Breast feeding provides advantages to the infant of adequate and appropriate nutrition, increased resistance to infection, and improved maternal bonding. The quality and quantity of breast milk can be maintained by increasing nutrient intake slightly above that needed for pregnancy. Vitamin and mineral supplementation is not necessary for successful lactation in the healthy, well-nourished woman.

references

1. NEUMANN, C. G., and M. ALPAUGH. "Birthweight Doubling Time: A Fresh Look." *Pediatrics* 57 (1976): 469.
2. CRAIG, G. J. *Human Development.* Englewood Cliffs, N.J.: Prentice-Hall, 1976.
3. AMBRON, S. R., and D. BRODZINSKY. *Lifespan Human Development.* New York: Holt, Rinehart and Winston, 1979.
4. SMITH, D. W., and E. L. BIERMAN. *The Biologic Ages of Man.* Philadelphia: Saunders, 1973.
5. FOMON, S. J. *Infant Nutrition,* 2nd ed. Philadelphia: Saunders, 1974.
6. FOMON, S. J., E. E. ZIEGLER, and L. V. THOMAS. "Excretion of Fat by Normal Full-term Infants Fed Various Milks and Formulas." *American Journal of Clinical Nutrition* 23 (1970): 1299.
7. SARGENT, D. *An Evaluation of Basal Metabolic Data.* Home Economics Research Report #8. Washington, D.C.: U.S. Department of Agriculture, 1962.
8. Food and Nutrition Board. *Recommended Dietary Allowances,* 9th ed. Washington, D.C.: National Research Council, National Academy of Sciences, 1980.
9. FAO/WHO, *Handbook on Human Nutritional Requirements.* FAO Nutritional Studies, No. 28, WHO Monograph No. 61, Rome, 1974.
10. FOMON, S. J., L. N. THOMAS, L. J. FILER, JR., E. E. ZEIGLER, and M. T. LEONARD. "Food Consumption and Growth of Normal Infants Fed Milk-based Formulas." *Acta Paediatrica Scandinavica* (Supplement 223), 1971.
11. Joint FAO/WHO Expert Group. *Energy and Protein Requirements.* WHO Technical Report Series No. 522. Rome: Food and Agriculture Organization of the United Nations, 1973.
12. HEIRD, W. C., and R. W. WINTERS. "Total Parenteral Nutrition: The State of the Art." *Journal of Pediatrics* 86 (1975): 2.
13. KIELANOWSKI, J. "Estimates of the Energy Cost of Protein Deposition in Growing Animals." *Proceedings of the Third Symposium on Energy Metabolism,* ed. K. L. Blaster, New York: Academic Press, 1969.
14. PAYNE, P. R., and J. C. WATERLOW. "Relative Energy Requirements for Maintenance, Growth, and Physical Acitivity." *Lancet* 2 (1971): 210
15. ASHWORTH, A., R. BELL, W. P. T. JAMES, and J. C. WATERLOW. "Calorie Requirements of Children Recovering from Protein-Calorie Malnutrition." *Lancet* 2 (1968): 600.
16. MACLEAN, W. C., and G. GRAHAM. "The Effect of Level of Protein Intake in Isoenergetic Diets on Energy Utilization." *American Journal of Clinical Nutrition* 32 (1979): 1381.

17. HOLT, L. E., JR., and S. E. SNYDERMAN. "The Amino Acid Requirements of Infants." *Journal of the American Medical Association* 175 (1961): 100.

18. FOMON, S. J., and L. F. FILER, JR. "Amino Acid Requirements for Normal Growth." In *Amino Acid Metabolism and Genetic Variation,* ed. W. L. Nyhan. New York: McGraw-Hill, 1971.

19. FOMON, S. J., L. N. THOMAS, L. J. FILER, T. A. ANDERSON, and K. E. BERGMANN. "Requirements for Protein and Essential Amino Acids in Early Infancy: Studies with a Soy-Isolate Formula." *Acta Paediatrica Scandinavica* 62 (1973): 33.

20. RAIHA, N. C. R., K. HEINONEN, D. K. RASSIN et al. "Milk Protein Quantity and Quality in Low Birthweight Infants. 1. Metabolic Responses and Effects on Growth." *Pediatrics* 57 (1975): 659.

21. Committee on Nutrition, American Academy of Pediatrics. "Commentary on Breast-Feeding and Infant Formulas, including Proposed Standards for Formulas." *Pediatrics* 57 (1976): 279.

22. CUTHBERTSON, W. F. J. "Essential Fatty Acid Requirements in Infancy." *American Journal of Clinical Nutrition* 29 (1976): 599.

23. ALFIN- SLATER, R. B., and L. AFTERGOOD. "Essential Fatty Acids Reinvestigated." *Physiological Review,* 48 (1968): 758.

24. WINICK, M., J. A. BRASEL, and P. ROSSO. "Nutrition and Cell Growth." In *Current Concepts in Nutrition.* Vol 1, *Nutrition and Development,* ed. M. Winick. New York: Wiley, 1972.

25. HANSEN, A. E., R. A. STEWART, G. HUGHES, and L. SODERHJELM. "The Relation of Linoleic Acid to Infant Feeding." *Acta Paediatrica Scandinavica* (supplement 137), 51 (1962): 1.

26. AAES, E. "Essential Fatty Acids." *Physiological Review* 41 (1961): 1.

27. ISSELBACHER, K. J. "Mechanisms of Absorption of Long and Medium Chain Triglycerides." In *Medium Chain Triglycerides,* ed. J. R. Senior. Philadelphia: University of Pennsylvania Press, 1968.

28. BERENBERG, W., F. MANDELL, and F. X. FELLERS. "Hazards of Skimmed Milk, Unboiled and Boiled." *Pediatrics* 44 (1969): 734.

29. ALFIN- SLATER, R. B., and D. B. JELLIFFE. "Nutritional Requirements—With Special Reference to Infancy." *Pediatric Clinics of North America* 24 (1977): 3.

30. FOMON, S. J. *Nutritional Disorders of Children: Prevention, Screening, and Followup.* DHEW Publication No. (HSA) 76-5612. Rockville, Md.: Health Services Administration, Bureau of Community Health Services, 1976.

31. Committee on Nutrition, American Academy of Pediatrics. "Iron Supplementation for Infants." *Pediatrics* 58 (1976): 765.

32. WINTERS, R. W., ed. *The Body Fluids in Pediatrics.* Boston: Little, Brown, 1973.

33. HAYCOCK, GEORGE B. "Water and Electrolytes." In *Textbook of Paediatric Nutrition,* eds. D. S. McLaren and D. Burnam. London: Churchill Livingstone, 1976.

34. ZIEGLER, E. E., and S. J. FOMON. "Fluid Intake, Renal Solute Load, and Water Balance in Infancy." *Journal of Pediatrics* 78 (1971): 561.

35. EDIDIN, D. V., L. L. LEVITSKY, W. SCHEY, N. DUMBOVIE, and A. CAMPOS. "Resurgence of Nutritional Rickets Associated with Breast-Feeding and Special Dietary Practices." *Pediatrics* 65 (1980): 232.

36. KENNELL, J. H., M. H. KLAUS, R. SOSA et al. "Early Neonatal Contact: Effect on Growth, Breast Feeding and Infection in the First Year of Life." *Pediatric Research* 10 (1976): 426.

37. HANNSON, L. A., and J. WINBERG. "Breast Milk and Defense against Infection in the Newborn." *Archives of Diseases of Children* 47 (1972): 845.

38. JELLIFFE, D. B., and E. F. P. JELLIFFE. *Human Milk in the Modern World.* Oxford: Oxford University Press, 1978.

39. JACKSON, R. L. et al. "Growth of 'Well-born' American Infants Fed Human and Cow's Milk." *Pediatrics* 33 (1964): 642.

40. JACKSON, R. L. "Long-term Consequences of Suboptimal Nutrition Practices in Early Life—Some Important Benefits of Breast Feeding." *Pediatric Clinics of North America* 24 (1977): 63.

41. JELLIFFE, D. B., and E. F. P. JELLIFFE. "The Uniqueness of Human Milk." *American Journal of Clinical Nutrition* 24 (1971): 1015.

42. NEWTON, M. "A Test for Lactation Success." *American Journal of Obstetrics and Gynecology* 64 (1952): 397.

43. PITKIN, R. M. "Nutritional Support in Obstetrics and Gynecology." *Clinical Obstetrics and Gynecology* 19 (1976): 489.

44. POTTER, M. J., and J. P. NESTEL. "The Effects of Dietary Fatty Acids and Cholesterol on the Milk Lipids of Lactating Women and the Plasma Cholesterol of Breast Fed Infants." *American Journal of Clinical Nutrition* 2 (1976): 5.

45. FILER, L. J., JR., F. H. MATTSON, and S. J. FOMON. "Triglyceride Configuration and Fat Absorption by the Human Infant." *Journal of Nutrition* 99 (1969): 293.

46. HALL, B. "Changing Composition of Human Milk and Early Development of Appetite Control." *Lancet* 1 (1975): 779.

47. ATKINSON, S. A., M. H. BRYAN, and G. H. ANDERSON. "Human Milk: Difference in Nitrogen Concentration of Milk from Mothers of Term and Premature Infants." *Journal of Pediatrics* 93 (1978): 67.

48. LONNERDAL, B., E. FORSUM, and L. HAMBRAEUS. "The Protein Content of Human Milk. 1. A Transversal Study of Swedish Normal Material. *Nutrition Reports International* 13 (1976): 125.

49. MCMILLAN, J. A., S. A. LANDAU, and F. A. OSKI. "Iron Sufficiency in Breast-Fed Infants and the Availability of Iron from Human Milk." *Pediatrics* 58 (1976): 686.

50. SAARINEN, V. M., M. A. SUMES, and P. R. DALLMAN. "Iron Absorption in Infants: High Bioavailability of Breast Milk Iron as Indicated by the Extrinsic Tag Method of Iron Absorption and by the Concentration of Serum Ferritin." *Journal of Pediatrics* 91 (1977): 36.

51. WEST, K. D., and A. KIRKSEY. "Influence of Vitamin B_6 Intake on the Content of the Vitamin in Human Milk." *American Journal of Clinical Nutrition* 29 (1976): 961.

52. THOMAS, M. R., J. KAWAMOTO, S. M. SNEED, and R. EAKIN. "The Effects of Vitamin C,

Vitamin B_6 and Vitamin B_{12} Supplementation on the Breast Milk and Maternal Status of Well-nourished Women." *American Journal of Clinical Nutrition* 32 (1979): 1679.

53. LAMPKIN, B. C., and E. F. SAUNDERS. "Nutritional Vitamin B_{12} Deficiency in an Infant." *Journal of Pediatrics* 75 (1969): 1053.

54. KIRKSEY, A., J. A. ERNST, J. L. ROEPKE, and T. L. TSAI. "Influence of Mineral Intake and Use of Oral Contraceptives before Pregnancy on the Mineral Content of Human Colostrum and of Mature Milk." *American Journal of Clinical Nutrition* 32 (1979): 30.

55. ROE, D. A. *Alcohol and the Diet.* Westport, Ct.: AVI Publishing, 1979.

56. KEISANIEMI, Y. A. "Ethanol and Acetaldehyde in the Milk and Peripheral Blood of Lactating Women after Ethanol Administration." *Journal of Obstetrics and Gynecology of the British Commonwealth* 81 (1974): 84.

57. TAYLOR, L. E., and B. S. WORTHINGTON. "Guidance for Lactating Mothers." In *Nutrition in Pregnancy and Lactation,* eds., B. S. Worthington, J. Vermeersch, and S. R. Williams. St. Louis: C. V. Mosby, 1977.

58. SAVAGE, R. L. "Drugs and Breast Milk." *Journal of Human Nutrition* 31 (1977): 459.

59. FOMON, S. J., L. J. FILER, JR., T. A. ANDERSON, and E. E. ZIEGLER. "Recommendations for Feeding Normal Infants." *Pediatrics* 63 (1979): 52.

60. Committee on Nutrition, American Academy of Pediatrics. "Fluoride Supplementation: Revised Dosage Schedule." *Pediatrics* 63 (1979): 150.

61 HALES, D., J. KENNEL, and R. ROSA. "How Early is Early Contact? Defining the Limit of the Sensitive Period." *Pediatric Research* 10 (1976): 448.

62. JELLIFFE, E. F. P. "Infant Feeding Practices: Associated Iatrogenic and Commerciogenic Diseases." *Pediatric Clinics of North America* 25 (1977): 49.

63. Committee on Nutrition, American Academy of Pediatrics. "The Feeding of Solid Foods to Infants." *Pediatrics* 21 (1958): 685.

64. ILLINGSWORTH, R. S., and J. LISTER. "The Critical or Sensitive Period, with Special Reference to Certain Feeding Problems in Infants and Children." *Journal of Pediatrics* 65 (1964): 839.

65. ANDERSON, T. A. "Commercial Infant Foods: Content and Composition. *Pediatric Clinics of North America* 24 (1977): 37.

66. TAITZ, L. S. "Obesity in Pedatric Practice: Infantile Obesity." *Pediatric Clinics of North America* 24 (1977): 107.

CHAPTER 3

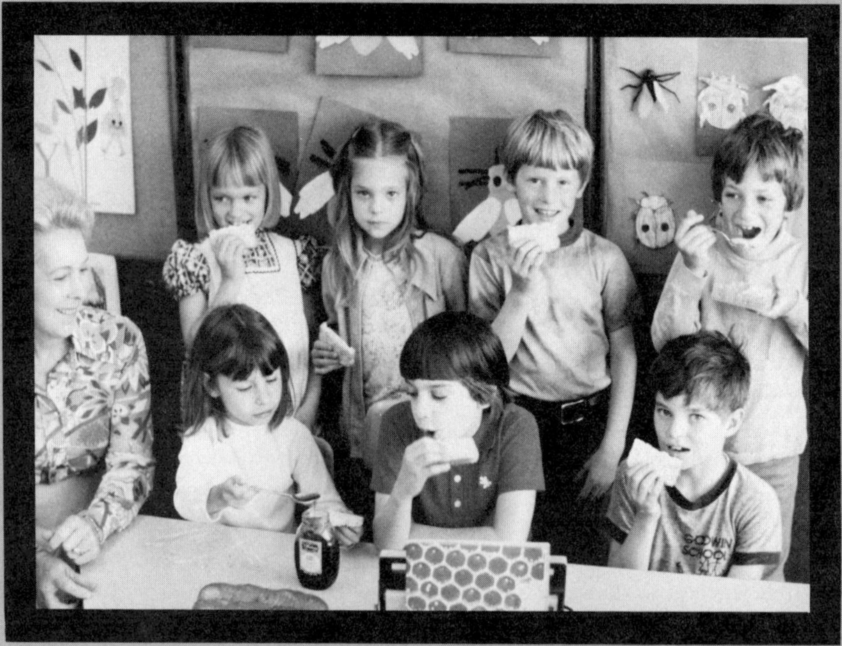

Photo by Kenneth P. Davis

nutrition during childhood

CHILDHOOD, INCLUDING THE PREPUBESCENT PERIOD, IS USUALLY CONSIDERED THE PERIOD FROM 1 THROUGH 9. This period is characterized by learning, exploration, socialization, increased physical activity, and slower growth in comparison to the first year. Changes in physical growth and nutritional needs are much more subtle than before. Individual differences begin to emerge more sharply, which makes assessing and assigning specific nutrient requirements much more difficult.

Requirements for nutrients for this period have been derived from a few studies with children, animal models, and adult studies with extrapolation for size. Boys and girls are similar in size, and physical activity and nutritional needs are similar. A child may have growth spurts at different times and then go for long periods with such slight growth that it is not noticeable. A mother who becomes concerned that her child has "stopped growing" may then see the same child outgrow two sizes of pants as the long bones lengthen and mineralize and muscle growth accelerates. Nutrition recommendations should be made according to physical size rather than age because of the great variation among children of the same chronological age.

Social and Psychological Needs

Socialization is continuous in childhood. As the child's world expands outside the home, he or she develops new means of interacting. Small children have a limited range of emotions including fear and anger. As the child grows older, the range of emotions increases. Family and peer groups identify what is acceptable and what is not. A child learns to achieve goals and win respect without alienating others. The peer group often provides more realistic feedback than the family, and allows the child to become more aware of strengths and weaknesses. Peer groups can also have a great influence on food intake and on the acceptance or rejection of foods.

The large number of working mothers and increasing numbers of single parents have placed many preschool children in day care. This means eating one or two meals away from home with peer groups. Group feeding may contribute from 50 to 75 percent of a child's total intake in a day. Types and amounts of foods served and the attitudes of other children will greatly influence nutrient intake and the establishment of food habits that may be quite different from those of the family.

The social pressures of working parents have also increased the frequency with which families eat at fast food restaurants, where typically foods are higher in calories and salts than foods consumed at home. More convenience foods or ready-to-eat items are used at home, which may confuse children about original sources of foods and turn them away from such foods as vegetables, which require more preparation time and usually have to be eaten at the table.

School-age children are involved in so many group activities after school and during summers that little time is reserved for eating. In our fast-moving society, family meals are almost nonexistent. The influence of parents' example is diminishing, with family members eating at different times and usually on the run. Peer groups begin to have greater influence on food habits than families because of the greater amount of contact children have with peers.

Physiological Changes and Growth

Growth in childhood is primarily linear. Each child has his or her own pattern of growth, and each system of the body has a different rate of growth, as shown in Figure 3–1. During this period, as in others, it is best to chart each child's growth individually instead of comparing him or her to other children (see Appendix for growth charts of the National Center for Health Statistics).

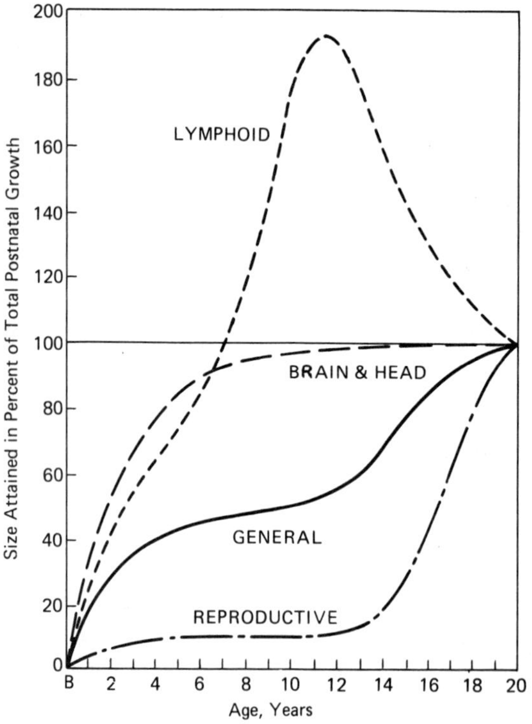

FIG. 3–1. Postnatal system growth. *Source:* R. E. Scammon, "The Measurement of the Body in Childhood." In *The Measurement of Man,* by J. A. Harris, C. M. Jackson, and R. E. Scammon (University of Minnesota Press, 1927).

age, height, and weight

An individual child's pattern of growth is predictable once his or her channel has been established. It is more important to know that a child is maintaining a given relationship of weight to height than to know that he or she is short or heavy for his or her age (1). Deviations from the pattern are of greater significance than actual percentile rankings. A sudden change in pattern, either up or down, may indicate nutritional imbalances and/or illnesses that require further attention.

Rates of growth decrease during childhood. During the second year the child gains approximately 3 kg (.25 kg/mo) in weight and 10 to 12 cm in height. From age 3, weight increments are 2.0 to 2.5 kg per year, and height increases by 5 to 7 cm until puberty. Weight gains may fluctuate through the year, but small losses are not considered significant. Many studies on children's growth have been summarized in Robert's *Nutrition Work with Children* (2), and additional in-depth reports and data are listed in Reed and Stuart (3) and Stuart (4).

One of the early graphs showing the relationship of growth to age, height, and weight was the **Wetzel grid** (5), which included measures of basal metabolism and maturity ratings. The grid was complex and required skill in recording, as well as interpretation. It was followed by graphs published by Jackson and Kelly, which used percentiles for height and weight from physical measurements obtained in Meredith's Iowa growth studies (6). Stuart and Stevenson followed these with charts that combined the Iowa data with data from the Harvard School of Public Health Studies and were known as the **Stuart-Meredith tables** (7). These were used until the late 1970s, when the National Center for Health Statistics (NCHS) charts were published (8); see Appendix.

other growth characteristics

In addition to growth as measured by height and weight, certain other growth characteristics have nutritional significance in childhood. Different portions of the body increase in length at different rates and at different times (see Figure 3–2). In fetal life the head is the fastest growing portion of the body. During the first year after birth, the trunk is the fastest growing portion. From 1 year to puberty, the legs grow faster than any other portion.

The brain grows rapidly in childhood. At age 2 it is approximately 50 percent of adult size; it is 75 percent at age 4, and 100 percent by 6 to 10 years of age. The central nervous system is especially vulnerable to nutrition insults from birth to 2 years. Lack of adequate food may impair synthesis of the fatty compounds that form myelin (9) and cause irreversible damage. Myelination proceeds rapidly until 2 years of age, but is not complete until approximately age 10.

Muscle growth prior to puberty is affected by the pituitary growth hormone (PGH), the thyroid hormones, and insulin (metabolism). The sex hormones play little part in growth until puberty, which explains the fact that there are few

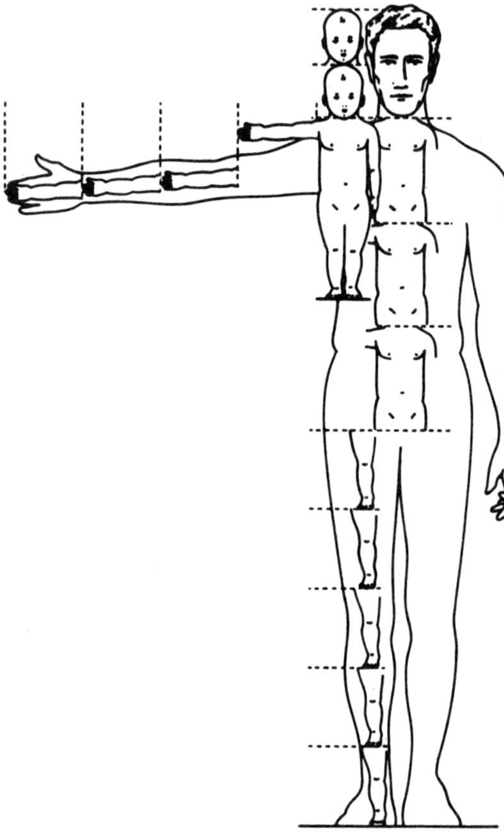

FIG. 3–2 Changes in body proportions. *Source:* I. Valadian and D. Porter, *Physical Growth and Development from Conception to Maturity: A Programmed Text* (Boston: Little, Brown, 1977).

differences in the growth of girls and boys prior to puberty. The number of voluntary muscle fibers is roughly the same for all ages in childhood; differences, if any, are due to the increase in size of individual muscles. Muscle strength is correlated with the total amount of muscle tissue. The child with larger muscles is generally stronger than the one with smaller muscles. During childhood, age seems to be the most important factor in the development of muscle strength. When children of the same height and weight are tested for muscle strength, the older children generally perform better—probably because of greater experience and training. Muscles that are not used lose both strength and bulk; muscles that are used and trained get stronger and larger.

There is rapid accumulation of adipose (fat) tissue during the first six months of life. Then fat thickness begins to decrease, and the slimming generally continues to age 6. From age 6 to puberty there is a slow, gradual accumulation of fat (see Figure 3–3) in both girls and boys. The total amount of fat accumulated depends on the number and size of existing adipose cells. Research is continuing on the factors related to the development of fat cells (see Chapter 9 for more details). Obese children have more fat cells and often larger fat cells than nonobese children at any given age. For example, a fat 6-year-old boy may have ten times the number of fat cells as a slender boy of the same height and age.

In childhood, the skeleton passes through successive stages of development: connective tissue, cartilage, and bone. Cartilage is found in all parts of the skeleton, even where bone is to be laid down directly in membrane, such as in the clavicle and cranial vault. The duration of the cartilaginous stage is a measure of speed of development: the more rapidly a bone is growing, the less time in the cartilaginous phase.

From 1 to 4 years, the cut surface of a long bone shows a pink texture of trabeculae with red marrow. From 4 to 7 years, fat gradually accumulates in droplets and by 7 years the bony trabeculae are replaced with real marrow. Between 12 and 14 years, there is fat in the midlength of the bone extending toward both ends. Changes in the epiphyses are similar to those in the shaft. The epiphysis is cartilaginous material at each end of the long bones. Ossification of the epiphysis develops from a separate center and not by penetration from the main center of ossification for the bone (see Figure 3–4 for resorption remodeling). Usually, epiphyses that ossify early unite with the shafts late. The relationship between age and physical maturation of the skeleton are as follows:

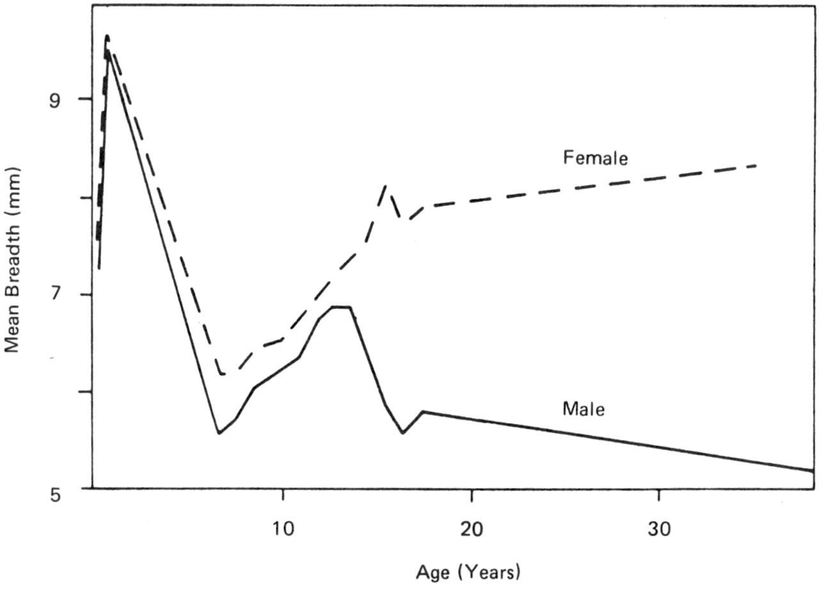

FIG. 3–3. Fat accumulation between childhood and adolescence. The distribution of subcutaneous fat for males and females in childhood and adolescence, estimated from mean breadth of fat in calf. *Source:* I. Valadian and D. Porter, *Physical Growth and Development from Conception to Maturity: A Programmed Text* (Boston: Little, Brown, 1977).

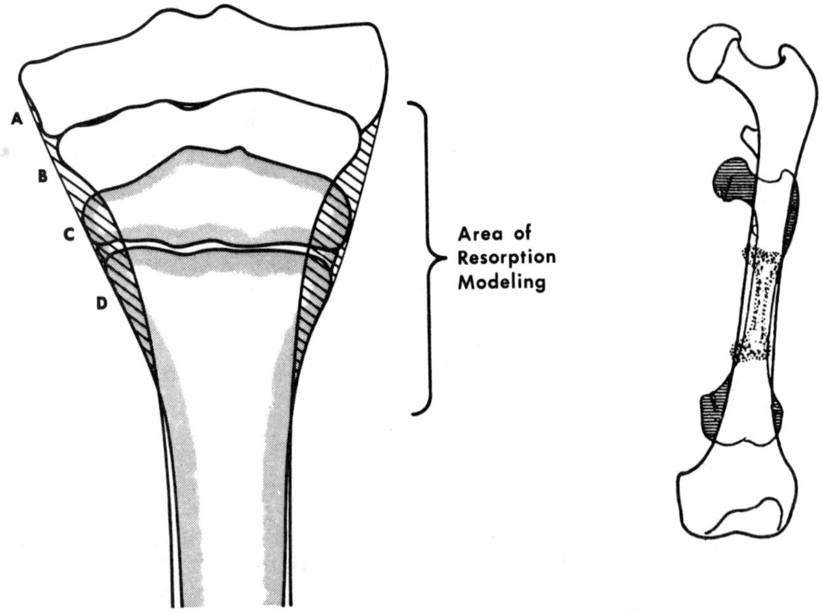

FIG. 3–4. Resorption modeling of long-shafted bone. As the bone grows in length the shape and width changes. The process is called resorption modeling. Bone is resorbed from some areas while deposition of minerals and ossification occurs in other areas.

1. *Birth to 5 years: appearance of ossification centers.*
2. *Five to 14 years: bony penetration of cartilaginous areas.*
3. *Fourteen to 25 years: epiphyseal-disphyseal union.*

The sequence of stages in skeletal maturation follows a fairly definite pattern. Because of high correlation between skeletal maturity (bone age), sexual maturity, and overall physical growth, X rays of certain portions of the skeleton are a reliable method of assessing physical maturation. Usually the hand and wrist are X-rayed because they contain large numbers of shafted and nonshafted bones that show progression in development at every age to maturity. Bone age is read by comparing X rays of a child with a standardized set that show bone development at six-month intervals (10). Racial and sexual variations in bone age do exist, with blacks showing earlier maturation than whites and girls being ahead of boys by several months during early childhood. There is considerable individual variation, with bone age varying from chronological age by one year without signs of abnormality. (Figure 3–5 illustrates the wide range of normal for the appearance of secondary ossification centers.)

Severe and prolonged malnutrition and disease can cause retardation in the maturation of bone (11, 12). Bone scars or lines of arrested growth may show up

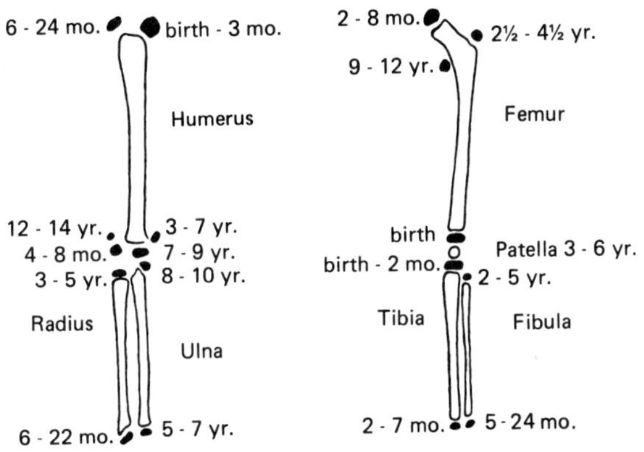

FIG. 3–5. Secondary ossification centers showing average time of appearance.

on X rays. These transverse lines along the shaft of long bones are visible because of increased density of the bone ends during periods of slowed growth. Normal density bone shows up once the period of slowed growth is over. Ordinarily, disturbances of the endocrine system have a much greater effect on bone maturation than infections or malnutrition.

A very low or inadequate protein intake may affect the formation of normal bone. Excessive intake of protein may interfere with the retention of calcium, thereby decreasing mineralization. Abnormal mineralization of the bony matrix may be related to malnutrition. In the complex interrelationship between nutrition and growth, the following factors must be considered: amount of protein, calcium to phosphorous ratio, blood pH, fat metabolism, adequate vitamin D, parathyroid hormones, and deficiencies of vitamin C.

Nutrient Requirements and Recommended Allowances

The recommended amounts of various nutrients, which are considered to give a 50 to 100 percent margin of safety, are listed in the RDA table in the Appendix. Here we will discuss only the more important ones.

The determination of nutrient requirements and subsequent recommendations for adequate levels of nutrients for good health in children are complicated by the implications of growth. Children need food for energy, regulation of body processes, and growth. Assessment of growth in childhood continues to be the best method of evaluating the influence of nutrition, particularly measurements of height and weight (see growth charts in the Appendix). Accurate measurement is essential for reliable interpretation. Errors in measurement of length are more common than errors in weight (13, 14). (The procedures for accurate measurement will be discussed in Chapter 7.)

energy

Energy needs are difficult to assess in children because of differences in body size and activities. Calorie requirements are more realistically based on body size (surface area) and physical development than on chronological age or sex. The recommendations for energy needs are based on observations of the caloric intakes of healthy children growing normally (15, 16). These needs are estimated in Table 3–1. The factors to be considered in determining energy needs in children are: 1) growth; 2) physical activity; 3) specific dynamic action (SDA) of food; 4) basal metabolic needs; and 5) calories lost in excreta.

Caloric requirements for growth are 5 to 10 kcal per kg/day after the first year and prior to puberty. The energy needed for physical activity varies with body size and intensity and duration of activity, but in general the requirement is less than 20 kcal per kg/day after the first year. Energy expenditures have been calculated for specific activities (see Chapter 9). The SDA requires 5 to 7 kcal per kg/day in the average diet; if food intake contains a large proportion of protein, the SDA may be doubled. Insufficient food intake will use fewer kcal and overfeeding may increase caloric need by as much as 40 percent. After the first year, the caloric requirements for basal metabolism are 25 to 30 kcal/kg/day. Approximately 10 percent of the body energy intake is lost each day through excretion.

In overweight and undernourished children, total energy needs should be calculated on the expected rather than actual weight of the child. That weight may

TABLE 3–1. Estimated Energy Needs of Children

age (years)	kcal/kg/day		total kcal/day for reference child	
	FAO/WHO[a]	RDA[b]	FAO/WHO[a]	RDA[b]
1–3	101	100	1360	1300
4–6	91	90	1830	1800
7–9	78	80[c]	2190	2400[c]

[a] Joint FAO/WHO ad hoc Expert Committee, *Energy and Protein Requirements*, Food and Agriculture Organization of the United Nations Nutrition Meetings Report Series No. 52, and WHO Technical Report Series No. 522. (Rome: Food and Agriculture Organization of the United Nations, 1973).

[b] Food and Nutrition Board, *Recommended Dietary Allowances*, 9th ed. (Washington, D.C.: National Research Council, National Academy of Sciences, 1980). Reproduced by the permission of the National Academy of Sciences, Washington, D.C.

[c] Age range for RDA is 7 to 10 years.

be calculated using the height measurement and the 50th percentile for weight at that height.

protein

Some estimates of protein needs have been based on nitrogen balance studies that utilize the lowest protein intake at which nitrogen retention and growth occurs (17). Some of these studies have been criticized because they involved previously undernourished children, so the nitrogen retention associated with growth may be overestimated and result in misleadingly high values. Balance study information is not available for all ages and sizes, so extrapolations have been made for some ages based on the available studies in which nitrogen balance has been attained on a low protein intake using high-quality protein (18).

Another method is the factorial approach, which depends on the computation of obligatory nitrogen losses observed on a minimum protein diet. This loss is about 1.4 mg/basal calorie in urine; 0.4 mg/basal calorie in feces; and a total with other routes of 2 mg/basal calorie daily. Data collected by the factorial method are 30 percent lower than that of the balance method. FAO/WHO data are computed from balance and factorial methods with a safety factor for individual variation. Most of the estimates are based on the assumption that proteins of high biological value are used.

For some children on strict vegetarian diets, there have been reports of less than optimal growth (19, 20). Adequate growth is possible, but the variety and total amount of vegetables eaten must be closely monitored in growing children (21). Quantitative information on amino acid needs during childhood is incomplete, but it should become available as our technology improves. The current information relates primarily to boys aged 10 to 12 years (22, 23).

Table 3–2 shows a comparison of the estimated amounts of protein necessary for children. Again, it should be used as a guide, and adjustments made as necessary for individual children. Note that the lower figures from FAO/WHO are presented as "requirements" or "safe levels," whereas the RDA figures are calculated with margins for optimal intakes. Most authorities agree that the higher figures must be used for mixed diets that include proteins of lesser quality. Nitrogen retention is not usually achieved if the intake of protein is less than 4 percent of total calories. Studies have shown that in most instances, protein intake will be adequate if energy intake is adequate (24).

vitamins and minerals

For children, there is a safe range of intake for fat-soluble vitamins and some minerals, especially the trace elements. Too little results in deficiency signs or

TABLE 3-2. Recommended Protein Intakes for Children

age (years)	g/kg/day		total g/day		percentage of total calories	
	FAO/WHO[a]	RDA[b]	FAO/WHO[a]	RDA[b]	FAO/WHO[a]	RDA[b]
1–3	1.19	1.77	16	23	4.7%	7.1%
4–6	1.01	1.50	20	30	4.4	6.0
7–9[c]	0.88	1.20	25	36	4.6	6.7

[a] Joint FAO/WHO ad hoc Expert Committee, *Energy and Protein Requirements*, Food and Agriculture Organization of the United Nations Nutrition Meetings Report Series No. 52, and WHO Technical Report Series No. 522. (Rome: Food and Agriculture Organization of the United Nations, 1973).

[b] Food and Nutrition Board. *Recommended Dietary Allowances*, 9th ed. (Washington, D.C.: National Research Council, National Academy of Sciences, 1980). Reproduced by the permission of the National Academy of Sciences, Washington, D.C.

[c] 7 to 10 years for RDA.

symptoms; too much results in toxic responses. Evidence exists for hypervitaminosis A and D, so supplementation with high doses can be harmful, although experimental data on the vitamin and mineral needs of children are limited.

The RDAs for vitamin A, vitamin E, folacin, B_{12}, and riboflavin have been extrapolated from infant and adult values, and the values for niacin have been arbitrarily set. For calcium and magnesium, the allowances have been estimated from limited data. Per kilogram of body weight, the vitamin C requirement appears to be higher for children than for adults. For children up to age 11 the requirement is 45 mg/day; for older children, it is 60 mg/day.

The thiamin allowance for children is based on studies of urinary excretion and whole blood levels of thiamin. About 0.3 mg/1000 kcal is the requirement, and the RDA is 0.5 mg/1000 kcal. For vitamin B_6, the allowances range up to 2.0 mg daily based on an intake of 0.02 mg of vitamin B_6 per gram of dietary protein intake. Ritchey et al. found an intake of 1.25 mg per day adequate for 7- to 9-year-olds (25).

Iron requirements are computed by considering iron losses and the increase in body stores of iron during growth. Other components of the diet also influence iron absorption, so the amount of iron needed is estimated to be 1 mg/day of absorbed iron for children. Zinc is necessary for sexual maturity and growth. Hambidge et al. (26) have identified retarded growth related to marginal zinc deficiency in children in one part of the United States. The minimum zinc requirement for growing children appears to be 6 mg/day, with the allowance set at 10 mg/day to allow for dermal losses and availability.

nutrition surveys

In the Preschool Nutrition Survey done from 1968 to 1970, those children with inadequate energy intakes also had less than adequate intakes of other nutrients (27). The nutrients most frequently reported as inadequate in other studies were iron, calcium, and vitamins A and C (28, 29, 30). Even though intakes were low, few deficiency diseases were seen, with the exception of iron deficiency anemia. This deficiency occurs most frequently in the child under 3 who consumes excessive amounts of milk to the exclusion of iron-containing foods. The Nutrition Canada National Survey (1973) reported values for hemoglobin, mean corpuscular hemoglobin concentration (MCHC), and transferrin saturation indicating widespread iron deficiency in the children surveyed. A third of the infants and toddlers and 25 percent of children 5 to 9 years of age had low biochemical values. Limited amounts of iron in the food intakes of children were marked and spread throughout the general population (31).

The first HANES Survey (1971–1972) indicated that median nutrient intakes of elementary school-age children were at or above the RDA, in contrast to those of younger or older children (32). Except for iron deficiency, other vitamin and mineral deficiencies are almost nonexistent in the United States because of food fortification programs, school food programs, improved food processing techniques, and public interest in nutrition. This is not true in developing countries, where food supplies are so limited that multiple deficiency diseases are common.

The Ten-State Nutrition Survey (1968–1970) noted low vitamin A intakes, particularly in Spanish-American children in the low-income areas (33). This same trend regarding low-income groups was also noted in the Canadian survey (31). Serum levels of vitamin A were classified as marginal although no clinical deficiency symptoms were seen. Low vitamin A intake is regarded as a potential problem for all children that can be prevented with increased intakes of vitamin A-rich or carotene-containing foods. The survey reported evidence of retarded growth and development in children from the low-income areas. But despite lower reported incomes, black children were taller than white children and were more advanced in skeletal and dental development.

Meeting Nutrition Needs

During childhood, certain characteristics of physical appearance and behavior have been suggested as indicative of adequate or less than adequate nutrition. Some of these characteristics are noted in Table 3–3. Poorly nourished children may be disadvantaged in educational and learning situations because these characteristics lead to negative responses and/or being ignored by peers and teachers. Numerous studies have shown that malnourished children show psychological disturbances, such as apathy and irritability, accompanied by loss of curiosity and exploratory behavior (34). Some authorities use interest in and response to environmental stimuli as reliable indications of improvement in nutritional status. Although malnutrition is only one of the complex factors affecting learning, it seems that undernourished and malnourished children make up a sizable number of those who do poorly in school.

Learning and behavior have been reported to improve as a result of feeding in school or day care programs. Data are mixed and inconclusive from controlled studies, but indications are that the child who has eaten at school (either breakfast or lunch) is more attentive, and therefore able to make better use of learning opportunities, than the child who is hungry (35). However, any specific

TABLE 3-3. Comparison of Characteristics Indicative of Adequate and Less than Adequate Nutrition

adequate (good)	less than adequate (poor)
General appearance of vitality, well-being, and alertness.	Strained expression; dull and listless; apathetic.
Bright, clear eyes; smiling, happy expression; no dark circles under eyes.	Sad looking; dark circles under eyes; no smile; prone to tears.
Recovers quickly from fatigue; endurance during activity.	Chronic fatigue; tires easily; takes excessive time to bounce back from physical activity; lack of endurance.
Full of energy; vigorous.	Lack of energy; weakness.
Smooth, glossy hair.	Dry, brittle, easily "pluckable" hair.
Good appetite; curious and eager to try new foods.	Poor appetite; unwilling to try new foods; may have many food dislikes.
Good posture; stands erect; well-developed muscles.	Poor posture; slumping; muscles weak and underdeveloped.
Skin is firm, resilient, and "feels alive"; subcutaneous fat layers, rosy hue.	Skin is dry; has little or no tone; pale; little or no subcutaneous fat.
Interested in environment; curious; responsive.	Irritable, nervous, slow to react; indifferent, passive, unresponsive; unable to cope with stimuli.
Good growth, adequate weight and height for age.	Stunted growth; thin, small for age; overweight for height.
Attentive, eager to learn and experiment.	Shortened attention span; reduced capacity to concentrate.

SOURCE: *Roberts' Nutrition Work with Children*, 3rd ed., revised by E. A. Martin (Chicago: University of Chicago Press, 1954).

effect on learning or behavior must be considered in relation to the total diet (36).

As growth slows during the second year, appetite decreases, allowing for food intake to correspond with decreased needs for growth. Some of the changes in childhood are shown in Table 3–4. Feeding problems may develop as a result of this natural phenomenon, particularly if mothers do not understand what is happening. If a mother begins to force the child to eat more, the child may rebel and eat nothing. Many children are brought to a physician with the mother complaining of poor appetite, refusal to eat, and no weight gain.

At 18 months to 2 years of age the child may become very independent and refuse to allow anyone to help with feeding. It is necessary for mothers to be aware of how much the child has eaten so that sufficient quantities are consumed. Not only is capacity still small, but attention spans are short and interest in food and feeding is of short duration. More than three meals per day are needed during this time to meet nutrient needs. For example, a 28-month old girl refused food when given adult portions. As the mother forced the girl to eat, she became more determined. The entire family joined the argument. When small portions were provided, the child began eating. A 2- or 3-year-old who is expected to eat only at mealtime with adults cannot consume enough food in three settings. When part of the food is offered between meals, the total amount consumed increases.

food consumption patterns

Children vary considerably in appetite between days and even meals. Capacity is small, so feedings should be frequent, with small servings. Too often the child's efforts at eating are judged by an adult according to what an adult would eat, rather than what a child should eat. Large servings tend to overwhelm the small child, who may then not even attempt to eat the food. Children would rather eat all of a serving and ask for more with encouragement. A rule of thumb for amounts of food to be consumed is one tablespoon of each food per year of age for the preschool years. Table 3–5 lists amounts of various foods needed during a 24-hour period and shows gradual increases as the child gets older. The nutrient content of the specified amounts of food will meet the recommended levels of nutrients (see RDA chart in the Appendix) for children at these different ages if a variety of foods is chosen. Using the same food from each group habitually could lead to nutrient deficiencies, for no single food contains all the nutrients, or in the proportions needed by children. Many children will attempt to consume one food to the exclusion of others. For instance, the child may drink excessive amounts of milk and then not have any appetite for other foods. Since milk is such a poor source of iron, anemia may result. This is a rather common occurrence in the 2- to 4-year age group. Bread is another food young children like to fill up on.

TABLE 3-4. Progressive Development of Children and Relation to Feeding

age	activity	related food behavior
15 months	Gross motor drive under better control.	Can sit through meals.
	Limited ability to feed self.	Prefers finger feeding; uses spoon, but often turns spoon on way to mouth. With fatigue accepts assistance in feeding or for certain meals, and may demand to feed self for other meals. Enjoys feeding parents or caretakers.
	Grasping.	Holds cup between thumb and forefinger. Tilts cup with fingers.
	Bottle feeding.	Some children still have a bottle before bedtime (bottles in bed should be avoided).
15–18 months	Sleep.	Regular time established—6–8 P.M., with 12 hours of sleep. Afternoon nap following lunch.
18 months	Appetite decreasing.	Reduced food consumption; refusals and perferences fluctuate.
	Improved ability in self feeding.	Some children can handle all meals; uses a spoon.
	Discovery of everything.	Will eat dangerous substances (medicine, liquid soaps) unless locked out of reach.
2 years	Moderate appetite.	Small breakfast; noon usually best meal.
	Marked food preferences—"finicky."	Prefers food not to be mixed up. Preferences related to taste, form, consistency, color. Repeats demand for one food; drops that food and selects another.
	Grasp of spoon begins to change to thumb and index finger.	Self feeding becomes easier, and child will not accept help. (A few children still need help, and most children will accept help when tired.)
	Sleep and naps.	Usually 12 hours; some children eliminate naps.
3 years	Appetite improving.	Best meals, breakfast and evening meal.
	Preferences and refusals less pronounced.	Wider variety of food accepted. Developing desire for sweets. Vegetables slowly accepted, may prefer raw.
	Spoon feeding.	Some, especially girls, hold spoon in adult fashion.
	Desire for attention.	Eats well alone, but may have difficulty with the family or in groups.
	Sleep.	About 12 hours daily.
4 years	Improved appetite.	All meals consumed equally. Food jags and food strikes prior to 4½ years.
	Much talking.	Usually does not interfere with meals.
	Likes to plan and help prepare meals.	May encourage eating a new food.
	Sleep.	About 11½ hours.
5 years	Good appetite.	Good noon and evening meal; poor breakfast. Feeds self slowly. May ask for help in feeding when hungry. Likes plain food rather than casseroles.
	Composure and observation.	Influenced by preferences and refusals of others.
	Sleep.	About 11 hours.

TABLE 3-4. (Continued)

age	activity	related food behavior
6 years	An active age.	
	Good increasing appetite.	Similar to 5-year old; may return to finger feeding.
	Variation in sleep patterns.	About 10½ hours.
7 years	More cautious approach. Appetite decreases.	Fewer refusals, overcoming aversions. May eat disliked food at beginning or end of meal.
	Sleep.	About 10 hours.
8–9 years	Improved appetite.	Eats rapidly; larger amounts. Some food dislikes remain. More willing to try new food. Handles a fork; some can use a knife to cut meat.
	Sleep.	Amount variable usually, 8–10 hours.
10 years and over	There is great diversity at any age, but it becomes more evident by this age, based on habits, culture, economic status, style of living, and media influences.	

SOURCES: E. Hurlock, *Developmental Psychology*, 5th ed. (New York: McGraw Hill, 1980). A. Gesell and F. L. Ilg, *Child Development* (New York: Harper and Row, 1949).

Food jags are common throughout childhood. Children get in a rut; they want to eat the same foods over and over, sometimes in large quantities. Peanut butter jags are typical; the child will want peanut butter every time food is offered. The jags are usually short-lived and do not present a problem unless there is excessive attention or disturbance which lets the child use this behavior to get his or her way or to control the caretaker's behavior.

For the younger, smaller children, foods need to be divided into small meals and/or snacks distributed throughout the day. Because of children's limited capacity and comparatively great nutrient needs, foods must be carefully chosen. Snacks or between-meal feedings must be of high quality and contribute to the overall nutrient needs. There is no place for "empty calories," even though adequate energy is a concern in this age group. Observations in day care and child development centers indicated that when intervals of approximately two hours separate feeding times, appetite and therefore food intake remains high. Rest or relaxation periods should immediately precede feeding times. If a child is allowed to become tired or too hungry, he or she may become irritable, with decreased appetite and decreased food intake.

building good food habits

In addition to meeting nutrient needs, foods and feeding times contribute to the development of good food habits. The developmental levels of children affect the kinds of foods offered and the preparation procedures used. For instance,

TABLE 3–5. Recommended Food Intake for Good Nutrition According to Food Groups and Average Size of Serving at Different Age Levels

food group	servings per day	average size of serving: 1 YEAR	2–3 YEARS	4–5 YEARS	6–9 YEARS	10–12 YEARS	13–15 YEARS
Milk and cheese (1 oz cheese = 1 c milk)	4	½ c	½–¾ c	¾ c	¾–1 c	1 c	1 c
Meat group (protein foods)	3 or more						
Egg		1	1	1	1	1	1 or more
Lean meat, fish, poultry (liver once a week)		2 tbsp	2 tbsp	4 tbsp	2–3 oz (4–6 tbsp)	3–4 oz	4 oz or more
Peanut butter			1 tbsp	2 tbsp	2–3 tbsp	3 tbsp	3 tbsp
Fruits and vegetables	At least 4, including:						
Vitamin C source (citrus fruits, berries, tomato, cabbage, cantaloupe)	1 or more (twice as much tomato as citrus)	⅓ c citrus	½ c	½ c	1 medium orange	1 medium orange	1 medium orange
Vitamin A source (green or yellow fruits and vegetables)	1 or more	2 tbsp	3 tbsp	4 tbsp (¼ c)	¼ c	⅓ c	½ c
Other vegetables (potato and legumes) *or*	2	2 tbsp	3 tbsp	4 tbsp (¼ c)	⅓ c	½ c	¾ c

Other fruits (apple, banana)		¼ c	⅓ c	½ c	1 medium	1 medium	1 medium
Cereals (whole-grain or enriched)	At least 4						
Bread		½ slice	1 slice	1½ slices	1–2 slices	2 slices	2 slices
Ready-to-eat cereals		½ oz	¾ oz	1 oz	1 oz	1 oz	1 oz
Cooked cereal (including macaroni, spaghetti, rice)		¼ c	⅓ c	½ c	½ c	¾ c	1 c or more
Fats and carbohydrates	To meet calorie needs						
Butter, margarine, mayonnaise, oils		1 tbsp	1 tbsp	1 tbsp	2 tbsp	2 tbsp	2–4 tbsp
Desserts and sweets: 100 calorie portions as follows. 1/3 c pudding or ice cream 2–3 cookies, 1 oz cake,. 11/3 oz pie, 2 tbsp jelly, jam, honey, sugar		1 portion	1½ portions	1½ portions	3 portions	3 portions	3–6 portions

[a]Prepared in collaboration with Mildred J. Bennett, Ph.D., from "Four Food Groups of the Daily Food Guide," Institute of Home Economics, USDA, and Publication 30, Children's Bureau of the United States Department of Health, Education, and Welfare.

C = 1 cup = 8 oz = 240 g.

SOURCE: From V. C. Vaughn III and R. J. McKay, *Nelson's Textbook of Pediatrics*, 10th ed. (Philadelphia: Saunders, 1975), p. 159.

the 2- to 3-year-old who is trying to be very independent—wanting to do everything for himself—needs finger foods or foods that cling easily to a spoon (see Table 3–6). Appropriate and functional use of the fork—spearing first and then as a lift—comes later, at 4 to 5 years. Use of a knife for cutting rather than spreading begins at approximately 6 to 8 years if the child has had opportunities to experiment. Just as the infant is gradually weaned from sucking the bottle to drinking from a glass, so the child progresses gradually from spoon to fork and finally to knife and fork for cutting. The progression is from a fisted grasp of the utensils to appropriate holding of spoon, fork, and knife.

Preschool and elementary age children are often described as "picky" or "particular" about the foods they eat. Rejection of foods that are difficult to chew, such as some meats, is common because chewing skills develop slowly and are related to position and timing of tooth eruption, sore gums, and food experience. Some may chew inadequately and then not be able to swallow the bolus, resulting in their spitting the food back into the plate. Mothers may see this as a dislike for certain foods, when in fact it merely has to do with the tenderness of the food

TABLE 3–6. Suggested Snacks and Finger Foods

fruits	vegetables
Apple wedges	Cabbage wedges
Banana slices	Carrot sticks
Berries	Caulifloweretts
Dried apples	Celery sticks[a]
Dried apricots	Cherry tomatoes
Dried peaches	Cucumber slices
Dried pears	Green pepper sticks
Fresh peach wedges	Tomato wedges
Fresh pear wedges	Turnip sticks
Fresh pineapple sticks	Zucchini or summer squash strips
Grapefruit sections (seeded)	
Grapes	**meats**
Melon cubes or balls	Cheese cubes
Orange sections (seeded)	Cooked meat cubes
Pitted plums	Hard-cooked eggs
Pitted prunes	Small sandwiches (quartered)
Raisins	Toast fingers
Tangerine sections	Whole grain crackers

[a]May be stuffed with cheese or peanut butter.

SOURCE: *A Planning Guide for Food Service in Child Care Centers*, USDA, FNS-64, Food and Nutrition Service, Washington, D.C., revised 1976.

or the size of the bite. Unfamiliar textures (crisp or hard, stringy or lumpy) may also be rejected at first. Children reject more foods on the basis of undesirable or unfamiliar textures than on the basis of taste. This concept is important to remember in making recommendations to mothers of children. Single items that can be carefully scrutinized for smell, texture (both in hands and mouth), and taste are more readily accepted by children than are mixtures which are not easily identified. The child may methodically pick familiar items out of a mixture, leaving those he or she cannot recognize.

Food acceptances and rejections change rapidly during these years. A food that has been consistently rejected through the preschool years may suddenly be accepted as the child starts school and sees others eating the rejected foods. Children are great imitators, something caretakers should remember in attempting to introduce new foods. If mother and/or father eats a food, the child may be motivated to try it. The teacher in nursery or elementary school becomes the role model for imitative behavior.

Children are curious and want to experiment. These traits should be emphasized in teaching good food habits. Childhood should be the preparation period for adolescence, when nutritive needs will be greater. Storage of nutrients occurs during childhood. In addition, lifelong food habits can be established at a time when a child is eager to learn and learns well and easily from repetition and experience.

group feeding

As more and more women enter the work force, larger numbers of preschool children are being cared for in group settings away from home. This may offer nutritional advantages to many children. One study has shown that greater amounts of nutrients are consumed at day care centers than at home by some children, particularly those in day care for more than eight hours daily (37). Because of the importance of feeding for overall nutritional status and growth, menu selection and food preparation techniques in preschool centers become even more important. Regulations must be imposed and monitored by appropriate governmental agencies for the protection of the children. In some states at present, only centers receiving federal reimbursement for meals served are under any scrutiny, so parents are well advised to check the center to which they send their children to be sure a qualified nutrition expert has been consulted in planning the menu. The pattern followed by a good day care center (see Table 3–7) may help parents as well (38).

The school food service program may offer these same advantages to older children. In the United States, group feeding of children to improve nutritional status dates back to early 1900. Some schools introduced a hot noon meal for students who lived too far to go home for lunch as early as 1915. The most significant changes have occurred since the enactment of the National School Lunch Act in 1946. Its purpose was "to safeguard the health and well being of

TABLE 3-7. Pattern of Feeding

breakfast	children 1 to 3 years	children 3 to 6 years
Milk, fluid[a]	1/2 cup	3/4 cup
Juice or fruit	1/4 cup	1/2 cup
Cereal or bread, enriched or whole grain[b]		
cereal, or	1/4 cup[c]	1/3 cup[d]
bread	1/2 slice	1/2 slice
midmorning or midafternoon supplement		
Milk, fluid[a]; or juice; or fruit; or vegetable	1/2 cup	1/2 cup
Bread or cereal, enriched or whole grain[b]		
bread, or	1/2 slice	1/2 slice
cereal	1/4 cup[c]	1/3 cup[d]
lunch or supper		
Milk, fluid[a]	1/2 cup	3/4 cup
Meat and/or meat alternate[e]		
Meat, poultry, or fish, cooked[f]	1 ounce	1 1/2 ounces
Cheese	1 ounce	1 1/2 ounces
Egg	1	1
Cooked dry beans and peas	1/8 cup	1/4 cup
Peanut butter	1 tablespoon	2 tablespoons
Vegetables and fruits[g]	1/4 cup	1/2 cup
Bread, enriched or whole grain[b]	1/2 slice	1/2 slice

[a] Includes whole milk, lowfat milk, skim milk, cultured buttermilk, or flavored milk made from these types of fluid milk which meet State and local standards.

[b] Or an equivalent serving of an acceptable bread product made of enriched or whole grain meal or flour.

[c] 1/4 cup (volume) or 1/3 ounce (weight), whichever is less.

[d] 1/3 cup (volume) or 1/2 ounce (weight), whichever is less.

[e] Or an equivalent quantity of any combination of foods listed under Meat and Meat Alternates.

[f] Cooked lean meat without bone.

[g] Must include at least *two* kinds.

SOURCE: *A Planning Guide for Food Service in Child Care Centers.* USDA, FNS-64, Food and Nutrition Service, Washington, D.C., revised 1976, p. 5.

the Nation's children and to encourage the domestic consumption of nutritious agricultural commodities and other foods." Not until the 1960s was the school lunch program operational in all fifty states. In 1966, the Child Nutrition Act strengthened and expanded the program to include child care institutions as well as schools. Nutrition education experiences were mandated in the programs in the late 1970s, and attention was focused on increasing the numbers of breakfast and summer feeding programs.

The National School Lunch Program (NSLP) is administered by the Food and Nutrition Service of the U.S. Department of Agriculture. A lunch pattern has traditionally been used to plan and evaluate meals served in these programs. In the 1970s studies were undertaken to evaluate plate waste, use of donated surplus foods (commodities), and alternative methods of meal planning (39, 40). New recommendations were made for giving students a choice of foods, smaller serving sizes for younger children, use of nutrient standards for planning, and the availability of competitive foods (see Table 3–8). Students and parents were encouraged to become involved in menu planning and other phases of the program. Food service personnel and teachers have become involved in programs of practical nutrition education with students at all grade levels. Demonstration projects have been begun to teach children the preventive aspects of nutrition and its relationship to health through improved food habits. The results of such programs should be shown in healthier adults in the future.

The school-age child, 6 to 10 years old, generally has a good appetite and tends to look up to teachers as authorities on all things, including what foods are good to eat. The teacher and the worker in the school food service become primary nutrition educators, and have opportunities to establish and strengthen food habits by example (41). Encouraging children to participate in food preparation activities at the preschool and elementary levels will take advantage of their curiosity and interest in food. Studies have shown that children do consume more foods and a greater variety if they have had an opportunity to help with preparation. Using the school food service facility as a laboratory for introducing new foods has helped to increase consumption of nutritious foods.

More recently, group feeding of children is being used to teach specific therapeutic regimens for obesity and diabetes. These programs have used summer camps with children assembled in groups for varying periods of time. The actual feeding of appropriate foods gives the children an opportunity to practice concepts while they learn them, which results in better retention of information (41, 42).

future needs and implications

Lack of specific information about nutrient requirements for different ages of childhood should be emphasized in the selection of research projects for the future. We need improved methods of nutrition education for children and teachers. We need creative experiments with individuals and in group feeding if we are to accomplish the goal of improved nutritional status for all Americans (38).

TABLE 3-8. School Lunch Patterns for Various Age/Grade Groups (U.S. Department of Agriculture, National School Lunch Program)

(USDA recommends, but does not require that you adjust portions by age/grade group to better meet the food and nutritional needs of children according to their ages. If you adjust portions, Groups I–IV are minimum requirements for the age/grade groups specified. If you do not adjust portions, the Group IV portions are the portions to serve all children.)

components		minimum quantities				recommended quantities[a]	specific requirements
		PRESCHOOL		GRADES K–3	GRADES 4–12[b]	GRADES 7–12	
		Ages 1–2 (group I)	Ages 3–4 (group II)	Ages 5–8 (group III)	Ages 9 & over (group IV)	Ages 12 & over (group V)	
Meat or Meat Alternate	A serving of one of the following or a combination to give an equivalent quantity:						Must be served in the main dish or the main dish and one other menu item. Textured vegetable protein products, cheese alternate products, and enriched macaroni with fortified protein may be used to meet part of the meat/meat alternate requirement. Fact sheets on each of these alternate foods give detailed instructions for use. NOTE: The amount you must serve of a single meat alternate may seem too large for the particular age group you are serving. To make the quantity of that meat alternate more reasonable, use a smaller amount to meet part of the requirement and supplement with another meat or meat alternate to meet the full requirement.
	Lean meat, poultry, or fish (edible portion as served)	1 oz	1 1/2 oz	1 1/2 oz	2 oz	3 oz	
	Cheese	1 oz	1 1/2 oz	1 1/2 oz	2 oz	3 oz	
	Large egg(s)	1	1 1/2	1 1/2	2	3	
	Cooked dry beans or peas	1/2 cup	3/4 cup	3/4 cup	1 cup	1 1/2 cup	
	Peanut butter	2 tbsp	3 tbsp	3 tbsp	4 tbsp	6 tbsp	

Vegetable and/or Fruit	Two or more servings of vegetable or fruit or both to total.	1/2 cup	1/2 cup	1/2 cup	3/4 cup	3/4 cup	No more than one-half of the total requirement may be met with full-strength fruit or vegetable juice. Cooked dry beans or peas may be used as a meat alternate or as a vegetable but not as both in the same meal.
Bread or Bread Alternate	Servings of bread or bread alternate. A serving is: 1 slice of whole-grain or enriched bread A whole-grain or enriched biscuit, roll, muffin, etc. 1/2 cup of cooked whole-grain or enriched pasta products, or other cereal grains such as bulgar or corn grits A combination of any of the above	5 per week	8 per week	8 per week	8 per week	10 per week	At least 1/2 serving of bread or an equivalent quantity of bread alternate for Group I, and 1 serving for Groups II–V, must be served daily. Enriched macaroni with fortified protein may be used as a meat alternate or as a bread alternate but not as both in the same meal. NOTE: *Food Buying Guide for School Food Service*, PA-1257 (1980) provides the information for the minimum weight of a serving.
Milk	A serving of fluid milk	3/4 cup (6 fl oz)	3/4 cup (6 fl oz)	1/2 pint (8 fl oz)	1/2 pint (8 fl oz)	1/2 pint (8 fl oz)	At least one of the following forms of milk must be offered: Unflavored lowfat milk Unflavored skim milk Unflavored buttermilk NOTE: This requirement does not prohibit offering milks, such as whole milk or flavored milk, along with one or more of the above.

[a] Group specifies recommended, not required, quantities for students 12 years and older. These students may request smaller portions, but not smaller than those specified in Group IV.

[b] Group IV is the one meat pattern which will satisfy all requirements if no portion size adjustments are made.

Summary

Growth slows after the first year of life and becomes linear. Growth charts, which measure growth of long bones and trunk, are a means of determining progress. Organs, muscles, and adipose tissues also increase in size.

Most of the values for nutrient needs are derived from data on other age groups, although a number of surveys provide information on the general needs of children. School feeding programs also make a major contribution.

Peer groups contribute to food patterns as well. Habits and likes vary and become unpredictable. Nutritional needs are more related to physical size than age. Social and psychological development is affected by the home, school, and community.

references

1. HAMILL, P. V., et al. "Physical Growth: National Center for Health Statistics Percentiles." *American Journal of Clinical Nutrition* 32 (1979): 607–629.
2. MARTIN, E. A., and V. A. BEAL. *Robert's Nutrition Work with Children,* 4th ed. Chicago: University of Chicago Press, 1978.
3. REED, R. B., and H. C. STUART. "Patterns of Growth in Height and Weight from Birth to Eighteen Years of Age." *Pediatrics* 24 (1959): 904.
4. STUART, H. C. "Need for Observations of Growth in Appraising Adequacy of Nutrition in Childhood." *Journal of Pediatrics* 7 (1935): 320.
5. WETZEL, N. C. "Physical Fitness in Terms of Physique, Development and Basal Metabolism." *Journal of the American Medical Association* 116 (1941): 1187.
6. JACKSON, R. L., and H. G. KELLY. "Growth Charts for Use in Pediatric Practice." *Journal of Pediatrics* 27 (1945): 215.
7. STUART, H. C., and H. V. MEREDITH. "Use of Body Measurements in the School Health Program." *American Journal of Public Health* 36 (1946): 1365.
8. National Center for Health Statistics. *NCHS Growth Charts, 1976. Monthy Vital Statistics Report.* DHEW Publication No. (HRA) 76–1120, Vol. 25, No. 3 (supplement). Washington, D.C.: U.S. Government Printing Office, 1976.
9. YUSUF, H. K. M., J. W. T. DICKERSON, and J. C. WATERLOW. "Changes in Content and Composition of Brain Phospholipids in Malnourished Children." *American Journal of Clinical Nutrition* 32 (1979): 2227.
10. GRUELICH, W. W., and S. I. PYLE. *Radiographic Atlas of Skeletal Development of the Hand and Wrist,* 2nd ed. (Palo Alto: Stanford University Press, 1959).
11. SONTAG, L. W., and J. LIPFORD. "The Effect of Illness and Other Factors on the Appearance Pattern of Skeletal Epiphyses." *Journal of Pediatrics* 23 (1943): 391.
12. DREIZEN, S., C. N. SPIRAKIS, and R. E. STONE. "A Comparison of Skeletal Growth and Maturation in Undernourished and Well-nourished Girls before and after Menarche." *Journal of Pediatrics* 70 (1967): 256.
13. Committee on Nutrition Advisory to CDC of National Academy of Sciences. *Comparison of Body Weights and Lengths or Heights of Groups of Children.* Atlanta: U.S. DHEW, Public Health Service Center for Disease Control, 1974.
14. FOMON, S. J. *Nutritional Disorders of Children. Prevention, Screening, and Followup.* Washington, D.C.: DHEW Publication No. (HSA) 76–5612, 1976.
15. BEAL, V. A. "Nutritional Intake of Children. 1. Calories, Carbohydrates, Fat and Protein." *Journal of Nutrition* 50 (1953): 223.

16. WAIT, B., R. BLAIR, and L. J. ROBERTS. "Energy Intakes of Well-nourished Children and Adolescents." *American Journal of Clinical Nutrition* 22 (1969): 1383.

17. HEGSTED, D. M. "Theoretical Estimates of the Protein Requirements of Children." *Journal of the American Dietetic Association* 33 (1957): 225.

18. HOWAT, P., M. KORSLAND, R. P. ABERNATHY, and S. J. RITCHEY. "Sweat Nitrogen Losses by and Nitrogen Balance of Preadolescent Girls Consuming Three Levels of Dietary Protein." *American Journal of Clinical Nutrition* 28 (1975): 879.

19. Committee on Nutrition, American Academy of Pediatrics. "Nutritional Aspects of Vegetarianism, Health Foods and Fad Diets." *Pediatrics* 59 (1977): 460.

20. SHULL, M., R. B. REED, I. VALADIAN, R. PALOMBO, H. THORNE, and J. T. DWYER. "Velocities of Growth in Vegetarian Preschool Children." *Pediatrics* 60 (1977): 410.

21. VYHMEISTER, I., U. D. REGISTER, and L. SONNENBERG. "Safe Vegetarian Diets for Children." *Pediatric Clinics of North America* 24 (1977): 203.

22. HOLT, L. E., JR. and S. E. SNYDERMAN. "Protein and Amino Acid Requirements of Infants and Children." *Nutrition Abstracts and Reviews* 35 (1965): 1.

23. NAKAGAWA, I., T. TAKAHASHI, T. SUZUKI, and K. KOBAYASHI. "Amino Acid Requirements of Children: Nitrogen Balance at the Minimum Level of Essential Amino Acids." *Journal of Nutrition* 83 (1964): 115.

24. MACY, I. G., and H. A. HUNSCHER. "Calories—A Limiting Factor in the Growth of Children." *Journal of Nutrition* 48 (1951): 189.

25. RITCHEY, S. J., F. S. JOHNSON, and M. K. KORSLAND. "Vitamin B_6 Requirements in the Preadolescent and Adolescent." in *Human Vitamin B_6 Requirements.* Washington, D.C.: National Academy of Sciences, 1978.

26. HAMBIDGE, K. M., C. HAMBIDGE, M. JACOBS, and J. D. BAUM. "Low Levels of Zinc in Hair, Anorexia, Poor Growth, and Hypogensia in Children." *Pediatric Research* 6 (1972): 868–874.

27. OWEN, G. M., K. M. KAM, P. J. GARRY, J. E. LOWE, and A. H. LUBIN. "A Study of Nutritional Status of Preschool Children in the United States, 1968–70." *Pediatrics* 53, supplement 4, part 2 (1974): 597.

28. CHASE, H. P., V. KUMAR, J. M. DODDS, H. E. SAUBERLICH, R. M. HUNTER, R. S. BURTON, and V. SPALDING. "Nutritional Status of Preschool Mexican-American Migrant Farm Children." *American Journal of Diseases of Children* 122 (1971): 316.

29. EPPRIGHT, E. S., H. M. FOX, B. A. FRYER, G. H. LAMKIN, V. M. VIVIAN, and E. S. FULLER. "Nutrition of Infants and Preschool Children in the North Central Region of the United States of America." *World Review of Nutrition and Dietetics* 4 (1972): 269.

30. BEAL, V. A. "Dietary Intake of Individuals Followed through Infancy and Childhood." *American Journal of Public Health* 51 (1961): 1107.

31. Nutrition Canada National Survey. *Nutrition: A National Priority.* Ottawa: Department of National Health and Welfare, 1973.

32. ABRAHAM, S., F. W. LOWENSTEIN, and C. L. JOHNSON. *United States Department of Health, Education and Welfare, National Center for Health Statistics: Preliminary Findings of the First Health and Nutrition Examination Survey, United States 1971–72; Dietary Intake and Biochemical Findings.* Washington, D.C.: DHEW Publication (HRA) 74-1219-1, 1974.

33. *Ten-State Nutrition Survey (1968–1970).* Vol. V, *Dietary.* Washington, D.C.: DHEW Publication No. (HSM) 72–8133, 1973.

34. BIRCH, H. G., and J. D. GUSSOW. *Disadvantaged Children: Health, Nutrition and School Failure.* New York: Harcourt Brace Jovanovich, 1970.

35. READ, M. S. "Malnutrition, Hunger and Behavior: II. Hunger, School Feeding Programs and Behavior." *Journal of the American Dietetic Association* 63 (1973): 386.

36. SCRIMSHAW, N. S., and J. E. GORDON, eds. *Malnutrition, Learning and Behavior.* Cambridge, Mass.: MIT Press, 1968.

37. BROWN, PATRICIA C. "The Nutritional Status of 4–6-Year-Old Children in Day Care Centers." Unpublished master's thesis, Texas Women's University, 1975.

38. JUHAS, L. "Nutrition Education in Day Care Programs: A New Challenge to Our Profession. *Journal of the American Dietetic Association* 63 (1973): 134.

39. PAIGE, D. M., A. CORDANO, and S. S. HUANG. "Nutritional Supplementation of Disadvantaged Elementary School Children." *Pediatrics* 58 (1976): 697.

40. JANSEN, R. J., J. M. HARPER, A. L. FREY, R. H. CREWS, C. T. SHIGETOMI, and J. B. LOUGH. "Comparison of Type A and Nutrient Standard Menus for School Lunch: III. Nutritive Content of Menus and Acceptability." *Journal of the American Dietetic Association* 66 (1975): 254.

41. BLAKEWAY, S. F., and M. E. KNICKREHM. "Nutrition Education in the Little Rock School Lunch Program." *Journal of the American Dietetic Association* 72 (1978): 389.

42. LUM, B. L. "Preventing Ketoacidosis in the Child with Juvenile-Onset Diabetes Mellitus: II. The Learning Environment." *Journal of the American Dietetic Association* 69 (1976): 289.

CHAPTER 4

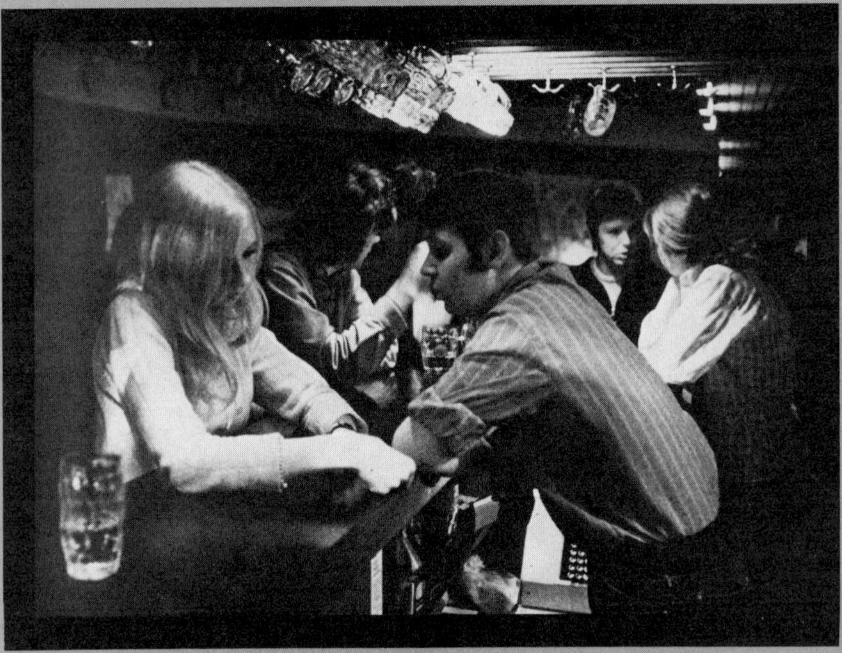

WHO photo by E. Mandelmann

nutrition during adolescence

THE PERIOD OF ADOLESCENCE IS GENERALLY ACCEPTED TO BE APPROXIMATELY 12 TO 21 YEARS. The precise chronologic timing of onset, progression, and completion varies from individual to individual and between the sexes. In addition, changes in weight, height, and secondary sexual development also vary from individual to individual and between males and females (1). In the age groups discussed so far, there were few if any nutritional consequences that could be related to sexual differences. During adolescence, physiological changes parallel endocrine and hormonal changes in each individual and are partly responsible for determining nutritional needs (2). Adolescence is a unique period: the maturation process is characterized by rapid physical and psychological growth, and accompanied by socialization activities necessary to develop and maintain the adult role.

Social and Psychological Needs

Sociologically, the child is becoming an adult with the resultant rejection of authority and assumption of independence. This means severing childhood relationships and forming new ones. Now the peer group becomes most important. Seeking peer acceptance is a high priority as the young adolescent begins to move away from home and parental authority. As puberty progresses, the peer group establishes the standards of behavior. Adolescents frequently demand more freedom than they can control. In the older adolescent, the opposite sex begins to have more influence on behavior than peers or parents. Dating replaces much previous group activity that included both sexes. The adolescent has increased enthusiasm, interest, and energy which may be channeled into a variety of social activities such as athletics, community projects, and cultural and intellectual pursuits.

The major psychological task at this time is the establishment of an identity and an adult personality. Development of the self-image is related to both social and physical growth. Overlapping of development and variation among individuals in the psychological maturational process often causes much anxiety and frustration for adolescents, parents, teachers, and friends. At a time when being like others is of utmost importance to the individual, the many individual differences must be carefully explained to the adolescent to prevent the development of unacceptable behavior patterns.

Daniel has described the psychological or emotional development of the adolescent in three stages—early, middle, and late. These categories include areas of concern: self-image, independence, acting out, peer relationships, opposite sex relationships, and intellectual and vocational achievement (3). The early adolescent is characterized as more unstable, restless and unsure of self. There is great desire to prove normalcy, and much time is spent in thinking, which is frequently mistaken for lack of interest or "daydreaming." The middle adolescent period shows great intensity and inconsistency of behavior. Adolescents are more secure with peers of the same sex, but may be at the peak of their struggle with adult authority. The late adolescent is more stable and has developed some consistency of behavior and some self acceptance. Thought processes are directed more toward others, toward career and adult life, than toward the self.

Physiological Changes

The physiological changes of adolescence are referred to as **puberty,** and their result is the capacity to reproduce. All adolescents are concerned about physical changes: they want to achieve age-appropriate height, weight, and secondary sexual development. They need much reassurance that there are great individual differences in these physical changes. Growth has an effect on psychological and sociological development. For instance, the rapid growth spurt may create problems in physical performance, such as awkwardness in athletics, until skills catch up with physical size and strength. Differences in height may make an individual more susceptible to being singled out by peers. But physical differences between the sexes appear to be more significant during adolescence: for example, the tall boy is much more socially acceptable than the tall girl.

Teenagers have a high degree of interest in their bodies and are frequently dissatisfied with their shape (4, 5). Both males and females may have unrealistic views about their fatness or thinness. In general, boys want to be bigger and heavier, while girls want to lose weight, and increase some dimensions and decrease others. Society currently dictates that adolescent boys be tall, strong, and muscular, while girls should be small and thin. Biologically these concepts are not achievable at will. Most girls normally get deposits of fat just prior to and early in puberty. Some boys may be very late in entering puberty compared to peers, so no amount of weight lifting and/or excessive eating will put on weight or muscle.

In general, the sex differences show as greater shoulder width or chest breadth in males, and increased hip width in females. Leg length relative to trunk length is usually greater in males. But for both sexes rate of growth is accelerated as it has not been since the first six months of life.

onset of puberty

The major period in the sexual development of the human occurs in adolescence and is called **puberty.** The process of puberty is associated with marked changes in somatic development, accompanied by alterations in body composition. The interrelated factors initiating the onset of puberty are highly complex. Onset in humans is associated with increased luteinizing hormone (LH) secretion during sleep and later during the daytime. This secretion probably stimulates the gonads to produce the steroids that initiate puberty. Endocrine rhythms that seem related to the sleep-wakefulness cycle and the light-darkness schedule may also be significant in the timing of puberty (6). Adequate nutrition is important for puberty to occur at a normal age.

Body weight and composition at puberty can be altered by dietary manipulations. After weaning, a variety of dietary and other factors can alter weight and timing of puberty. Severe undernutrition before weaning will delay onset. After weaning, undernutrition delays puberty through its influence on hormonal levels or by increasing the time needed to reach the critical body weight for puberty. There is controversy over the importance of the amount of adipose tissue in the initiation of puberty. If body fat is important, the mechanism of influence may be estrogen metabolism. Extreme leanness may be related to the production of anti-estrogens. Frisch presents evidence in favor of the view that a certain level of adipose tissue in the body acts as a signal for puberty (7). Other studies indicate that a high-fat diet speeds the onset of puberty (8). Puberty occurs at a younger age and at a lighter weight with a high-fat diet. Alteration of amino acids in the diet also alters body weight at puberty. Clearly, regulation of the time of onset and weight at puberty is complex and depends upon growth rate, diet, and other factors.

growth

During puberty, the percentage of body fat increases in females and decreases in males. The body of the adolescent female averages approximately 25 percent fat content, which is twice that of the adolescent male. Females have a greater percentage of fat prior to puberty and sustain this fat throughout adolescence and adulthood. Males gain some fat in adolescence, only to lose it later for greater gains in muscle mass. Therefore, weight cannot be used as the only measure of nutritional status. Figure 4–1 shows weight differences for males and females between ages 6 and 18. A better measure is the ratio of lean body mass to height. This ratio changes during adolescence for both males and females, with the ratio being considerably less for females (9). Maximum weight increments also occur earlier in females than in males, with the female depositing more fat and males having a greater percentage of lean body mass (muscle). Figure 4–2 illustrates

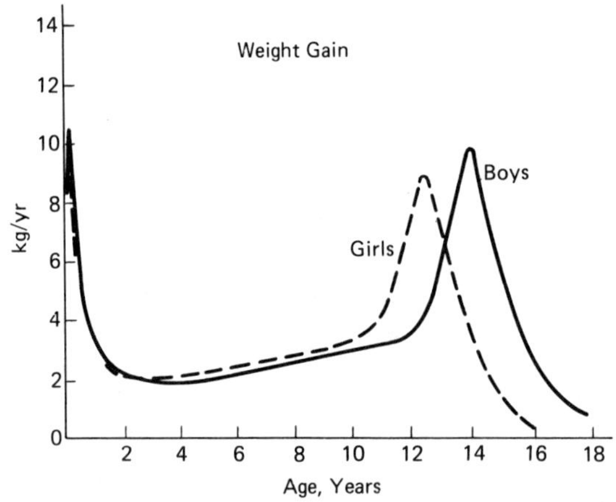

FIG. 4–1. Mean weight gain for age of males and females between infancy and 18 years of age. *Source:* P. V. V. Hamill, F. E. Johnston, and S. Lemeshow, *Heights and Weights of Youths 12–17 Years, United States, 1966–1970.* Vital and Health Statistics, Series II, No. 124. DHEW Publication No. (HSM) 73-1606 (Washington, D.C.: Government Printing Office, 1973).

these differences in body fat as measured by the triceps skinfold, or subcutaneous fat (10).

The pattern of growth is different for males and females, with females entering prepubescence at a younger chronological age (7.5 to 14.5 years). Males enter later (9.5 to 16.5 years) and have a more intense growth spurt that lasts longer than for females. In both, a slight deceleration in rate of growth occurs just prior to puberty and this slowed rate of growth is more pronounced in males and females who experience a late onset of puberty.

Growth spurts occur prior to puberty. For girls, the average age of beginning the growth spurt is 10 years, whereas, the mean age of onset of puberty is 10.5 years, with a range of 9 to 12 years. There is no direct relationship between puberty onset and skeletal age in females. At the skeletal age of 10 years, the female has attained 84 percent of her height, with the additional 16 percent coming during puberty. Very little increment in height is seen after **menarche** (first menstruation), so that 95 percent of adult female height is attained by the skeletal age of 13 years (11). Females who experience menarche early will reach their adult height at a younger age. Those females who mature later may attain a taller final height due to the longer prepubescent period (12). Female height increases from approximately 138 cm at 10 years to 162 cm at 18 years; male height increases from 140 cm at 10 years to 174 cm at 18 (13).

In general, males enter puberty at a later chronological age than females and take longer to complete the process (four to six years as compared to three years for females). Males achieve 84 percent of their adult height by the skeletal age of 12 years and 95 percent by the skeletal age of 15 years (see Figure 4–3). The Health and Nutrition Examination Survey (HANES) of the late 1960s indicated that females were usually taller than males from approximately 9 years to 13 years and were heavier for almost the same period, 8 to 14 years (14).

The differences in height and weight between males and females during their respective adolescent growth spurts do not cause any radical change in

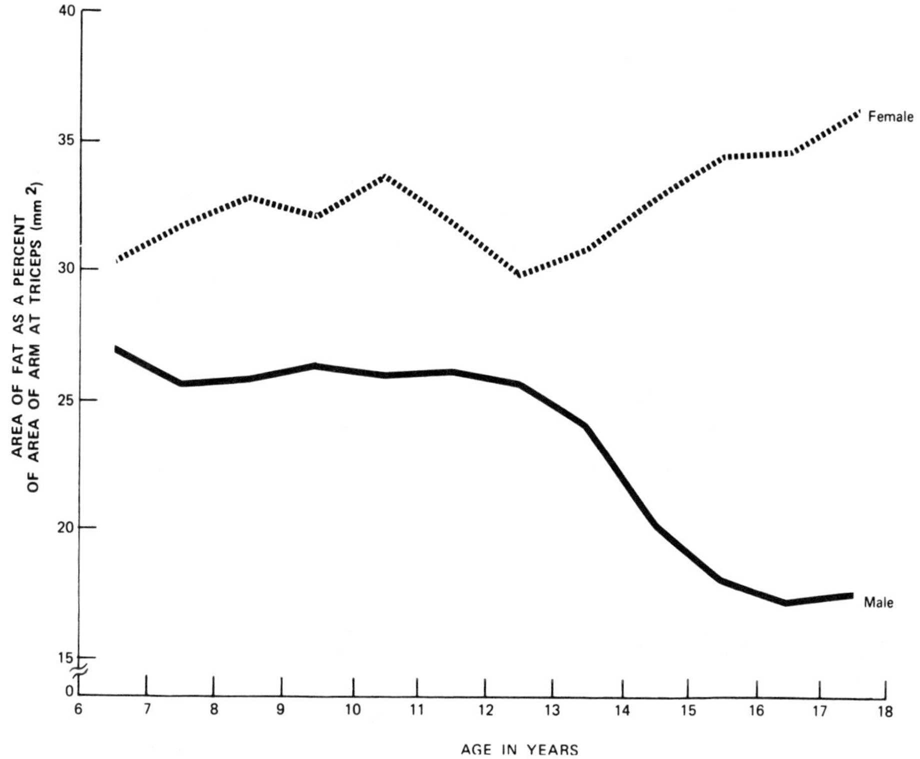

FIG. 4–2. Percentage of cross-sectional area of arm comprised of fat by age and sex. *Source:* National Center for Health Statistics, *Skinfold Thickness of Youths 12–17 Years, United States.* Vital and Health Statistics, Series II, No. 132, DHEW Publication No. (HRA) 74-1614 (Washington, D.C.: Government Printing Office, 1974).

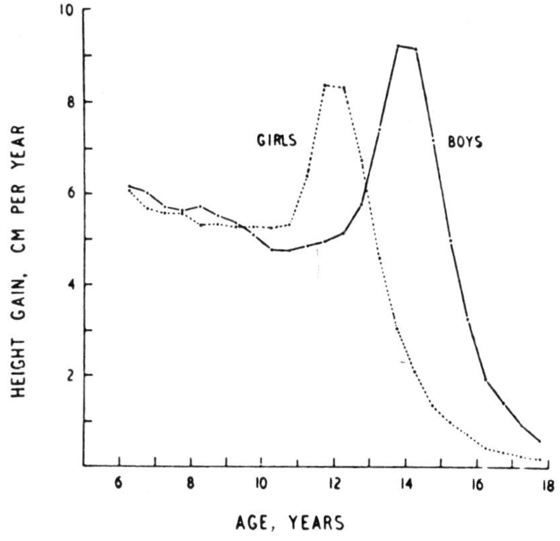

FIG. 4–3. Mean heights for males and females between 6 and 17 years of age, National Health Survey Cycles I and II. *Source:* P. V. V. Hamill, F. E. Johnston, and S. Lemeshow, *Height and Weight of Youths 12–17 Years, United States, 1966–1970.* Vital and Health Statistics, Series II, No. 124. DHEW Publication No. (HSM) 73-1606 (Washington, D.C.: Government Printing Office, 1973).

individual body build. Growth merely adds to the already established physique, with early maturers of both sexes usually being heavier and taller at all ages than their late-maturing counterparts (15).

Factors affecting the growth spurt of adolescence include individual heredity, season of the year, nutrition, socioeconomic factors, and other environmental circumstances such as illness. It is difficult to separate these interdependent factors as individual causes of problems, nor is it possible to specify their relative importance quantitatively. However, in studies associated with postwar famines, it appears that malnutrition had more influence on delaying the beginning of puberty than on slowing or decreasing total growth (16, 17, 18). Therefore, *timing* of the growth spurt may be a more sensitive indicator of malnutrition than growth itself. These concepts have been demonstrated directly in animal experiments (19, 20). Humans and animals also have the power to catch up if the periods of malnutrition are not too severe or too prolonged.

Females appear to have the ability to withstand malnutrition with less significant effect on rates of growth than do males (21, 22, 23, 24). In most instances severely malnourished children are retarded in height, weight, and skeletal maturity relative to well-nourished children, but females are less retarded in each area than males after periods of malnutrition. The same phenonemon occurs in rats (25, 26). Food consumption surveys point out that teenage girls eat less and get fewer nutrients than boys of the same age. The effect is quantitative in most instances rather than qualitative. Because of peer pressure, boys and girls of this age eat the same kinds of foods. Girls reduce their total intake to preserve the small, thin image. Boys increase their intake to get the big, strong, athletic look. None of these food choices appear to be made on the basis of nutrition knowledge, however.

Some writers have proposed that exercise can accelerate the rate of growth in adolescence (27, 28). But we need more data and controlled studies in order to reach definite conclusions. Such data are difficult to collect because of the many variables that affect the results—age, sex, appetite, sleep and rest, food intake, and environmental temperatures. A study from the Netherlands reports that exercise or physical activity makes a difference in body composition. Male adolescents who were physically active had less subcutaneous fat and greater muscle mass, as determined by anthropometric measurements (29). Females in that study reflected the same trend, with female office workers having more subcutaneous fat and less lean muscle than female athletes.

Psychological influences on the growth of infants and young children have been well documented, but they are not often thought to be contributory in adolescence (30). However, adverse emotional conditions can affect growth in this age group as well. Widdowson reports on changes in the growth of children and teenagers living in an orphanage run by a stern woman who meted out punishment to some while favoring others (31). All groups were supplemented with additional calories at varying times, and each supplemented period was supervised by the same stern person. Weight gains corresponded to her absence rather than to supplementation with extra calories, which would have been expected. Her favorites gained more than all the others. Effects on height were also noticeable, but to a lesser extent than weight. Other studies have been reported where psychological factors in part explained delays or slowed growth during periods of emotional stress (32, 33, 34). As in younger children, the intake of food may be adequate without positive effects on growth if the psychological climate is poor.

Nutrition Requirements and Recommendations

When the growth spurt starts, it is necessary to determine how long it lasts and its intensity in order to relate recommendations to need without underestimating or creating excesses in food intake. Nutrient needs for adolescents must be related to sexual maturity stages rather than to chronological age (1). There is no animal model of adolescent growth, so animal experiments for estimating requirements are not easily structured. Popular opinion is that nutrient requirements are high for this group because of the growth spurt, extra activity, and less rest. But few data are available to support estimates of the quantities needed. In addition, teenagers are reluctant to cooperate in food intake surveys or metabolic studies. So our information about what and how this group eats is limited and frequently raises more questions about reliability than it answers about nutrient intake. The vulnerability of this age group to fads and peer pressure is still another factor in the difficulty of making adequate and accurate estimates of what teenagers actually need in terms of nutrition.

Females are less vulnerable to inadequate nutrient intakes because of their lower energy needs and smaller muscle mass. The desire to be slim and the individual limiting of food choices creates inadequate nutrient intake in many girls; in fact, surveys have reported inadequate intakes of total calories, iron, and some vitamins. When compared to intakes of food by males, the difference is quantitative rather than qualitative. Caloric intakes for boys have been estimated to exceed those for girls on a daily basis by as much as 1000 to 1500 calories.

Many factors contribute to the food intake patterns of adolescents. In evaluating intake, each adolescent must be assessed individually, because in spite of their being peer-oriented, adolescents do eat at times with other people, and intakes can vary. Here we will focus on the group as a whole, but evaluations and recommendations should be made on an individual basis, taking into consideration stage of development and rate of growth. The following is a partial list of the factors affecting the food intake patterns of adolescents:

1. *Lack of time—involved in many activities.*
2. *Priority of peer activities over eating.*
3. *Lack of supervision in selection of meals away from home.*

4. *Most food eaten outside the home.*
5. *Concern that certain foods cause or aggravate acne.*
6. *Fear of obesity.*
7. *Fear of underweight and lack of muscle.*
8. *Desire to excel in athletics.*
9. *Exclusion of certain foods such as milk from diet.*
10. *Skipping meals.*

The adolescent's life style is one of skipping regular mealtimes and eating snacks. Most teenagers admit to snacking, and studies have shown that between-meal eating for this group is advantageous for their nutritional status (35, 36). Estimates are that from one-fourth to one-third of the adolescent's total calories come from snacks, which indicates that a significant amount of other nutrients may also come from this source. The adolescent needs guidance in making appropriate food choices. Educating teenagers about the nutritive value of snack foods would seem to be easier than attempting to modify their schedules or eating times and habits.

The Berkeley study, done in the early 1970s, indicated that the increased appetite of most teenagers was a positive force to ensure adequate intake (5). One-third of the girls and approximately one-half of the boys in the ninth grade reported being hungry most of the time. In general, teenagers who ate more often tended to have adequate intakes of nutrients, whereas those who skipped meals and ate less frequently had poorer intakes or decreased appetite in the morning.

Researchers in two studies have attempted to relate increased appetites and increased food intake to the growth spurt (37, 38). But in both studies it was difficult to identify a significant, sudden increase in food intake that corresponded with the growth spurt. The greatest intake of calories for girls was between 12 and 14 years, whereas boys continued their increased intake to 17 or 18 years and continued to gain weight. Data from the Ten-State Nutrition Survey were similar, showing some differences in income levels related to girls' intake (35). Highest intakes of calories and protein occurred in low-income girls 12 to 14 years old, with declining intakes thereafter. Girls in higher income ranges continued to increase caloric intake with increasing age. Boys of all income groups tended to increase intakes through 16 years, which was the last age documented. A recent study by Lacey et al. reported marked daily variation in calorie intakes for females 16 to 17 years of age, with the largest intakes being four times the lowest (39). This tends to support the irregularity of food intake of adolescent females reported by others. So it would appear from the limited data available that the increased food intake of adolescents does somewhat parallel the growth spurt.

By this age, eating patterns are well established and have been influenced by personal experiences, educational level of the mother, cultural concepts, and family life style. Nevertheless, some changes in interests and concerns may be reflected in attitudes toward food. Adolescents are aware that they can use food to achieve some of the goals they perceive as necessary, such as feeling energetic; being the "right" size; becoming independent of parents; and using food socially (with peers) for fun.

Since we have little or no research data on nutrient requirements for adolescents specifically, the figures in the RDA charts are the result of a few animal experiments or have been interpolated from adult maintenance figures, with an additional amount added for growth (40, 41). This lack of specific information has undoubtedly led to overestimation of some nutrients and underestimation of others. See the RDA chart in the Appendix for specific recommendations, and note that because of technical difficulties, recommended amounts are listed by chronological age rather than physiological or developmental age or sexual maturation, all of which have more direct impact on nutrient needs than chronological age.

energy

The recommended range of kcal for males is 2000–3700 (11–14 years) and 2100–3900 (15–18 years) or approximately 60 kcal to 45 kcal/kg. For females the range is 1500–3000 (11–14 years) and 1200–3000 (15–18 years), or approximately 50 kcal/kg and 40 kcal/kg, respectively. The Joint FAO/WHO ad hoc Expert Committee on Energy and Protein Requirements made recommendations similar to the RDA figures but used some younger ages where the estimates were higher (see Table A–2 in the Appendix). Because of the marked variation in energy expenditures for both boys and girls, recommendations must be individually adjusted.

protein

Protein requirements for adolescents are based on calculations derived from studies of infants and adults. Quality of protein (ratio and amounts of essential amino acids available) must be taken into consideration when discussing protein needs. Most adolescents eat a mixture of plant and animal proteins and are assured of adequate intakes of essential amino acids. Table 4–1 presents the amounts of protein recommended as safe by RDA and FAO/WHO. The FAO/WHO amounts are somewhat less at all ages than the RDAs.

Based on energy recommendations already noted, the protein to energy ratio seems less than that ordinarily recommended for adequate growth. Studies in other periods of growth, especially infancy, recommend that 10 percent of total calories come from protein (42, 43). With a mixed diet using proteins of varying quality, the percentage of total calories should not be less than 8. Table 4–2 shows the recommendations of RDA and FAO/WHO for protein-energy ratios. The recommendations of FAO/WHO for all age groups and both sexes are for less than 8 percent of total calories from protein sources. The RDA recommends at

TABLE 4-1. Recommended Level of Protein

	Age (years)	g Protein per kg per day RDA[a]	g Protein per kg per day FAO/WHO[b]
MALES			
	10–12	—	0.8
	11–14	1.0	—
	13–15	—	0.7
	15–18	.8	—
	16–19	—	0.6
FEMALES			
	10–12	—	0.8
	11–14	1.0	—
	13–15	—	0.6
	15–18	.8	—
	16–19	—	0.6

[a]From Committee on Dietary Allowances, *Recommended Dietary Allowances*, 9th rev. ed. (Washington, D.C.: Food and Nutrition Board, National Research Council, National Academy of Sciences, 1980). Reproduced by the permission of the National Academy of Sciences, Washington, D.C.

[b]From Joint FAO/WHO ad hoc Expert Committee, *Energy and Protein Requirements*. Food and Agriculture Organization of the United Nations Nutrition Meetings Report Series No. 52, and WHO Technical Report Series No. 522 (Rome: Food and Agriculture Organization, 1973).

least 8 percent of total calories from protein for all groups except 11- to 14-year-old males. These recommendations are estimates for groups, so they may be low for some individuals during the extremely rapid growth spurt. But most adolescents consume far greater amounts of protein than these recommendations would indicate. An individual who is not growing appropriately must have a careful evaluation of protein intake as well as energy to be sure which is the factor related to food intake.

vitamins and minerals

Recommendations for vitamins and minerals during the adolescent period are based on very little data, primarily food consumption surveys of growing adolescents. The nutrients most likely to be low in adolescent diets are iron, calcium, vitamin A, riboflavin, and ascorbic acid (5, 44, 45).

The RDA for iron is the same for adolescent boys and girls—18 mg/day, assuming the average availability of food iron to be 10 percent. The increased amount for males is to cover the increased blood volume associated with increases

TABLE 4-2. Estimates of Protein/Energy Ratios

	Age (years)	Total Energy (kcal/day)	Protein (g/day)	Percentage of Total Energy as Protein
MALES				
	10–12[a]	2600	30	4.5%
	11–14[b]	2700	45	6.7
	13–15[a]	2900	37	5.0
	15–18[b]	2800	56	8.0
	16–19[a]	3070	38	5.0
FEMALES				
	10–12[a]	2350	29	5.0
	11–14[b]	2200	46	8.0
	13–15[a]	2490	31	5.0
	15–18[b]	2100	46	8.8
	16–19[a]	2310	30	5.0

[a]From Joint FAO/WHO ad hoc Expert Committee, *Energy and Protein Requirements.* Food and Agriculture Organization of the United Nations Nutrition Meetings Report Series No. 52, and WHO Technical Report Series No. 522 (Rome: Food and Agriculture Organization, 1973).

[b]From Committee on Dietary Allowance, *Recommended Dietary Allowances,* 9th rev. ed. (Washington, D.C.: Food and Nutrition Board, National Research Council, National Academy of Sciences, 1980). Reproduced by the permission of the National Academy of Sciences, Washington, D.C.

in muscle mass, and in females to cover the blood losses of menstruation. The source of iron (heme form or nonheme) and the presence or absence of ascorbic acid must be considered in evaluating the availability of iron from food. An individual's iron stores affect absorption: an individual with good iron stores will absorb less iron than an individual who is iron-deficient.

The allowance for calcium is controversial and based on no real adolescent studies. Maximum retention of calcium is not achieved until 1 to 1.5 g/day is consumed. Therefore, for adolescent males and females, the recommended amount is 1.2 g/day. The recommendation for phosphorus is the same as for calcium, or a ratio of Ca:P of 1.0.

Few, if any, primary vitamin deficiency diseases are seen in adolescents. For the most part, the recommendations are based on energy or protein intake. Riboflavin, thiamin, and niacin values are based on calorie levels. Pyridoxine or B_6 recommendations are based on protein levels. As protein levels increase, so should amounts of B_6. Vitamin A recommendations are based on body weight. Therefore, recommended amounts of vitamin A for females during adolescence are approximately 80 percent of those for males.

Nutrition-Related Problems

A number of nutrition problems are typical in adolescence: dental caries, obesity and weight control, iron deficiency anemia, and acne (46, 47, 48). In recent years, teenage pregnancy, alcoholism and drug abuse, and disorders such as anorexia nervosa have also become common, as have fads like vegetarianism and the macrobiotic diet. Here, we will discuss iron deficiency anemia, acne, and pregnancy; obesity and anorexia are discussed in Chapter 9, and dental problems are covered in Chapter 11.

iron deficiency anemia

Iron deficiency anemia is a significant nutritional problem of adolescence. The biological age of the teenager, rather than chronological age, must be considered with regard to iron needs. As noted earlier, both males and females need significant amounts of iron daily to fulfill the needs of increasing blood volume in males and menstrual losses in females. The RDA for both sexes is 18 mg iron daily, which is difficult to achieve, particularly with the irregular food intake patterns of some teenagers. Most studies have reported that few teenagers even approach adequate intakes of iron (49, 50). Males do far better than females because they tend to eat more of all foods and are able to build up iron stores.

In determining iron deficiency anemia, body stores of iron, as well as circulating iron in the form of hemoglobin and hematocrit, must be assessed. Most authorities agree that measurements of serum iron and total iron binding capacity must be taken so that the percentage of transferrin saturation can be determined as an indication of stores. Transferrin saturation of 16 percent or less is usually considered indicative of deficient body stores (51, 52). More recently, measures of serum ferritin are being used as signs of iron stores (53).

Each individual must be evaluated separately. On any given day a teenager may have adequate iron intake, normal hemoglobin and hematocrit, and deficient body stores of iron. Using only one of these parameters, incorrect counseling could be given. In addition, some racial differences are evident in normal hematocrit levels, with black adolescents having lower normal values than white adolescents (54). Gaines and Daniel reported differences in dietary intakes of iron to be significant between white and black males by the end of sexual maturity (52, 55). Differences in intake for white and black females occurred prior to onset of puberty only, with black girls having greater iron intakes than white girls. Black males also had greater intakes of iron prior to onset of puberty (56); see Figure 4-4.

Folic acid is also important for the adolescent. Folate is necessary to support growth and the rapid increase of cells occurring with that growth. Daniel's studies showed that boys had higher intakes of folate than girls and their plasma folate levels decreased more with sexual maturity than those of girls, presumably because of greater muscle mass (55). Again, this points up the usefulness of compar-

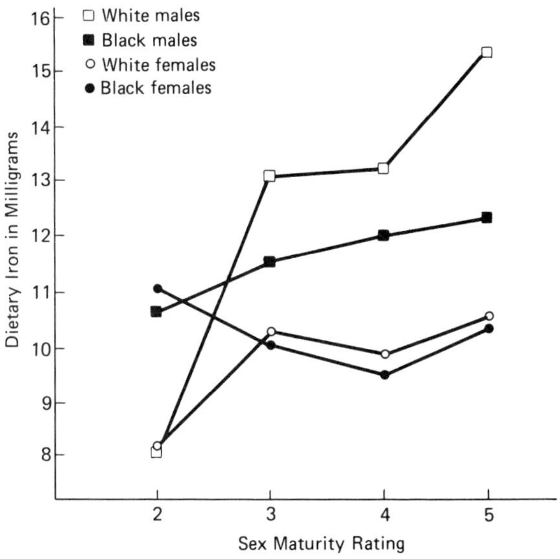

FIG. 4–4. Dietary iron intake according to sex, race, and age. *Source:* E. G. Gaines and W. A. Daniel, Jr., "Dietary Iron Intakes of Adolescents," *Journal of the American Dietetic Association* 65 (1974): 275–280. Copyright The American Dietetic Association.

ing nutrient needs and intakes to biological age (sexual maturity) rather than chronological age.

acne

Acne is another problem of adolescence frequently associated with nutrition by the layperson and teenager. Even some physicians and nutritionists believe that certain foods, notably chocolate, fat, greasy fried foods, cola beverages, nuts, milk, and iodine-containing foods aggravate acne (57).

Chocolate has received the most publicity, but in controlled, double blind clinical studies no clear-cut effects could be noted (58). In fact, some complexions appeared to be improved with eating chocolate, possibly because of increasing maturity. There is also no evidence that fats significantly influence acne. In a study that compared the responses of teenagers with acne on high carbohydrate and moderate carbohydrate diets, no differences in the course of the acne were noted (59).

The relationship of iodine-containing foods to acne has also been examined under controlled study conditions (57). The results were inconclusive, but it was doubtful that iodine in foods caused precipitation or aggravation of acne. There are no specific foods that have been shown to have adverse effects on acne. Although vitamin A has been used topically and as a food supplement in the treatment of acne, most physicians have found it to be ineffective. In addition, large doses of the fat-soluble form can be toxic, particularly if taken over a long period of time. Cleanliness and a balanced diet help keep the skin healthy and are the recommended advice for teenagers suffering from skin problems.

pregnancy

Pregnancy can occur in adolescence or even before. Because most of the studies are of adults, our discussion of pregnancy is included in Chapter 5. There are a few special concerns for pregnant adolescents. Although the major growth spurt is achieved prior to conception, some growth remains to be completed. There can be some competition between maternal and fetal needs. Inadequate nutrient intakes and pregnancy among young teenagers (under 16) are more likely to occur under poor socioeconomic conditions. Well-nourished and older adolescents demonstrate no great complications in pregnancy.

SUMMARY

Nutrition evaluation, care, and status of the adolescent are tied to the increased needs associated with the sudden growth spurt occurring just prior to and during puberty. Needs increase, particularly for calories and protein, but also for vitamins and minerals. The nutrition needs of pubertal growth are complicated by the great individual variations in energy expenditure, and by lack of adequate sleep and rest brought about by an active life style.

Social changes, particularly the importance of peer group pressures, affect food habits and therefore food intake. Even though the adolescent is beginning to reject parental authority, food habits up to this point have been influenced by the family group. During adolescence, the peer group becomes the dominant influence. The group spends more time together and less time at home, thereby eliminating much family supervision of food choices. The drive for independence influences food consumption since the adolescent begins to eat more snack and fast foods that can be prepared or obtained independently.

Establishment of identity and self-image is the main psychological thrust behind many fad diets and/or concepts such as vegetarianism, weight reduction, "muscle building," and experimenting with alcohol and other drugs. Before evaluation of nutritional status and/or plans for nutrition care and education can be successful, the counselor or physician must determine how the adolescent feels about his or her body.

The adolescent period is difficult to define. In this chapter we have attempted to illustrate the complex nature of adolescence and how social and psychological needs affect physiological changes. The internal pressures of puberty are associated with numerous hormonal changes and rapid physical growth. External pressures come mostly from the peer group.

There are considerable gaps in our knowledge of the nutrient requirements for adolescents. Available information is related primarily to chronological age, whereas nutrition and growth need to be related to developmental age and sexual maturation for both males and females (1). Research needs to be focused directly on this group, instead of extrapolating from adult studies.

references

1. *Adolescent Health Care: A Guide for BCHS-Supported Programs and Projects.* DHEW Publication No. (HSA) 79-5234. Rockville, Md.: HEW, PHS, BCHS, 1979.
2. BARNES, H. V. "Physical Growth and Development during Puberty." *Medical Clinics of North America* 59 (1975):1305.
3. DANIEL, W. A., JR. "An Approach to the Adolescent Patient." *Medical Clinics of North America* 59 (1975):1283.
4. DEISCHER, R. W., and C. A. MILLS. "The Adolescent Looks at His Health and Medical Care." *American Journal of Public Health* 53 (1963):1928.
5. HUENEMANN, R. L., M. C. HAMPTON, A. R. BEHNKE, L. R. SHAPIRO, and B. W. MITCHELL. *Teen-age Nutrition and Physique.* Springfield, Ill.:Charles C Thomas, 1974.
6. OJEDA, S. R. "The Endocrinology of Sexual Development." *Federation Proceedings* 39 (1980):2353–2354.
7. FRISCH, R. E. "Pubertal Adipose Tissue." *Federation Proceedings* 39 (1980):2395–2400.
8. GLASS, A. R., and R. S. SWERDLOFF. "Nutritional Influences on Sexual Maturation of the Rat." *Federation Proceedings* 39 (1981) 2360–2364.
9. Forbes, G. B. "Relation of Lean Body Mass to Height in Children and Adolescents." *Pediatric Research 6* (1972): 32.
10. National Center for Health Statistics. *Skinfold Thickness of Youths 12–17 Years."* U.S. Vital and Health Statistics, Series 11, No. 132; DHEW Publication No. (HRA) 74–1614. Washington, D.C.: Government Printing Office, 1974.
11. TANNER, J. M., R. H. WHITEHOUSE, W. A. MARSHALL, and B. S. CARTER. "Prediction of Adult Height from Height, Bone Age and Occurrence of Menarche at Ages 4–16 with Allowance for Midparent Height." *Archives of Diseases of Children* 50 (1975):14.
12. ONAT, T., and B. ERTE. "Adolescent Female Height Velocity: Relationships to Body Measurements, Sexual, and Skeletal Maturity." *Human Biology* 46 (1974):199.
13. TANNER, J. M., and R. H. WHITEHOUSE. "Clinical Longitudinal Standards for Height, Weight, Height Velocity, Weight Velocity, and the Stages of Puberty." *Archives of Diseases of Children* 51 (1976):170.
14. HAMILL, P. V. V., F. E. JOHNSTON, and S. LEMESHOW. *Height and Weight of Youths 12–17 Years, United States 1966–1970.* Vital and Health Statistics Series 11, No. 124; DHEW Publication No. (HSM) 73-1606. Washington, D.C.: U.S. Government Printing Office, 1975.

15. WOLFF, O. H. "Obesity in Childhood: A Study of the Birth Weight, the Height, and the Onset of Puberty." *Quarterly Journal of Medicine* N.S. 24 (1955): 109.

16. LAPORTE, M. "Effect of War-imposed Dietary Limitations on Growth of Paris School Children." *American Journal of Diseases of Children* 71 (1946): 244.

17. MARSHALL, W. A. "Interrelationships of Skeletal Maturation, Sexual Development and Somatic Growth in Man." *Annals of Human Biology* 1 (1974): 7129.

18. WOLFF, G. "A Study of the Trend of Weight in White School Children from 1933–36. Material Based on the Examination of Pupils of the Elementary Schools in Hagerstown, Maryland." *Child Development* 11 (1940): 159.

19. JACKSON, C. M. "Recovery of Rats upon Refeeding after Prolonged Suppression of Growth by Underfeeding." *Anatomical Records* 68 (1937): 37181.

20. NISSEN, H. W., and A. H. REISEN. "Retardation in Onset of Ossification in Chimpanzee Related to Various Environmental and Psychological Factors." *Anatomical Records* 105 (1949): 665.

21. DREIZEN, S., C. N. SPIRAKIS, and R. E. STONE. "A Comparison of Skeletal Growth and Maturation in Undernourished and Well-nourished Girls before and after Menarche." *Journal of Pediatrics* 70 (1967): 256.

22. GREULICH, W. W. "The Growth and Development Status of Guamanian School Children in 1947." *American Journal of Physical Anthropolgy* N.S. 9 (1951): 55.

23. GREULICH, W. W., C. S. CRIMSON, and M. L. TURNER. "The Physical Growth and Development of Children Who Survived the Atomic Bombing of Hiroshima or Nagasaki." *Journal of Pediatrics* 43 (1953): 121.

24. TRULSON, M. F., C. COLLAZOS, and D. M. HEGSTED. "Growth and Development of Peruvian Children. I. Carquin and San Nicholas." *Pediatrics* 17 (1956): 510.

25. JONES, D. B. "Sex Differences in the Growth of Young Rats and Survival of Adult Rats Fed Protein-deficient Diets." *Journal of Nutrition* 44 (1951):465.

26. SCHULTZE, M. O. "Effects of Malnutrition in Early Life on Subsequent Growth and Reproduction of Rats." *Journal of Nutrition* 56 (1955): 25.

27. SCHWARTZ, L., R. H. BRITTEN, and L. R. THOMPSON. "Studies in Physical Development and Posture. 1. The Effect of Exercise on the Physical Condition and Development of Adolescent Boys. 2. Bodily Growth with Age. 3. Physical Fitness as Reflected in Tests of Muscular Strength." *Public Health Bulletin* 179 (1928): 124.

28. TANNER, J. M. "The Effect of Weight-Training on Physique." *American Journal of Physical Anthropology* N.S. 10 (1952): 427.

29. LUYKEN, R., J. F. DEWIJN, and G. B. POST. "Studies of Adolescents in the Netherlands with Special Reference to Training." In *Nutrient Requirements in Adolescence,* eds. J. I. McKigney and H. N. Munro. Cambridge, MA: MIT Press, 1976.

30. WHITTEN, C. F., "T.L.C. and the Hungry Child." *Nutrition Today* 7 (1972): 10.

31. WIDDOWSON, E. M. "Mental Contentment and Physical Growth." *Lancet* 1 (1951): 1316.

32. WIDDOWSON, E. M., and R. A. MCCANCE. "Growth at Home and at School." *Lancet* 2 (1944): 152.

33. FRIEND, G. E., and E. R. BRANCH. "Physique and Growth of School Boys." *Lancet* 2 (1947): 677.

34. HOWE, P. E., and M. SCHILLER. "Growth Responses of the School Child to Changes in Diet and Environmental Factors." *Journal of Applied Physiology* 5 (1952): 51.

35. THOMAS, J. A., and D. A. CALL. "Between Meal Eating: A Nutrition Problem Among Teen-Agers?" *Nutrition Reviews* 31 (1973): 137.

36. U.S. Department of Health, Education and Welfare. *Ten-State Nutrition Survey 1968-1970: V. Dietary.* DHEW Publication No. (HSM) 72-133. Washington, D.C.: Government Printing Office, 1972.

37. BEAL, V. A. "Nutritional Intake," In *Human Growth and Development,* Ed. R. W. McCammon. Springfield, Ill.: Charles C Thomas, 1970.

38. BURKE, B. S., R. B. REED, A. S. VAN DER BERG, and H. C. STEWART. "Caloric and Protein Intakes of Children between 1 and 18 Years of Age." *Pediatrics* 24 (supplement, part 2) (1959): 922.

39. LACEY, J. H., C. CHADBUND, A. H. CRISP, J. WHITEHEAD, and J. STORDY. "Variation of Energy Intake of Adolescent Schoolgirls." *Journal of Human Nutrition* 32 (1979): 419.

40. MUELLER, J. F. "Current Recommended Dietary Allowances for Adolescents." In *Nutrient Requirements for Adolescence,* eds. J. I. McKigney and H. N. Munro. Cambridge, MA: MIT Press, 1976.

41. Food and Nutrition Board, *Recommended Dietary Allowances,* 9th ed. Washington, D.C.: National Research Council, National Academy of Sciences, 1980.

42. MACLEAN,, W. C., and G. G. GRAHAM. "The Effect of Level of Protein Intake in Isogenergetic Diets on Energy Utilization." *American Journal of Clinical Nutrition* 32 (1979): 1381.

43. HEGSTED, D. M. "Assessment of Nitrogen Requirements." *American Journal of Clinical Nutrition* 31 (1978): 1669.

44. LEE, C. J. "Nutritional Status of Selected Teenagers in Kentucky." *American Journal of Clinical Nutrition* 31 (1978): 1453.

45. KIES,, C. and M. CAST. "Nutritional Status and Food Patterns of American and Moroccan Adolescents." *Federation Proceedings* 37 (1978): 846.

46. U.S. Department of Health, Education and Welfare. *Ten-State Nutrition Survey, 1968-70: III. Clinical, Anthropometry, Dental.* DHEW Publication No. (HSM) 72-8131. Washington, D.C.: Government Printing Office, 1972.

47. KELLY, J. E., and C. R. HARVEY. *Decayed, Missing and Filled Teeth among Youths 12–17 Years.* U.S. Vital and Health Statistics, Series 11, No. 144; DHEW Publication No. (HRA) 75-1626. Washington, D.C.: Government Printing Office, 1974.

48. HUENEMANN, R. L., L. R. SHAPIRO, M. C. HAMPTON, and B. W. MITCHELL. "Food and Eating Practices of Teenagers." *Journal of the American Dietetic Association* 53 (1968): 17.

49. U.S. Department of Health, Education and Welfare. *Preliminary Findings of the First Health and Nutrition Examination Survey, U.S. 1971–72: Dietary Intake and Biochemical Findings.* DHEW Publication No. (HRA) 74-1219. Washington, D.C. Government Printing Office, 1974.

50. Food and Nutrition Board, National Research Council, National Academy of Sciences, Committee on Nutrition of the Mother and Preschool Child. *Iron Nutriture in Adolescence.* DHEW Publication No. (HSA) 77: 5100, 1976.

51. DANIEL, W. A., E. G. GAINES, and D. L. BENNETT. "Iron Intake and Transferrin Saturation in Adolescents." *Journal of Pediatrics* 86 (1975): 299.

52. GAINES, E. G., and W. A. DANIEL. "Dietary Iron Intakes of Adolescents." *Journal of the American Dietetic Association* 65 (1974): 275.

53. LIPSCHITZ, E., et al. "A Clinical Evaluation of Ferritin and an Index of Iron Stores." *New England Journal of Medicine* 290 (1974): 1213.

54. HEALD, F. P., P. S. LEVY, P. V. V. HAMILL, and M. ROWLAND. "Hematocrit Values of Youths 12–17 Years." *National Center for Health Statistics Data from the National Nutrition Health Survey,* Series 11, No. 146, DHEW Publication No. (HRA) 75-1628, 1974.

55. DANIEL, W. A. "Hematocrit: Maturity Relationship in Adolescence." *Pediatrics* 52 (1973): 388.

56. GARN, S., et al. "Race Differences in Hemoglobin Levels." *Ecology of Food and Nutrition* 3 (1974): 299.

57. REISNER, RONALD M. "Acne Vulgaris." *Pediatric Clinics of North America* 20 (1973): 851.

58. FULTON, J. G., and A. KLIGMAN. "Effect of Chocolate on Acne Vulgaris." *Journal of the American Medical Association* 210 (1969): 2071.

59. CORNBLEET, T., and I. GIGLI. "Should We Limit Sugar in Acne?" *Archives of Dermatology* 83 (1961): 968.

CHAPTER 5

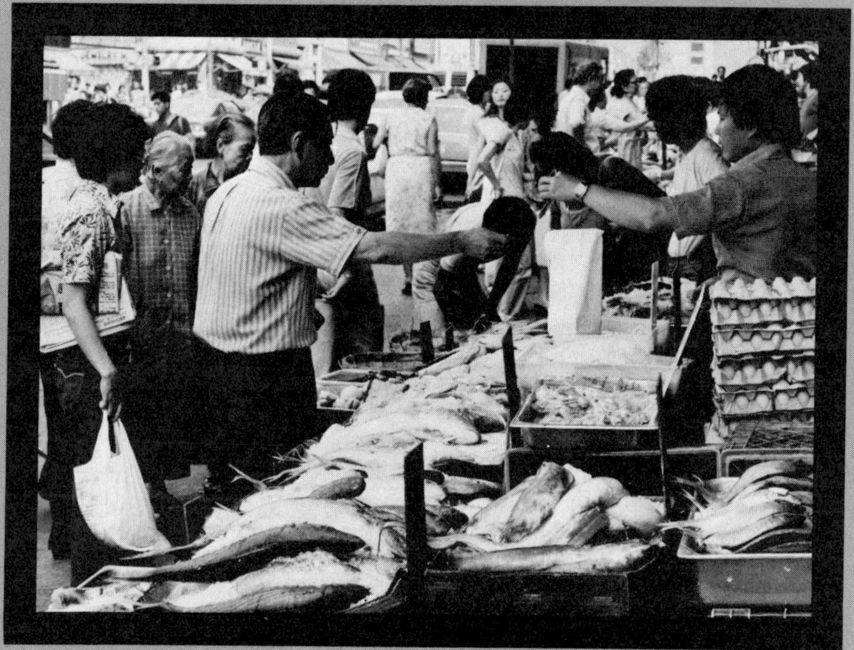

Photo by Marc Anderson

nutrition in the adult years

Adulthood is generally agreed to begin at the completion of skeletal growth and the attainment of sexual maturity. Its end is not so clear: usually it continues until the end of what we call "middle age," which corresponds in most individuals to ages 19 to 50. In addition, these ages correspond to those used in the RDA for adults. This will be the approximate time frame of this chapter. It will include a discussion of the recommendations currently available for adults in general, as well as the food habits recommended for good nutrition and the role of nutrition in preventing certain chronic diseases. We will also look at one of the functions of the adult—reproduction—and the role of nutrition in this process.

Social and Psychological Needs

It has been said that any of us can achieve optimal health and body functioning by maintaining our ideal body weight, exercising regularly and in moderation, eating a variety of foods in moderation, and minimizing stress. But it is not at all this simple. Physiological needs ensure that we eat, but psychosocial needs determine what we choose to eat. The foods we choose may have little to do with food itself, but rather be symbols with emotional meanings such as reward, punishment, or celebration. For many adults, food can become a substitute for affection, attention, or emotional gratification. Food can satisfy in many ways—it can give sensory pleasure and allow the expression of creativity. For a mother, food can symbolize security and caring for her family.

In addition, how and what we eat has much to do with our culture. No matter how nutritious (or physiologically appropriate) certain plants and animals are, cultural taboos may prohibit their consumption (1). In our culture it has been socially acceptable for the male adult to eat more than the female and to be bigger. Therefore, most food consumption surveys indicate that adult men come closer to meeting their physiological needs through food than women. Certain foods are considered masculine (meat and potatoes), others, feminine (salads, fancy desserts) (2).

Such social factors as availability of food are also important in influencing the adult's food intake (3). For instance, rural, low-income adults may eat more nutritious foods than their urban counterparts because of their access to gardens. Lack of refrigeration may limit the dairy products available for consumption.

Even the season of the year and natural hazards or disasters may limit food choices.

So the challenge to persuade adults to make modest life style changes (primarily changes in food habits) to reduce the risk of disease is indeed a complex one. An understanding of the person's life style and psychosocial behaviors therefore is just as important in monitoring and improving nutritional status as is physiological need.

Physiological Changes

Adult is a period of slower change when compared to infancy, adolescence, and terminal old age. There are no dramatic points in physical development in the adult. Social and psychological factors probably have more influence on adult nutrition than physiological factors, except for disease. Stability is the major physiological characteristic of adulthood. This explains why so many studies are conducted with young adults.

Most body functions are fully developed by the mid-20's. Height, strength, coordination, health, efficiency, and endurance are at maximum levels. Only very gradual declines occur over the next 20 or 30 years. The change and rate of decline is very individual. Each adult has a somewhat different rate of decline which depends on nutrition, climate, exercise, and work.

By the early 20's maximum height has been achieved. Since the beginning of this century, the maximum and mean height of young adults has been increasing. Today's 20-year-old adults are taller by several inches than the 20-year-olds in 1945.

About five years after maximum height is reached, an adult demonstrates maximum strength. From this point there is a gradual but steady, loss of about 10 percent by age 60. Exercise helps to maintain muscle strength.

The systems of the body reach their peak efficiency and optimum functioning before age 30. The major systems of the body are the skeletal-muscular, the digestive, the urinary, the respiratory, the circulatory, the nervous, the cardiovascular and the reproductive. The process of digestion, distribution, and metabolism of the nutrients depends on a well-developed interaction and feedback mechanism. Enzymes and hormones act to balance the system to maintain homeostasis, the state of equilibrium of the body.

The composition of the adult body varies with degree of fatness, sex, and amount of muscular and skeletal development. Variations in gross body weight are due to fat, muscle, and water. In direct analysis of male cadavers, body composition was 56 to 68 percent water, 12 to 20 percent fat, 14 to 19 percent protein, and 5 to 6 percent mineral ash. The percentage of water in the fat-free weight varied from 69 to 78 percent (4). There was no constant composition of the fat-free portion of the body.

Even though for the adult physical growth is completed, the body's tissues and cells remain in a dynamic state. Catabolism slightly exceeds anabolism, resulting in a net decrease in the total number of cells. In the adult female, the anabolic rate will exceed the catabolic rate during pregnancy and lactation. But the same nutrients are essential at every age because the same body processes are taking place, although at a slower pace. There is no need to change the kinds or quality of foods in adulthood if appropriate intake patterns have been set. No single food or nutrient has been shown to increase longevity, but there is abundant evidence that the quality of nutrition throughout life has a significant influence on health and well-being. Adults who are well nourished subjectively feel better and healthier, have more energy, and are better able to withstand psychological and physiological stresses than those on inadequate food intakes. But well nourished may not mean too well fed. Animal studies have indicated a direct relationship between restricted energy intakes and longevity. Lean and chronically undernourished rats were shown to live longer than rats fed freely from early infancy into adulthood (5, 6). Whether these results would be true for humans is not clear, since such experiments cannot be duplicated with human groups. The implications, however, are interesting.

Nutrient Requirements and Recommendations

RDAs for adults are divided into amounts for males and for females primarily because of differences in body size and composition between the sexes. Only in the case of iron do females have an increased requirement over males because of appreciable losses during menstruation.

The adult body is adaptive; it has regulatory mechanisms that tend to conserve essential nutrients when dietary intake is reduced or inadequate. In addition, the body stores certain nutrients when amounts consumed exceed immediate needs. Even so, nutrient recommendations are expressed as daily allowances to provide a way to evaluate food intakes. With adequate stores, an adult can exist for varying periods without consuming every nutrient daily. But if the intake continues to be insufficient to meet needs long enough to deplete stores, the body's ability to withstand stress, trauma, or illness will be significantly reduced.

energy

The RDA for energy for adults is expressed in average needs rather than individual variations at specific ages. Average values mean that individuals may require considerably more or less than the stated value. But adults should also remember that adequate energy intake is necessary for efficient utilization of protein. Then too, many vitamins and minerals are widely distributed and in low concentration in some foods, making it difficult to assume nutritional adequacy at less than 1200 to 1400 kcal.

Many American adults are overweight; in addition, they lead very sedentary lives, thereby expending considerably less energy than the average. Energy intake for the obese adult should be less than the average, but monitored closely to ensure inclusion of adequate nutrients other than calories. Maintenance of desirable body weight in adults depends upon achieving a balance between energy intake and energy output. Even a small daily excess of kcal above energy need will result in the accumulation of several pounds of fat in a year's time (7). Body composition continues to change in adults because of loss of lean body mass, which is compensated by an increase in fat tissue (8). Basal metabolic rate is reduced in proportion to loss of lean body mass; the reduction is approximately 2 percent per decade after age 21.

Table 5–1 gives a summary of desirable weights for men and women based on insurance company statistics of weight in relation to longevity. Surveys by the National Center for Health Statistics in 1979 described the average American male adult as 178 cm (70 in.) tall, and the average female as 163 cm (64 in.) tall. The average desirable weights were described as 70 kg (154 lb) for the male and 55 kg (120 lb) for the female throughout adulthood. Table 5–2 lists the RDA for energy intake for both males and females during the adult years, with both an average figure and a range for differences in physical activity. The most variable factor in estimating energy needs for both men and women is level of physical

TABLE 5–1. Suggested Desirable Weights for Heights and Ranges for Adult Males and Females

height[a]		weight[b]							
		MEN				WOMEN			
in.	cm	lb		kg		lb		kg	
58	147		—		—	102	(92–119)	46	(42–54)
60	152		—		—	107	(96–125)	49	(44–57)
62	158	123	(112–141)	56	(51–64)	113	(102–131)	51	(46–59)
64	163	130	(118–148)	59	(54–67)	120	(108–138)	55	(49–63)
66	168	136	(124–156)	62	(56–71)	128	(114–146)	58	(52–66)
68	173	145	(132–166)	66	(60–75)	136	(122–154)	62	(55–70)
70	178	154	(140–174)	70	(64–79)	144	(130–163)	65	(59–74)
72	183	162	(148–184)	74	(67–84)	152	(138–173)	69	(63–79)
74	188	171	(156–194)	78	(71–88)		—		—
76	193	181	(164–204)	82	(74–93)		—		—

[a]Without shoes.

[b]Without clothes. Average weight ranges in parentheses.

SOURCE: G. A. Bray, *Obesity in Perspective*. DHEW Publication No. 75–708, National Institutes of Health, Washington, D.C.

TABLE 5-2. Mean Heights and Weights and Recommended Energy Intake

category	age (years)	weight (kg)	weight (lb)	height (cm)	height (in.)	energy needs (with range) (kcal)		(mj)
Infants	0.0–0.5	6	13	60	24	kg × 115	(95–145)	kg × 0.48
	0.5–1.0	9	20	71	28	kg × 105	(80–135)	kg × 0.44
Children	1–3	13	29	90	35	1300	(900–1800)	5.5
	4–6	20	44	112	44	1700	(1300–2300)	7.1
	7–10	28	62	132	52	2400	(1650–3300)	10.1
Males	11–14	45	99	157	62	2700	(2000–3700)	11.3
	15–18	66	145	176	69	2800	(2100–3900)	11.8
	19–22	70	154	177	70	2900	(2500–3300)	12.2
	23–50	70	154	178	70	2700	(2300–3100)	11.3
	51–75	70	154	178	70	2400	(2000–2800)	10.1
	76+	70	154	178	70	2050	(1650–2450)	8.6
Females	11–14	46	101	157	62	2200	(1500–3000)	9.2
	15–18	55	120	163	64	2100	(1200–3000)	8.8
	19–22	55	120	163	64	2100	(1700–2500)	8.8
	23–50	55	120	163	64	2000	(1600–2400)	8.4
	51–75	55	120	163	64	1800	(1400–2200)	7.6
	76+	55	120	163	64	1600	(1200–2000)	6.7
Pregnancy						+300		
Lactation						+500		

Note: The data in this table have been assembled from the observed median heights and weights of children, together with desirable weights for adults for the mean heights of men (70 in.) and women (64 in.) between the ages of 18 and 34 years as surveyed in the U.S. population (HEW/NCHS data).

The energy allowances for the young adults are for men and women doing light work. The allowances for the two older age groups represent mean energy needs over these age spans, allowing for a 2-percent decrease in basal (resting) metabolic rate per decade and a reduction in activity of 200 kcal/day for men and women between 51 and 75 years, 500 kcal for men over 75 years, and 400 kcal for women over 75 years. The customary range of daily energy output is shown in parentheses for adults and is based on a variation in energy needs of ± 400 kcal at any one age, emphasizing the wide range of energy intakes appropriate for any group of people.

Energy allowances for children through age 18 are based on median energy intakes of children of these ages followed in longitudinal growth studies. The values in parens are 10th and 90th percentiles of energy intake, to indicate the range of energy consumption among children of these ages.

SOURCE: *Recommended Dietary Allowances*, 9th rev. ed. (Washington, D.C.: National Academy of Sciences, 1980). Reproduced by the permission of the National Academy of Sciences, Washington, D.C.

activity. Most adults in this country are thought to follow light to sedentary activity patterns (see Table 5–3). Activity patterns must be taken into account when evaluating an individual's need. Some adults will work at a sedentary job but participate in strenuous daily recreational activity; others have no regular exercise at all. Adults of larger (or smaller) body size will require proportionally more (or less) total energy per unit of time for activities that involve moving mass over distance. Their resting metabolic rates will also vary accordingly, so that energy allowances must take into consideration differences in body size as well.

Energy requirements decline gradually after early adulthood, but are related to changes in lean body mass, decreased BMR, and decreased physical activity rather than increase in age per se. With increasing age, individual differences in physical activity become more pronounced, so there are greater individual variations in energy expenditures and needs. Calorie intake should therefore decrease in proportion to the decrease in energy expenditure. Because of these changes, food sources of energy must be chosen carefully, especially by women. Females need to consume smaller amounts of nutrients (with the exception of iron) than males; they must also consume fewer calories. Therefore, females should choose nutrient-dense foods rather than foods containing only calories (9). For adult women, complex carbohydrates (whole grains, enriched cereals, dried beans, legumes, potatoes) are better energy choices than sugars. No more than 5 to 10 percent of total calories should come from sugars. In addition, the complex carbohydrates contain more fiber, which is beneficial for regulation of bowel movements and the prevention of constipation and irritable bowel syndrome (10).

Although fats are a concentrated source of energy for adults, they have been linked to atherosclerosis and coronary heart disease (particularly saturated fats). Some experts feel fats should not comprise more than 30 to 35 percent of total calories. Serum triglycerides increase with age in both males and females; serum cholesterol levels are higher in men aged 50 to 59 and in women 60 to 69, and then decline. Elimination of all fats is not recommended, however, because many fat-containing foods are excellent sources of other essential nutrients. In addition, fats serve as vehicles for the fat-soluble vitamins, and provide satiety.

proteins

The rate of protein synthesis declines with age, although the efficiency of nitrogen utilization is maintained between the ages of 20 and 75. Young et al. recommend that protein intake should therefore be reduced by approximately 30 percent during this time (11). Decreased protein systhesis and decreased lean body mass would suggest that older adults need less protein than younger adults. Other studies have shown that in some adults with inadequate caloric intake, protein foods are metabolized for energy, and that increased amounts of protein might help prevent deterioration of muscle mass. The RDA for protein is 56 g and 44 g for men and women, respectively, from 23 to 50 years of age (see Table 5–4).

TABLE 5-3. Examples of Daily Energy Expenditures of Mature Women and Men in Light Occupations

activity category	TIME (hr)	man, 70 kg RATE (kcal/min)	man, 70 kg TOTAL [kcal (kJ)]	woman, 58 kg RATE (kcal/min)	woman, 58 kg TOTAL [kcal (kJ)]
Sleeping, reclining	8	1.0–1.2	540 (2270)	0.9–1.1	440 (1850)
Very light Seated and standing activities, painting trades, auto and truck driving, laboratory work, typing, playing musical instruments, sewing, ironing.	12	up to 2.5	1300 (5460)	up to 2.0	900 (3780)
Light Walking on level, 2.5–3 mph, tailoring, pressing, garage work, electrical trades, carpentry, restaurant trades, cannery workers, washing clothes, shopping with light load, golf, sailing, table tennis, volleyball.	3	2.5–4.9	600 (2520)	2.0–3.9	450 (1890)
Moderate Walking 3.5–4 mph, plastering, weeding and hoeing, loading and stacking bales, scrubbing floors, shopping with heavy load, cycling, skiing, tennis, dancing.	1	5.0–7.4	300 (1260)	4.0–5.9	240 (1010)
Heavy Walking with load uphill, tree felling, work with pick and shovel, basketball, swimming, climbing, football.	0	7.5–12.0		6.0–10.0	
Total	24		2740 (11,500)		2030 (8530)

SOURCE: *Recommended Dietary Allowances*, 9th rev. ed. (Washington, D.C.: National Academy of Sciences, 1980). Reproduced by the permission of the National Academy of Sciences, Washington, D.C.

TABLE 5-4. Recommended Dietary Allowance, Revised 1980, for Adults (Protein)

age and sex group	weight kg	weight lb	height cm	height in	protein gm
Males					
19–22 yr	70	154	177	70	56
23–50 yr	70	154	178	70	56
Females					
19–22 yr	55	120	163	64	44
23–50 yr	55	120	163	64	44
Pregnancy					+30

SOURCE: *Recommended Dietary Allowances*, 9th rev. ed. (Washington, D.C.: National Academy of Sciences, 1980). Reproduced by the permission of the National Academy of Sciences, Washington, D.C.

These recommendations are estimates for healthy adults; those suffering from chronic disease or on prolonged medication may, in fact, need even larger amounts of protein.

vitamins

Few controlled studies have been done to determine vitamin requirements for adults. Most adult estimates are based on observations of the amounts needed to relieve deficiency symptons or taken from animal studies, so our knowledge in this area of nutrition is not precise. Table 5–5 shows the RDAs for the vitamins and minerals for adults from 19 to 50.

FAT-SOLUBLE VITAMINS. Vitamins A, D, E, and K may be consumed in less than adequate amounts because of decreased fat intake, decreased bile or lipase (as in liver or gall bladder disease), or use of laxatives and other medications that interfere with fat digestion and/or absorption. Recent studies involving large numbers of adult subjects have confirmed earlier findings as to vitamin A requirements (12, 13). Both reports indicated 500 to 600 μg of retinol, or twice as much β-carotene, was a minimum requirement for adults to maintain adequate blood levels and prevent deficiency symptoms. An intake above requirement level would be necessary to maintain liver stores. Therefore, the RDA for vitamin A is 1000 RE (5000 IU) for adult males and 800 RE (4000 IU) for females. Women have been reported to have similar liver stores and adequate blood levels on lower intakes than males, presumably because of their smaller body size (14, 15).

Vitamin D is especially important for adults because of its role in calcium and phosphorus metabolism and bone mineralization. Although the precise re-

TABLE 5-5. Recommended Dietary Allowances, Revised 1980,[a] for Adults (Vitamins)

age and sex	weight		height		fat-soluble vitamins			water-soluble vitamins						
	kg	lb	cm	in	A (μg RE)[b]	D (μg)[c]	E (mg α TE)[d]	C (mg)	THIAMIN (mg)	RIBO-FLAVIN (mg)	NIACIN (mg NE)[e]	B_6 (mg)	FOLACIN[f] (μg)	B_{12} (μg)
MALES														
19–22 yr	70	154	177	70	1,000	7.5	10	60	1.5	1.7	19	2.2	400	3.0
23–50 yr	70	154	178	70	1,000	5.0	10	60	1.4	1.6	18	2.2	400	3.0
51 + yr	70	154	178	70	1,000	5.0	10	60	1.2	1.4	16	2.2	400	3.0
FEMALES														
19–22 yr	55	120	163	64	800	7.5	8	60	1.1	1.3	14	2.0	400	3.0
23–50 yr	55	120	163	64	800	5.0	8	60	1.0	1.2	13	2.0	400	3.0
51 + yr	55	120	163	64	800	5.0	8	60	1.0	1.2	13	2.0	400	3.0
Pregnancy					+200	+5.0	+2	+20	+0.4	+0.3	+2	+0.6	+400	+1.0
Lactation					+400	+5.0	+3	+40	+0.5	+0.5	+5	+0.5	+100	+1.0

[a] The allowances are intended to provide for individual variations among most normal persons as they live in the United States under usual environmental stresses. Diets should be based on a variety of common foods in order to provide other nutrients for which human requirements have been less well defined.

[b] Retinol equivalents; 1 retinol equivalent = 1 μg retinol or 6 μg β-carotene.

[c] As cholecalciferol: 10 μg cholecalciferol = 400 I.U. vitamin D.

[d] X tocopherol equivalents: 1 mg d-X -tocopherol = 1X TE.

[e] NE (niacin equivalent) = 1 mg niacin or 60 mg dietary tryptophan.

[f] The folacin allowances refer to dietary sources as determined by *Lactobacillus casei* assay after treatment with enzymes ("conjugases") to make polyglutamyl forms of the vitamin available to the test organism.

SOURCE: *Recommended Dietary Allowances*, 9th rev. ed. (Washington, D.C.: National Academy of Sciences, 1980). Reproduced by the permission of the National Academy of Sciences, Washington, D.C.

quirement for adults is not known, daily consumption of 7.5 μg (300 IU) of vitamin D from age 19 to 22, and 5 μg (200 IU) after age 22 is recommended. The requirement for most adults can be met by adequate exposure to sunlight. However, there is evidence that those with heavily pigmented skin, or those who live in areas where sunlight is limited or with considerable atmospheric pollution, need an additional dietary or supplemental source of vitamin D (16).

Evidence of vitamin E deficiency in adults has been observed only in persons with long-term fat malabsorption (17). There were no specific clinical symptoms, but laboratory studies showed increased fragility of red blood cells, increased urinary excretion of creatinine, and deposits of ceroid pigment in the musculature of the small intestine. In normal adults, the range of total plasma tocopherols is 0.5–1.2 mg/100 ml (18). It is assumed that a plasma level of less than 0.5 ml/100 ml is undesirable, although it has not been demonstrated that lesser amounts result in inadequate tissue concentrations.

Unlike the other fat-soluble vitamins, vitamin E has not been shown to be toxic in adults, even when given in large doses. However, some caution may be warranted in giving large doses over long periods of time. Food intake studies indicate great variation in the amount of vitamin E in adult diets (19), and estimates of adequate intake should be calculated from several days' intake. Animal studies have shown that the need for vitamin E increases when the intake of polyunsaturated fatty acids (PUFA) is increased (20). But this has little significance, since the primary food sources of PUFA are also the richest sources of vitamin E. The RDA for vitamin E for adults is a range of 7–13 mg alpha-tocopherol equivalent (10–20 IU), or that amount which maintains plasma levels of total tocopherols above 0.5 mg/ml.

Some synthesis of vitamin K occurs in the intestinal tract, which means that deficiencies in adults would occur only after elimination of dietary sources from malabsorption or antibiotic therapy. Because of this body synthesis, no specific recommended allowance is made. The range of 70–140 μg per day given for adults can easily be supplied by a varied diet (see Appendix Table A–1).

WATER-SOLUBLE VITAMINS. Intake of the water-soluble vitamins must be more closely monitored, since they are not stored and since many adults are often on weight-loss diets. Table 5–4 gives the RDAs for specific vitamins. The allowance recommended for vitamin C for adults of both sexes is 60 mg, which has been shown to be necessary to maintain a body pool of 1500 mg. Hodges et al. have reported that a pool of this size would prevent overt signs of deficiency in the adult male for a period of 30 to 45 days (21).

Thiamin deficiency does occur in adults, and has been observed in alcoholics and in those who existed primarily on unenriched white rice (22). Recent reports indicate that other adults at risk of deficiency are those on renal dialysis treatment programs or long-term intravenous feedings and those consuming large amounts of tea daily (23, 24, 25). Clinical symptons of deficiency involve the central nervous and cardiovascular systems and may appear gradually over a long period of time. The symptoms most frequently observed are anorexia, muscular weakness, mental confusion, ataxia, peripheral paralysis, edema, muscle wasting, tachycardia, and enlarged heart (26).

The requirement for thiamin is related to energy intake because it is essential for reactions in carbohydrate metabolism. Sauberlich et al. reported the thiamin requirement to be proportional to energy intake when calories ingested were primarily from carbohydrate (27). Tissue stores are rapidly depleted in adults when thiamin intake is zero (28), so a minimal intake of 1 mg thiamin per day is recommended for adults even when caloric intake is restricted. The RDA is 0.5 mg/1000 kcal, which means the daily intake recommended for females is less than that for males because of decreased energy needs (see Table 5–5).

Physical signs of riboflavin deficiency (cheilosis, angular stomatitis, scrotal skin changes, seborrheic dermatitis) have been observed in male and female adults consuming 0.25 mg or less of riboflavin per 1000 kcal and approximately 2000 kcal/day (29, 30). Therefore, the RDA for riboflavin is 0.6 mg/1000 kcal for all adults except those whose caloric intake may be less than 2000 kcal; in this case, a minimum intake of 1.2 mg/day is recommended.

Niacin deficiency in adults results in pellagra, which is characterized by dermatitis, inflammation of mucous membranes, and dementia (31). Estimation of niacin requirements in adults is complicated by the conversion of some tryptophan to niacin and by the limited number of studies. A dietary intake of 60 mg tryptophan is considered equivalent to 1 mg niacin and 1 niacin equivalent (NE) is comparable to either. Studies of adult men and women were used to arrive at these figures (32, 33, 34). The RDA for adults is 6.6 NE over 1000 kcal and not less than 13 NE at energy intakes of less than 2000 kcal.

In adults, vitamin B_6 deficiency may cause depression and confusion, and electroencephalographic abnormalities followed by convulsions (35, 36, 37). The establishment of allowances for vitamin B_6 in adults is complicated by the interaction with protein: the requirement seems to be increased on high-protein diets (38). The RDA for adult males is 2.2 mg/day; and for adult females, it is 2.0 mg.

Major characteristics of folacin deficiency (megaloblastic cytology) have been observed in adults after 16 weeks on low-folacin diets (39). Supplementing the diet with 100 μg of pteroylglutamic acid per day maintained the normal level of serum folacin; smaller amounts did not. Since only 25 to 50 percent of dietary folacin is nutritionally available, the RDA is set at 400 μg for adult males and females.

Symptoms of vitamin B_{12} deficiency in adults resulting from inadequate intake are rare. Deficiencies have been observed in adults on strict vegetarian diets that did not include any milk, eggs, or meat. The requirement seems to be met with a wide range of intakes and in quantities present in most mixed diets. The RDA is 3.0 μg of vitamin B_{12} for adult males and females.

minerals

The minerals are divided into the macroelements present in large amounts in the body, like calcium, phosphorus, magnesium, potassium, and iron, and the trace elements zinc, iodine, and copper, which are needed in very small amounts. The requirements for the macrominerals can be estimated from human balance studies. Requirements for trace elements also depend on the levels of intake that prevent deficiency, studies with radioisotopes, and cellular studies of body fluids.

The minerals chosen for discussion here are those for which more research data exists for determining recommendations (see Tables 5–6 and 5–7).

The adult body adapts to the level of calcium intake in order to maintain equilibrium. If an excessive amount is taken in, large amounts of the calcium will not be absorbed. When intakes are decreased the body eventually becomes more efficient, absorbing a greater percentage of the smaller amount to maintain equilibrium (40). Many aspects of food intake affect calcium absorption in adults: level of protein, phosphorus, available vitamin D, and fat intake. The evidence relating osteoporosis (loss of bone mass) to calcium intake is conflicting. Although some authorities recommend levels as high as 1500 mg daily for women, others say calcium balance can be maintained at less than half that amount. The RDA is 800 mg/day for adults of both sexes, and careful planning is necessary to include this amount daily if the person excludes dairy products from the diet.

Phosphorus depletion has been observed in adults taking excessive amounts of nonabsorbable antacids over a long period of time. The symptoms were weakness, anorexia, malaise, and pain in the bones; they were alleviated with discontinuation of the antacid and the provision of adequate phosphorus (41). The RDA for adults in milligrams per day is the same as for calcium, allowing for a Ca:P ratio of 1:1.

The role of magnesium deficiency in adults is not clear. There is no evidence that large oral intakes are harmful in those with normal renal function, although some people have reported a cathartic effect if they have taken in excess of 3 to 5 g magnesium salts per day (42). Deficiency in adults has been seen only in malabsorption syndromes and certain gastrointestinal diseases; the characteristics reported were neuromuscular dysfunction manifested by hyperexcitability with tremors and convulsions (43). The RDA for adult males is 350 mg/day and for adult females is 300 mg/day.

The iron requirements of female adults are higher during the years of menstruation, but after menopause women's need for iron is the same as that of men. The RDA for all adult males and adult females above 50 is 10 mg/day; for females 19 to 51, the allowance is 18 mg/day. In adult women, the iron loss in menstrual blood flow is approximately 0.5 mg/day averaged over one month (44) and both men and women lose approximately 1 mg iron/day through other routes (45). The main control of iron status in adults is at the site of absorption.

TABLE 5-6. Recommended Dietary Allowances, Revised 1980, for Adults (Minerals)

age and sex	weight		height		minerals					
	kg	lb	cm	in	CALCIUM (mg)	PHOSPHORUS (mg)	MAGNESIUM (mg)	IRON (mg)	ZINC (mg)	IODINE (μg)
MALES										
19–22 yr	70	154	177	70	800	800	350	10	15	150
23–50 yr	70	154	178	70	800	800	350	10	15	150
51 + yr	70	154	178	70	800	800	350	10	15	150
FEMALES										
19–22 yr	55	120	163	64	800	800	300	18	15	150
23–50 yr	55	120	163	64	800	800	300	18	15	150
51 + yr	55	120	163	64	800	800	300	10	15	150
Pregnancy					+400	+400	+150	*a*	+ 5	+25
Lactation					+400	+400	+150	*a*	+10	+50

[a] The increased requirement during pregnancy cannot be met by the iron content of habitual American diets or by the existing iron stores of many women; therefore, the use of 30 to 60 mg supplemental iron is recommended. Iron needs during lactation are not substantially different from those of nonpregnant women, but continued supplementation of the mother for 2 to 3 months after parturition is advisable in order to replenish stores depleted by pregnancy.

SOURCE: *Recommended Dietary Allowances*, 9th rev. ed. (Washington, D.C.: National Academy of Sciences, 1980). Reproduced by the permission of the National Academy of Sciences, Washington, D.C.

TABLE 5–7. Estimated Safe and Adequate Daily Dietary Intakes of Additional Selected Vitamins and Minerals for Adults

vitamins	trace elements[a]	electrolytes
K (70–140 μg)	Copper (2.0–3.0 mg)	Sodium (1,100–3,300 mg)
Biotin (100–200 μg)	Manganese (2.5–5.0 mg)	Potassium (1,875–5,625 mg)
Pantothenic acid (4–7 mg)	Fluoride (1.5–4.0 mg)	Chloride (1,700–5,100 mg)
	Chromium (0.05–0.2 mg)	
	Selenium (0.05–0.2 mg)	
	Molybdenum (0.15–0.5 mg)	

NOTE: Because there is less information on which to base allowances, these figures are not given in the main table of the RDAs and are provided here in the form of ranges of recommended intakes.

[a]Since the toxic levels for many trace elements may be only several times usual intakes, the upper levels for the trace elements given in this table should not be habitually exceeded.

SOURCE: *Recommended Dietary Allowances*, 9th rev. ed. (Washington, D.C.: National Academy of Sciences, 1980). Reproduced by the permission of the National Academy of Sciences, Washington, D.C.

Absorption of iron is a complicated process influenced by the intestinal mucosa, the amount and chemical nature of iron ingested, and a variety of dietary factors that increase or decrease the availability of iron (46). Because of this circumstance, a method has been proposed for calculating absorbable iron in each given meal to provide a more realistic estimate of the amount of iron available to the body (47) (see Table 5–8). Calculated amounts of absorbable iron can be related to the RDA by multiplying the value by a factor of 10, since the RDAs are based on the assumption that only 10 percent of total ingested iron is absorbed. In addition, medicinal substances commonly consumed by adults may further reduce the availability of iron. Some of these are antacids and calcium and phosphate salts, as well as phytates and tannic acid in tea. Unusually large amounts of these substances should be avoided if they affect the person's iron status.

In human metabolic studies, intakes of 12.5 mg of zinc per day were shown to maintain equilibrium or a positive balance in heatlhy adults (48). Allowing for absorption of 40 percent of dietary zinc, an intake of 15 mg/day is recommended for adults. The average zinc content of mixed diets consumed by adults has been reported as 10 to 15 mg/day (49). Animal meats and seafoods are better sources of zinc than vegetables, because fiber and phytate can adversely affect the availability of zinc.

Iodine deficiency is manifested in the adult by an enlarged thyroid gland (goiter), but its incidence has fallen dramatically since the introduction of iodized salt. The daily iodine requirement to prevent goiter in adults is 50 to 75 μg or, approximately 1 μg/kg of body weight (50). The RDA for all adults is set at 150

TABLE 5-8. Availability of Iron in Different Meals

type of meal	absorption of iron present in meal (%) NONHEME IRON	HEME IRON
LOW-AVAILABILITY MEAL	3%	23%
< 30 g meat, poultry, fish < 25 mg ascorbic acid		
MEDIUM-AVAILABILITY MEAL	5	23
30–90 g meat, poultry, fish or 25–75 mg ascorbic acid		
HIGH-AVAILABILITY MEAL	8	23
> 90 g meat, poultry, fish or > 75 mg ascorbic acid; or 30–90 g meat, poultry, fish plus 25–75 mg ascorbic acid		

SOURCE: *Recommended Dietary Allowances*, 9th rev. ed. (Washington, D.C.: National Academy of Sciences, 1980). Reproduced by the permission of the National Academy of Sciences, Washington, D.C.

μg to meet increased demands, to account for individual variation, and to counteract natural goitrogens. Only those adults who are strict vegetarians and thus eat no seafood or who refuse to use iodized salt may have deficiency problems.

Dietary copper deficiency has not been known in adults under normal circumstances, but may occur in certain cases of severe malnutrition or malabsorbtive disease states. The estimate of copper requirements for adult males and females has been based on balance studies. Intakes between 1.0 and 2.0 mg/day have been shown to maintain balance (51, 52), so the RDA for all adults is 2 to 3 mg/day. Most mixed diets of adults in the United States will supply more than 5 mg/day (53).

Reproduction and Nutrition

The ability to reproduce is affected by events early in the individual's life, although much more research support is needed to establish the relationship between diet and reproduction in humans. Most available information is from animal studies, retrospective studies during famine and wartime conditions, or survey studies in malnourished or low-income populations. The data we have are confusing and in some instances contradictory, but two generalizations may be made: 1) severe and acute malnutrition in a previously well-nourished population is associated with a drop in fertility rate and a less remarkable but significant drop in birth weight in infants; and 2) mild to moderate chronic malnutrition causes no impairment in fertility but has far-reaching negative effects on maternal and child health.

The childbearing competence of women is influenced long before the reproductive period (54). Nutrition cannot be separated from food intake, income level, educational attainment, health care, infection, age, parity, or hard physical work. Many studies are criticized because no direct, statistical cause and effect relationship can be demonstrated between nutrition and health, or food intake and nutritional status. But even with these ambiguities and uncertainties, there is general agreement with Mellanby's statement that "nutrition is undoubtedly the most important of all environmental factors in childbearing" (55)—and in the ability to reproduce healthy offspring—for both men and women.

general health and reproductive ability

FEMALES. Three stages in a woman's reproductive life are most vulnerable to nutritional imbalance: 1) prepubescence, 2) adolescence, and 3) pregnancy.

The nutritional vulnerability of the prepubescent period has been difficult to prove because retrospective information is almost never available, and dietary histories are subject to gross errors of memory. Longitudinal studies are also needed to observe the same individuals through childhood, conception, and pregnancy. Because of the lack of specific data on preconceptional nutritional status, some authorities have used shortness of stature as an indication of poor food intake and nutritional status during childhood (56). Thomson, for example, in a study done in Scotland, showed that shorter women, regardless of socioeconomic status, were more likely to be judged in "poor health." This study also reported that the association between decreasing stature and increased rates of prematurity, delivery complications, and deaths in the perinatal period continued for each parity and for age groups within parities. The author concluded that outcome of pregnancy was influenced more by events and circumstances in the mother's childhood and adolescence, which determine her general health and physiological efficiency, than by events during pregnancy (57).

There are no similar studies of women in the United States. However, in a recent review of data collected at Harvard, some of the same conclusions were reached (58). Taller women had better reproductive performance than did their shorter peers, as indicated by fewer premature infants and spontaneous abortions. Even more significant was the retrospective review of dietary data accumulated on the same women during their participation in a childhood nutrition study at Harvard years earlier. Eighty percent of the women who had daily intakes of 70 g protein or more between 8 and 12 years of age had healthy babies in all pregnancies, compared to only 30 percent of the women who had consumed lesser amounts of protein during childhood. Therefore, improving nutritional status during the prepubescent period may indeed be the best method of ensuring better reproductive records and healthier babies. (59)

During adolescence, there is rapid growth and physiological maturation of the reproductive system. The specific mechanisms that initiate this hormonally controlled state are not fully understood, as discussed earlier (Chapter 4), but a "critical" body weight or state of skeletal development may be necessary to initiate physiological sexual development. Frisch states that the percentage of body fat is responsible for the peaking of growth and the time of menarche, which occurs at a specific weight for each girl, regardless of age (60). Tanner has divided the reproductive development of the female into various stages of sexual maturity (64). In normal females, the initiation of the adolescent growth spurt begins before 10 years of age, and menarche occurs at approximately 12 years of age. Chronological age is not as important as reproductive or biological age—that is, chronological age minus menarchal age (65).

Nutritional status affects the rate of body development, including the distribution of muscle, fat, and other tissue components (61). There may be competition between height and weight for the available calories (62). Once cyclical ovulation and menses occur, the adolescent female is capable of childbearing. The Committee on Adolescence of the Academy of Pediatrics recently concluded that data show that adolescent pregnancy does not carry age-related nutritional risks except in physiologically or gynecologically immature girls. But other risks of teenage pregnancy related to socioeconomic class do include nutritional problems (66).

Ovulation is dependent on a complex hormonal system that can be related to nutritional status (63). The production of hormones depends on the availability of nutrients for synthesis. Both extremes, underweight and obesity, alter ovulation. Upon maturity, ovulation occurs about every 28 days as a result of the interaction of ovarian and pituitary hormones. The pituitary hormone, follicle stimulating hormone (FSH), influences an ovarian follicle (a small sac of supporting cells surrounding the ovum) to become mature and secrete greater amounts of the ovarian hormone estrogen. The estrogen stimulates a build-up of the uterine lining or endometrium. When the follicle ruptures, the mature ovum, surrounded by cells from the ruptured follicle and some fluids, breaks through the surface of the ovary. This is called ovulation and is triggered by a rapid increase in the levels of the pituitary luteinizing hormone (LH). The cells remaining in the follicle sink into the break in the surface of the ovary, and under the influence of LH develop a yellow endocrine body called the corpus luteum. The corpus luteum produces the ovarian hormone progesterone, which maintains the endometrium for implantation of a fertilized ovum (pregnancy). If pregnancy does not occur, the corpus luteum declines and the endometrium is sloughed off—that is, menses occurs (see Figure 5–1).

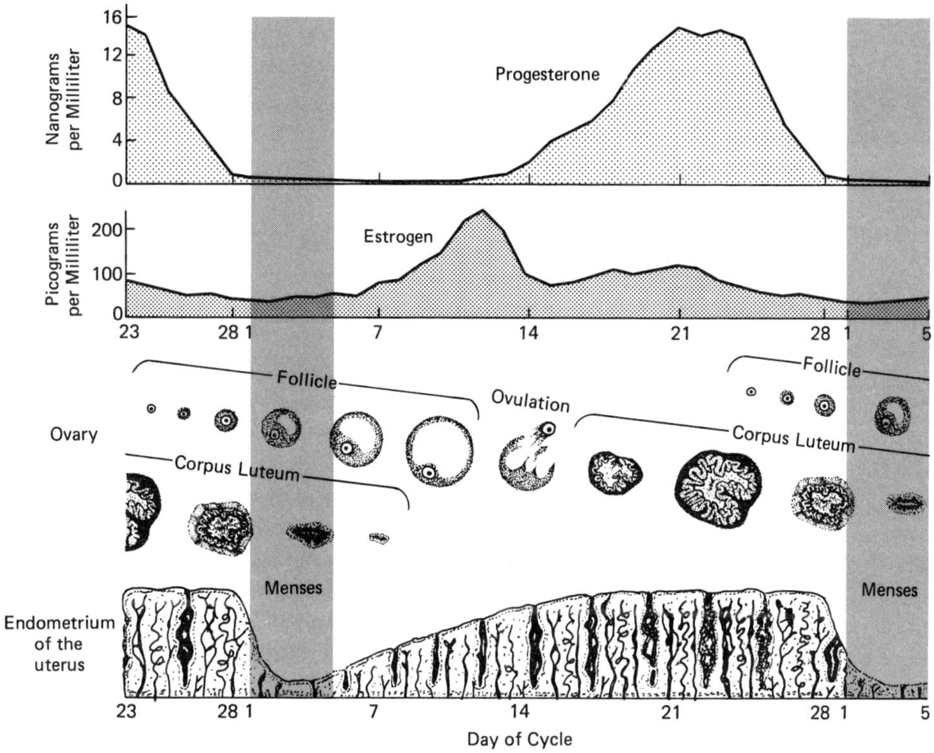

FIG. 5–1. The female reproductive cycle. *Source:* I. Valadian and D. Porter, *Physical Growth and Development from Conception to Maturity: A Programmed Text* (Boston: Little, Brown, 1977).

MALES. In the male, reproductive ability begins during the adolescent period, just as it does in females. Tanner describes this development according to stages of sexual maturity that the average male completes by 15 years of age (64). Progression from one stage to the next varies according to the rate of height and weight gain.

Pubertal emaciation due to various causes, including anorexia nervosa, can result in temporary pituitary insuffiency and has been shown to adversely affect growth and steroid hormone synthesis (67), although it is thought to be reversible with adequate dietary treatment. In the prepubescent period, undernutrition results in retardation of puberty, and in an arrest in the development of mature spermatocytes (68, 69).

Prasad and Ronaghy studied boys in Egypt and Iran suffering from dwarfism, hypogonadism, and iron deficiency anemia (70, 71). Additional studies also showed decreased zinc concentrations in various tissues. The anemia was completely corrected by the administration of oral iron supplements (ferrous sulfate) without zinc. When zinc supplements were given to some of the dwarfs, significant increases in height and maturation of the reproductive organs were noted. Poor nutrition may delay the beginning of adolescence and also have cumulative detrimental effects on earlier growth periods in childhood.

The evidence is inconclusive and controversial as to the specific role of nutrition in reproductive performance in males, although nutrition is, of course, necessary for all physiological functions. Excessive fatness (obesity) and severe undernutrition both cause decreased fertility in male animals, and some similarities have been noted in humans (72, 73). General malnutrition, as well as deficiencies in specific nutrients, may be related to reproductive failure in the male (74). Normal sperm must be produced in adequate amounts and must be actively mobile, and certain biochemical and metabolic reactions are necessary for the maintenance of viable sperm (75). Studies have shown that in adult men, semi-starvation has little effect on sperm count; however, motility of sperm was reduced (73). Severe nutrient deprivation depresses the function of all organs, including the sex organs (74, 76). During starvation, men appear to lose potency and libido. Decreased fertility results not only from severe famine conditions, but also from other environmental, social, economic and physiological factors.

The role of specific vitamins in relation to fertility in men is not clearly established, and there is little evidence to justify the administration of massive doses of vitamins to improve male fertility. Studies attempting to show the therapeutic effects of vitamin A, the B complex vitamins, and vitamin E do not provide conclusive evidence of their efficacy in treating male sterility.

conception

Usually conception occurs in the Fallopian tubes when one of the millions of sperm expelled during ejaculation migrate to the tubes and penetrate the ovum. Both sperm and ovum must be present in the tubes. The fertilized ovum then moves down the Fallopian tube and becomes attached to the uterine wall about six to seven days later (see Figure 5–2).

contraception

It is not possible to discuss reproduction without including a section on contraceptive techniques. When family planning methods are not accessible or may not be part of the individual's value systems, maternal and infant nutritional status are greatly jeopardized by uncontrolled fertility and concurrent marginal nutrition (77, 78). As an immediate benefit, effective birth control methods offer protection from pregnancy to women who are classified obstetrically and nutritionally in the high-risk group, including immature adolescents and women in the premenopausal and menopausal years. Contraception also allows mothers to space children for more complete physical and nutritional recovery, to time pregnancies at desired intervals, and to limit family size. Concurrent advantages

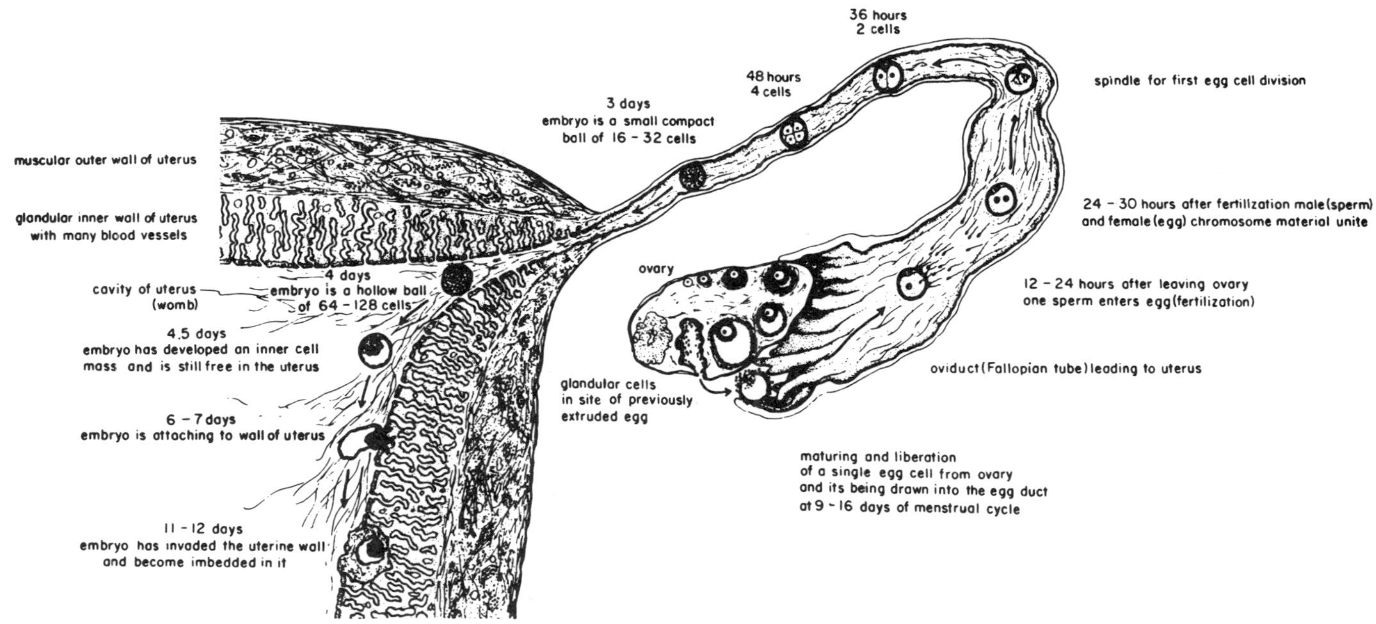

FIG. 5–2. Fertilization and implantation. *Source:* I. Valadian and D. Porter, *Physical Growth and Development from Conception to Maturity: A Programmed Text* (Boston: Little, Brown, 1977).

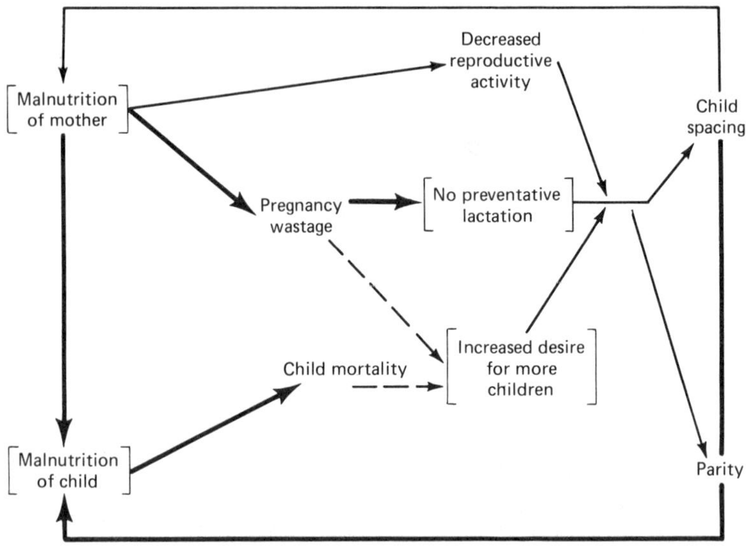

FIG. 5–3. Nutrition-fertility relationships. Width of line indicates relative impact; dotted lines indicate uncertain interaction; items enclosed in boxes indicate points appropriate for intervention. *Source:* Nutrition and Fertility Interrelationships. National Research Council Subcommittee on Nutrition and Fertility. Food and Nutrition Board, National Research Council, Washington, D.C.: National Academy of Sciences, 1975.

offer families better outcomes of pregnancies and increased neonatal and infant survival. Some of these interrelationships are illustrated in Figure 5–3.

Worldwide about 50 million women, including over 10 million in the United States, are currently using oral contraceptive agents (OCA) (79). Figure 5–4 shows the age and marital status of women using OCA in the United States; Table 5–9 lists the groups of OCA available. Generally OCA are combination or sequential in nature. Within each type, the hormone dosage and composition may vary. In general, the OCA inhibits ovulation and/or brings about a series of biochemical and physiological changes in the cervical mucosa and endometrium, making the implantation of the ovum in the uterine environment less favorable or inhibiting penetration of the sperm (80).

OCA: NUTRITIONAL EFFECTS. The nutritional effects of oral contraceptives have been reviewed by a number of investigators (81, 82). Many of the metabolic effects of OCAs are similar to those seen in normal pregnancies, and users with marginal nutrient status and/or body stores could be at greater risk. The OCA can cause an alteration of the body's metabolism of carbohydrates, lipids, proteins, vitamins, and minerals similar to the action of steroid hormones. The effects on carbohydrate metabolism vary with the type of hormone. Based on glucose tolerance tests (GTT), about 10 percent of women who have taken OCA for at least

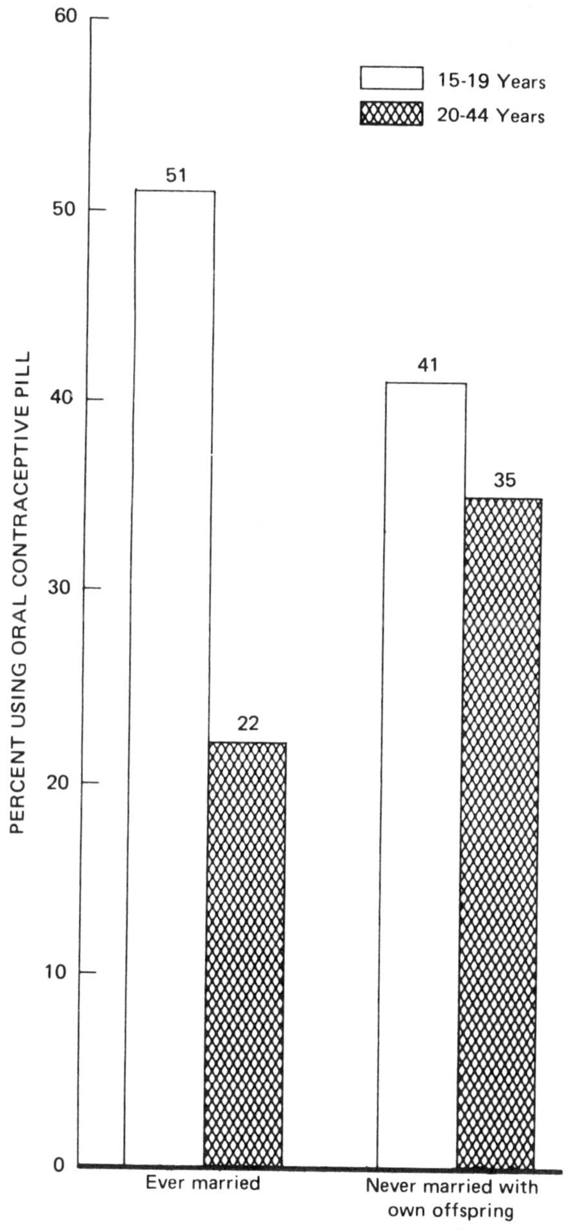

FIG. 5–4. Percentage of women 15–44 years of age using the oral contraceptive pill, by age and marital status: United States, 1976. *Source:* "Selected Demographic Characteristics of Teenage Wives and Mothers," Advance Data 61: 6, 1980. USDHHS, National Center for Health Statistics.

TABLE 5–9. Types of Oral Contraceptive Hormones Commercially Available

type of drug	hormones
Combination	Estrogen and a progestogen.
Sequential	Estrogen followed by a short course of both estrogen and progestogens.
Mini pills	Low dosage of progestogens.
Depot hormones	Either progestogens alone or a combination of progestogens and estrogens; parenterally administered.

a year have shown an increased frequency of elevated serum glucose levels. Discontinuation of the OCA for three months has generally been associated with GTT returning to normal (83). Other observations in healthy women, summarized in Table 5–10, indicate elevations in the fasting blood sugar, plasma insulin, and growth hormone levels. The risk of abnormal carbohydrate metabolism due to the effects of oral contraceptives significantly increases in women with histories of obesity, excessive weight gain, delivery of large infants, diabetes, or a family history of diabetes.

Some reports have associated the impaired glucose metabolism with changes in tryptophan metabolism, subclinical vitamin B_6 deficiency, or reduced blood levels of vitamin B_6. Increased excretion of tryptophan metabolites has been demonstrated in estrogen users (84); these urinary losses were reversed by giving large doses of vitamin B_6. Blood levels of pyridoxine are reported to be decreased in OCA users, but pyridoxine supplementation remains controversial. Since vitamin B_6 is involved in the metabolism of protein, animal studies need to be conducted to determine the effects of OCA and vitamin B_6 supplementation in conjunction with protein deficiencies. It could have a deleterious effect. The conversion of tryptophan to niacin may also be altered because pyridoxine is needed for the reaction. Some authors have suggested that this is the mechanism for the mental depression seen in many OCA users (85). Administration of large doses of vitamin B_6 has been shown to reverse this depression in some women.

Oral contraceptives may also affect protein metabolism, as shown in Table 5–7. Some of these changes appear to be the result of an estrogen effect on the endoplasmic reticulum of the liver that alters protein production, but clinical implications of the changes in protein metabolism have not been clearly established (86). Laboratory analyses for serum carrier proteins of thyroid hormones and certain minerals show altered levels (87), and studies using protein-deficient animals have raised concern because of the interaction of hormones, protein

TABLE 5–10. Alterations in Metabolism Related to Oral Contraceptive Agents (OCA)

biochemical test	effect[a]
CARBOHYDRATE	
Glucose tolerance test	Abnormal
Fasting blood sugar	Increased
Plasma insulin	Increased
Growth hormone	Increased
Urinary tryptophan metabolites	Increased
Plasma pyridoxine	Decreased
PROTEIN	
Serum proteins	Decreased
Serum coagulating factors	Increased
Serum amino acids	Decreased
Hepatic proteins	Increased
Other proteins	Increased
Carrier globulins	
LIPID	
Serum triglycerides	Increased
Serum cholesterol	Increased
Serum phospholipids	Increased
Serum lecithin	Increased
MINERAL	
Plasma calcium	Increased
Serum iron, TIBC	Increased
Plasma copper, ceruloplasmin	Increased
Plasma magnesium	Increased
Plasma zinc, erythrocyte zinc	Increased
VITAMIN	
Serum folacin	Decreased
Erythrocyte folacin	Decreased
Urinary metabolic excretion	Increased
Megaloblastic anemia	Rare
Serum vitamin B_{12}	Decreased
Erythrocyte riboflavin	Decreased
Vitamin B_6	Altered tryptophan metabolism
Plasma PLP	Decreased
	Depression
Leukocyte ascorbic acid	Decreased
Platelet ascorbic acid	Decreased
Urinary excretion (ascorbic acid)	Increased
Plasma vitamin A	Increased
Plasma carotene	Decreased
Liver vitamin A content (rats)	Decreased
Plasma vitamin E (rats)	Slightly decreased
Plasma vitamin K	Slightly decreased
Clotting factors	

[a] Effect does not necessarily indicate clinical significance.

deficiency, and liver injuries. Although interpretation of these studies may not have direct implications for humans, the questions they raise need careful study.

Table 5–10 indicates the changes in lipid metabolism noted in some OCA users. Although the risk of occlusive vascular disease has been demonstrated in a few women, the significance of the rise in serum lipids in normal, healthy women has not been established. The mechanism for such an association is not clear, but it would be a complex interrelationship of dietary fat intake, serum lipid levels, and dosages of estrogen (89). More study is needed to determine if the alteration in lipid metabolism is related to variations in dietary intakes of specific lipids.

The numerous interactions of OCA with vitamins are also summarized in Table 5–10. In some instances, studies showed greater vitamin depletion when OCA usage was associated with other factors such as alcoholism and other drugs, concurrent dietary deficiencies, malabsorption syndromes, and adverse socioeconomic conditions. When oral contraceptives are discontinued and pregnancy occurs without a sufficient time period for vitamin levels to readjust to normal values, the pregnant woman may need supplements to prevent clinical deficiencies. Vitamin imbalances have exerted teratogenic effects on the developing fetus in animal studies (90). Most of the reports noted the effects of OCA on minerals, including calcium, iron, copper, magnesium, and zinc (91, 92). But more definitive studies are needed to show the clinical significance, if any, of the metabolic changes.

OCA: RISKS. Risk of thromboembolic disease may be greater in OCA users because of increased levels of serum clotting factors. Increased risk in OCA users has been confirmed, but the exact mechanism is not clear. Factors associated with this risk include fat intake, clotting factors, and levels of estrogen dose. At present a relationship between nutrition, OCA, and thromboembolic disease is speculative, and further study is needed (88). Other factors, such as smoking, have an effect. The risk of developing hypertension is greater for OCA users, and the risk increases with duration of use. Nutritional relationships are only suggestive at this time, but excessive weight gain and alterations in carbohydrate and lipid metabolism have been implicated.

The side effects and metabolic complications observed in users are generally a function of the dosage levels, types of hormones, chemical properties, and/or duration of use. The side effects are more pronounced in women who are classified in the high-risk group, such as adolescents; lactating women; women with poor nutritional status; women with histories of diabetes, hypertension, and vascular diseases; and those with poor food intakes.

The metabolic and nutritional effects of intrauterine devices are probably due to the chemical composition of the devices. In some cases, the devices have caused increased menstrual blood losses, thus necessitating dietary iron supplementation (93).

To maintain optimum nutritional status for contraceptive users, the following steps are recommended:

1. *Assess the individual's current nutritional status (see Chapter 7).*
2. *Provide dietary counseling particularly to women in the high-risk group. See Table 5–11 for appropriate food sources.*

PREGNANCY

The placenta is a separate organ from the maternal body and the fetus or embryo. The organ develops in the uterus to sustain, support, and nourish the fetus; it is the site of hormone production, especially of estrogens and progesterone. The placenta begins developing in the first weeks of pregnancy. The maternal side of the placenta is part of the uterine mucosa. Villi merge into the chorion on the fetal side, and inside the chorion are vessels that connect with the vascular system coming from the fetus in the umbilical cord.

There is a linear increase in weight of the placenta with the weight gain of the fetus up to 3500 g of fetal weight usually about the 35th week of gestation. The normal cellular growth of the placenta proceeds through an orderly se-

TABLE 5–11. Food Items with Selected Nutrient Contents

nutrient	food group	food sources
Riboflavin	Bread	Enriched whole-grain breads and cereals.
	Vegetable/fruit	Green leafy vegetables.
	Milk	Milks and cheese.
	Meat	Organ meats and eggs.
Vitamin B_6	Bread	Whole-grain breads and cereals.
	Vegetable/fruit	Potatoes, sweet potatoes, cabbage, and other vegetables; bananas.
	Meat	Meat, liver, poultry, fish, eggs.
Folic acid	Bread	Whole-grain breads and cereals.
	Vegetable/fruit	Dark green leafy vegetables.
	Meat	Meats, organ meats, poultry, fish, eggs, nuts.
Ascorbic acid	Vegetable/fruit	Dark green leafy vegetables, green pepper, raw cabbage, citrus fruits and juices, tomatoes, melons.
Iron	Bread	Enriched or whole-grain breads and cereals.
	Vegetable/fruit	Dark green leafy vegetables, dried fruits (apricots, peaches, prunes, raisins).
	Meat	Meats, liver and most organ meats, egg yolk, shellfish, nuts, legumes.
Zinc	Bread	Wheat germ, whole grains.
	Meat	Meats, liver, other organ meats and fish.

quence of changes as gestation progresses. After the 36th week the placenta grows by an increase in the size of existing cells and not by further cell division.

Maternal malnutrition can reduce the transport of amino acids and certain sugars across the placenta. The cellular changes of severe prenatal food restriction are reflected in the placenta; placentas from malnourished mothers have fewer cells (94).

Nutrient transfer in the placenta employs mechanisms similar to those used in the gastrointestinal tract, such as diffusion and active transport, except that two completely separate blood supplies are maintained. Maternal and embryonic or fetal blood do not mix. Maternal and fetal capillaries are separated by layers of cells, and nutrient transfer to the fetus is a one-way process. The placenta exchanges oxygen between mother and fetus, and maternal hemoglobin affects the oxygen supply available to the fetus. Waste products are removed from fetal circulation and transferred to maternal circulation for disposal. The placenta is permeable to carbon dioxide, water, urea, creatinine, and uric acid.

development of embryo and fetus

Soon after conception (the fertilization of an ovum by a sperm), the cells begin to divide. The fertilized ovum moves slowly down the Fallopian tube to the uterus, floats freely in the uterus, and is implanted in the uterine wall. Fetal membranes begin forming—first is the amnion, which surrounds the embryo and attaches to the chorion that will ultimately carry nutrients to the embryo from the mother. Differentiation is occuring rapidly. At two weeks of age the embryo has attached to the uterine wall, developed membranes, and organized the germinal layers—the endoderm, the ectoderm, and the mesoderm. The gastrointestinal tract and its appendages and the respiratory organs will develop from the endoderm. From the mesoderm the gonads, kidneys, adrenal cortex, and abdominal cavity lining develop, and further differentiation produces the connective, vascular, skeletal, muscular, and hematopoietic tissues. The brain, nervous tissue, sense organs, and skin develop from the ectoderm. By three weeks, the embryo's heart appears and a vascular system develops. By the fourth week, circulation occurs within the embryo.

The embryo becomes a fetus by the end of the second month, with the heart beating in a regular rhythm. Skeletal muscles are present and arms and legs are forming. Viscera are formed and beginning to function. Organization is beginning for face, tongue, mouth, eyes, and ears. Fetal size is about an inch. By the third month, the fetus is about three inches in size and the neuromuscular system is developing rapidly. By this point the basic structure of the human is formed; the remainder of pregnancy is a period of further differentiation, growth, and refinement to prepare the fetus for life outside the uterus.

The influence of nutrients or drugs on the embryo or fetus is dependent on the period of development. Figure 5–5 shows these periods and major effects, as well as general embryonic and fetal development.

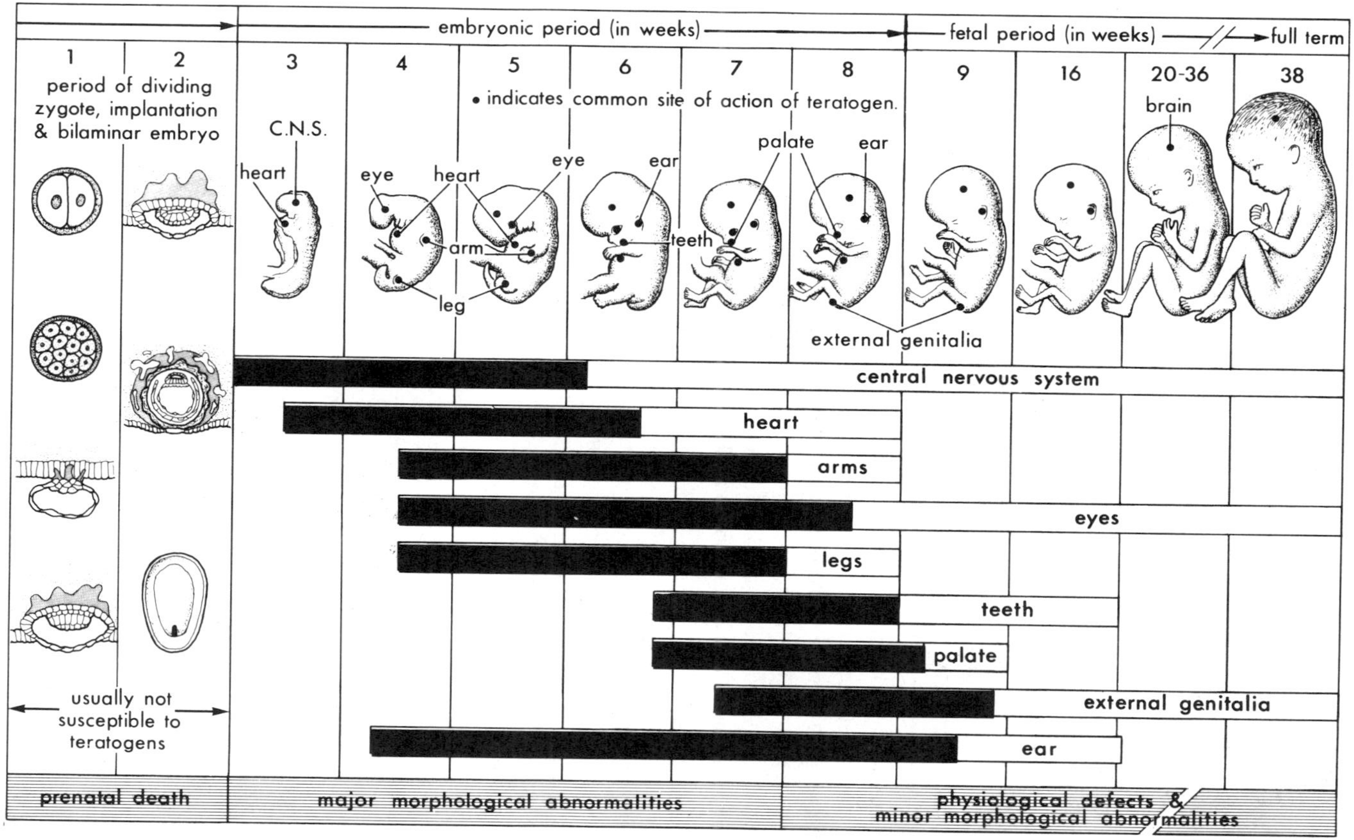

FIG. 5–5. Critical periods of development. Black bar denotes highly sensitive periods. *Source:* K. L. Moore, *The Developing Human,* 2nd ed. (Philadelphia: Saunders, 1977).

maternal nutrition and the outcome of pregnancy

Studies and reviews of previous work have directed new interest toward maternal nutrition and the outcome of pregnancy (59, 95, 96). Various researchers have shown that nutritional status of the mother prior to conception and during pregnancy directly influences the fetus (97, 98). Weight gain during pregnancy is thought by some to be the single most significant influence on weight of the fetus (99). In addition, animal studies have shown serious, even teratogenic effects of specific nutrient restriction as well as general restriction (Table 5-12). Observations on live births, information from autopsies of dead babies, and natural disasters such as wartime famines have provided evidence that the effects of maternal nutritional deprivation in humans and animals are similar.

Early reports by Burke showed a statistically significant relationship between diet during pregnancy and the condition of the infant at birth (100, 101). Mothers with poor diets produced smaller babies and had increased incidence of stillbirths. Retrospective studies on infants born to mothers during famines and sieges during World War II showed decreased birth rates, spontaneous abortions, premature births, stillborn infants, low birth weight infants, and increased neonatal death rates. In Holland, the women studied had previously been well nourished (prior to conception), and more food was available for their infants, allowing for weight gains and no consistent deleterious effects in adulthood (102, 103, 104). In Leningrad, the deprivation period was longer, and the quantity and quality of food available to women and infants was extremely inadequate (105). Stillbirths increased dramatically, as did premature births. Environmental conditions during these times were so stressful it is difficult to state that malnutrition alone was responsible for the outcome. However, poor nutrition is thought to have been a dominant factor.

TABLE 5-12. Results of Maternal Malnutrition in Animal Studies

general concepts
Malnutrition prior to mating and during gestation affects even second generation.
Decreased fertility—fewer pregnancies.
Fewer offspring per litter.
Smaller babies—lower birth rates.
Stunting of entire litter.
Increased maternal and fetal mortality.
Congenital anomalies.
Irreversible damage to learning capabilities.

As a result of these findings, dietary supplementation during pregnancy became popular. Supplementation has been shown to be advantageous for the poorly grown, as judged by short stature, and malnourished or underweight mothers (106, 107). Less conclusive benefits have been documented for those well nourished prior to and during pregnancy. Thomson demonstrated that the birth weight of infants increased as the energy value of the mother's diet increased, and also that the incidence of low birth weight babies decreased (57). However, when his data were corrected for prepregnancy nutritional status of the mothers, diet during pregnancy lost much of its significance. Tompkins and his associates also found that a low prepregnancy weight predisposed the mother to a premature birth regardless of weight gain during pregnancy (108). In addition, his data show a dramatic risk of prematurity associated with low prepregnancy weight interacting with a low weight gain during pregnancy. In Canada, Higgins has reported increased birth weights and decreased obstetrical complications for low-income women given energy and protein supplements (109). Weight gains during pregnancy were also increased. Similarly, in Guatemala birth weights increased and morbidity and mortality of newborns decreased when maternal diets were supplemented with protein and energy (107). Studies have shown positive relationships between maternal nutrition, prepregnancy weight, weight gain during pregnancy, and increased birth weights and decreased morbidity and mortality.

Based on these accumulated data, The American College of Obstetrics and Gynecology (ACOG) and The American Dietetic Association recently stated the nutritional risk factors of pregnancy (Table 5–13). The evidence for including as risk factors smoking, drugs, and alcohol has come from more recent studies (110, 111). Chronic alcoholics and drug addicts often have inappropriate food intakes. (See Chapter 10). Cigarette smoking inhibits normal gains in weight for the mother and retards fetal growth. The retardation of growth may be due to undernutrition, which is more common in smokers. Fetal and neonatal mortality are increased by cigarette smoking due to disorders of the placenta and congenital malformation of the fetus. The number of years the mother has smoked is important for some disorders. Even increasing the weight gain in pregnancy does not decrease the disorders, indicating that greater food intake by pregnant women may not protect their fetuses (59). We do not yet understand the mechanisms that relate smoking to the outcome of pregnancy.

The most appropriate amount of weight to gain during pregnancy has been the subject of much controversy. At one time it was considered appropriate to restrict weight gain during pregnancy (112), but now it is generally agreed that pregnancy is not the time for weight reduction, nor is restriction of gain appropriate. More important than the total amount of weight gained is the pattern or rate of gain. During the first weeks after conception, the fetus gains less than 1 g per day. After the first trimester, a steady gain in maternal weight should begin (see Figure 5–6). During the second and third trimesters, a gain of 400 g per week of 14 ounces is recommended. By the sixth month, the fetus is gaining only about 10 g per day; the rest of the gain is in maternal tissues. Almost half of the total

TABLE 5-13. Nutritional Risk Factors during Pregnancy

THE OBSTETRICAL PATIENT IS VERY LIKELY TO BE AT NUTRITIONAL RISK IF, AT THE ONSET OF PREGNANCY:

1. She is an adolescent (15 years of age or less).
2. She has had three or more pregnancies during the past two years.
3. She has a history of poor obstetric or fetal performance.
4. She is economically deprived (an income less than the poverty line or a recipient of local, state, or federal assistance, such as Medicaid or the USDA Food Programs, such as WIC).
5. She is a food faddist ingesting a bizarre or nutritionally restrictive diet.
6. She is a heavy smoker, drug addict, or alcoholic.
7. She has a therapeutic diet for chronic systemic disease.
8. She had a prepartum weight at her first prenatal visit of <85% or >120% of standard weight.

SHE IS VERY LIKELY TO BE AT NUTRITIONAL RISK IF, DURING PRENATAL CARE:

9. She has a low or deficient hemoglobin/hematocrit (low is Hb <11.0 gm, HCT <33; deficient is Hb <10.0 gm HCT <30).
10. She has inadequate weight gain (any weight loss during pregnancy or gain <2 pounds (1 kg) per month).
11. She has excessive weight gain during pregnancy (> 2 pounds (1 kg) per week).
12. She is planning to breast feed her infant.

SOURCE: *Task Force on Nutrition: Assessment of Maternal Nutrition.* Chicago: The American College of Obstetrics and Gynecologists and The American Dietetic Association, 1978. Reprinted by permission.

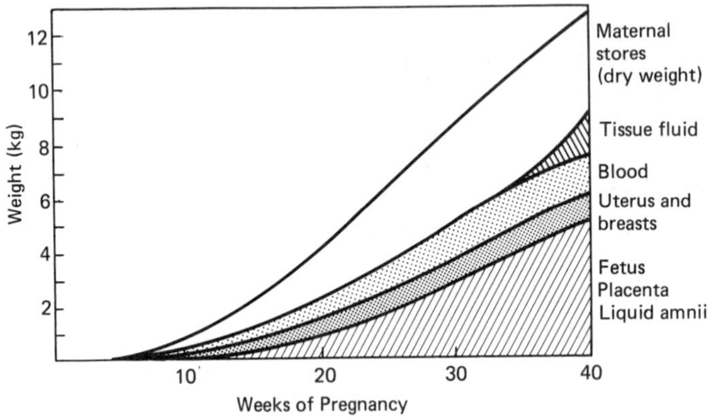

FIG. 5-6. The components of weight gain in normal pregnancy. *Source:* Committee on Maternal Nutrition, Food and Nutrition Board, National Research Council, National Academy of Sciences. Reprinted with permission of *Clinical Obstetrics.* J. B. Lippincott Co., 1953.

weight of the fetus is gained during the last two months of gestation, so that the six weeks just prior to delivery show the most rapid rate of gain for the fetus. This is why the fetus delivered prior to term is considerably underweight.

physiological changes

There is no opportunity for direct measurement of body composition during pregnancy, only indirect indices. Total body water increases progressively (113). The hormones produced during pregnancy affect the entire system, not just the reproductive process. Human chorionic gonadotropin (HCG) levels in serum increase rapidly in early pregnancy to peak values at 60 days, and then decline quickly to a low level. HCG provides hormonal support for the developing embryo or fetus until the placenta produces sufficient hormones and has little known effect on other tissues. Estrogens increase during pregnancy and have a generalized effect on the maternal body, the reproductive system, and carbohydrate and lipid metabolism. Progesterone levels increase during pregnancy and drop before labor begins.

Pulse rate increases, but blood pressure does not. In the kidney, the glomerular filtration rate increases by 50 percent, and renal plasma flow increases. The reabsorption of sodium is enhanced. The tone and mobility of the alimentary tract is reduced. Gastric emptying and intestinal transit times are prolonged. Gastric acid secretion is reduced.

Hemoglobin and hematrocrit values decline unless iron supplementation is provided for the mother. If blood volume expansion is great, the low values or physiologic anemia of pregnancy may persist even with iron supplementation. Urinary excretion of nitrogen is related to protein intake. There is a decrease in most plasma amino acids, and urinary excretion is increased. Total serum protein gradually decreases until the 28th week, when it levels off due to the fall in serum albumin. Some globulin fractions increase so the albumin falls more than the total protein. The serum values range from 2.30 to 3.74, compared to nonpregnant values of 3.42 to 4.63 g/100 ml.

Vitamin A and vitamin C status of the serum may reflect the nutritional status of the pregnant woman or hormonal adjustments to pregnancy. Serum folate levels fall during pregnancy due to increased demands for the vitamins and increased excretion.

increased nutrient recommendations

Table 5–14 shows the increased amounts of nutrients recommended during pregnancy compared to those for the nonpregnant adolescent and woman and the lactating woman. There are many reference sources for food and meal patterns and for the diet during pregnancy (120, 121). The most effective diets are based on modifications of the usual food habits of the individual woman.

TABLE 5-14. Recommended Dietary Allowances for Females

nutritive factors	women			adolescent, during pregnancy[a]	
	NON-PREGNANT (55 kg)	DURING PREGNANCY	DURING LACTATION	11–14 (YEARS)	15–18 (YEARS)
Energy, kcal	2100	2400	2600	2500	2400
Protein, gm	46	74	64	76	76
Calcium, mg	800	1200	1200	1600	1600
Phosphorus, mg	800	1200	1200	1600	1600
Magnesium, mg	300	450	450	450	450
Iodine, μg	150	175	200	175	175
Iron, mg	18	b	b	b	b
Zinc, mg	15	20	25	20	20
Vitamin A, μg R.E	800	1000	1200	1000	1000
Thiamin, mg	1.1	1.5	1.6	1.5	1.5
Riboflavin, mg	1.3	1.6	1.8	1.6	1.6
Niacin (equivalent) mg	14	16	19	17	16
Folacin, μg	400	800	500	800	0.8
Vitamin B_6, mg	2.0	2.6	2.5	2.4	2.6
Vitamin B_{12}, μg	3.0	4.0	4.0	4.0	4.0
Vitamin C, mg	60	80	100	70	80
Vitamin D, μg	7.5	12.5	12.5	15.0	15.0
Vitamin E, mg α T.E.	8.0	10.0	11.0	10.0	10.0

[a]Values are derived from RDA by adding the amounts recommended for the non-pregnant adolescent plus the increased amounts recommended for pregnancy.

[b]Statement on iron from RDA chart.

SOURCE: Ninth Revised Edition (1980) with the permission of the National Academy of Sciences, Washington, D.C.

CALORIES. The increase in recommended energy intake is not large—300 kcal/day—but increases in energy needs really parallel more closely the increases in fetal weight and maternal tissues. Therefore, the increase in calories should be greater in the third trimester than in the first. In addition, the energy cost of physical activity will be greater in the third trimester. The best monitor of adequacy of energy intake is the rate or pattern of maternal weight gain.

PROTEIN. Protein requirements are related to adequate energy intake. Calloway and associates showed a linear relationship between energy intake and nitrogen balance in pregnant women and concluded that part of the protein ingested is used for energy (114, 115, 116). The RDA for protein is 76 g per day during pregnancy, or approximately 1.3 g/kg/day and assumes mixed animal and vegetable sources. This is an increase of 30 g per day or 0.5 g per kg over the nonpregnant recommendation. Some authorities have suggested that only 10 g additional protein would be needed if utilization was complete. The need for adequate amounts of essential amino acids and therefore protein of high quality is stressed. The exact amount of additional protein needed remains controversial, as shown by the changes in RDA in 1968 (10 g increase) and in 1974 and 1980 (30 g increase).

MINERALS. Recommendations for sodium consumption have also been the subject of controversy. In the past, physicians recommended sodium restriction during pregnancy to reduce edema and weight gain, and to prevent toxemia. Recent studies have shown that some fluid retention is physiological and that some toxemias respond to increased sodium intake (117, 118). In addition, it seems inappropriate to restrict dietary sodium when the body is recycling and conserving sodium (119).

Maternal serum calcium falls during pregnancy even when the dietary intake is adequate. The increase recommended for pregnancy is 400 mg per day. Calcification of the fetal skeleton begins at about 8 weeks and by 40 weeks the fetus will have accrued approximately 30 g of calcium. Dietary intake must be adequate to replenish maternal stores and to meet fetal needs.

The recommended allowance for iron is more than 18 mg, and difficult to achieve in dietary intake alone. The amount of iron needed for pregnancy is increased because of the dramatic increases in maternal blood volume and erythrocytes and because of the need to supply the fetus and placenta with iron. Total erythrocyte increase will be 30 percent above the nonpregnant count if adequate iron is taken. The fetus will get the iron needed from maternal stores if dietary intakes are not adequate. This is shown by the fact that hematocrits of newborns fall within the normal range regardless of amount of maternal dietary iron intakes. However, their iron stores may be less than adequate, and they will need iron supplementation early to prevent anemia.

During the last half of pregnancy, the diet of the mother should be supplemented with iron, as it is nearly impossible for her to get adequate iron from food. The normal woman (with adequate stores at onset) needs approximately 800 mg additional iron during pregnancy. This would indicate a need to absorb 4 to 5 mg daily during the latter part of the pregnancy. Daily supplementation with elemental iron of 30 to 60 mg is recommended for all pregnant women, with the exception of those who have sickle cell disease. If iron deficiency occurs, a therapeutic dose of 120 mg elemental iron daily may be given.

Zinc, copper, and iodine need to be increased during pregnancy because of the needs of the fetus and decreased maternal plasma levels. Iodine needs are readily met by the use of iodized salt and other foods. Sandstead has estimated that the pregnant woman must ingest 750 μg of zinc daily during the latter two-thirds of pregnancy to meet needs of the fetus (49). Most women will consume adequate amounts of zinc if animal products are eaten. Those who consume clay, dirt (a condition called *pica*), or large amounts of fiber may need to be evaluated more closely in that absorption of zinc and other minerals as well as total nutrients may be decreased.

VITAMINS. Only moderate increases are needed for the fat-soluble vitamins, A and D. Large doses can be detrimental to the developing fetus. During pregnancy, the maternal blood levels of water-soluble vitamins fall. Fetal blood levels are 50 to 100 percent above the maternal levels. Thiamin, riboflavin, and niacin requirements are positively correlated to energy needs.

Folacin is needed for rapidly growing tissues and results in an increased folate requirement during pregnancy. Folate deficiency anemia, in fact, was first described in a pregnant woman (59). Pregnancy is still the most common cause of this type of anemia. The RDA is therefore doubled, from 400 to 800 μg. Intake of Vitamin B_6 needs to be increased with greater protein intake. Although maternal blood levels drop during pregnancy, this is probably a physiological adjustment, so the allowance is increased only from 2 to 2.5 mg.

Supplementation with vitamins during pregnancy is not necessary unless the food intake is inadequate. Even though all vitamin recommendations are increased during pregnancy, intake is usually adequate if protein and calories are adequate. Supplements are recommended only if vitamin deficiencies are actually demonstrated, and these are rare. A balanced diet is considered the best means of obtaining adequate vitamins.

CHRONIC DISEASES OF ADULTS

The role of nutrition in the prevention of disease and the promotion of health is important for adults. Although life expectancy has increased in terms of years, primarily because of better medical care and improved sanitation and nutrition, mortality from major chronic diseases has increased more than 250 percent (122). Treatment of these diseases had top priority in the 1950s and 1960s. During the 1970s information began to accumulate suggesting a strong relationship, if not cause and effect, between certain aspects of life styles and prevention of these diseases. Some major risk factors have now been identified (123), and we now have the scientific evidence to formulate recommendations for improved health.

Violence and accidents are the leading causes of death in early adulthood, followed by chronic illnesses in later adult years (See Figure 1–1). At each stage of the life cycle, different steps can be taken to prevent disease and promote health. Early eating habits and patterns of exercise, for example, may predispose a person to health problems in later life. There are many health problems that can destroy a person's life without causing death. And life expectancy for a man aged 45 is only five years greater than it was in 1900. In 1970, the death rate for 25- to 64-year-olds was higher than it had been in 1960. More than one-third of these deaths in adults are due to cardiovascular diseases, primarily coronary artery (heart) disease and strokes.

Heart disease not only causes deaths; it is the leading cause of permanent disability claims among workers under 65 and responsible for more days of hospitalization than any other single disorder. Strokes also produce significant disability; approximately 10 percent of nursing home admissions for persons under 65 years of age are the result of strokes. Both diseases are related to the process of atherosclerosis, in which arteries become narrowed by fatty deposits. The walls of the affected arteries thicken with plaque which usually consists of a core of fats and cholesterol. This thickening progressively narrows the artery, impairing circulation by reducing the amount of oxygen-carrying blood going to all parts of the body. Heart attacks occur when the coronary artery is blocked, shutting off blood flow to an area of heart muscle. A stroke occurs when the blood and oxygen supply to the brain is significantly reduced by these clogged arteries.

A strong association has been established between premature heart disease and elevated serum cholesterol levels. Heart attacks are five times as frequent in both men and women who have serum cholesterol levels above 265 mg/dl as among those with levels less than 220 mg/dl (122). Cholesterol carrier substances in the blood, called lipoproteins, have recently been found to play a role in atherosclerotic disease. Low-density lipoproteins (LDL) appear to accelerate cholesterol deposits in artery walls; high-density lipoproteins (HDL) may even protect against plaque formation. Exercise and dietary modification may increase the ratio of HDL to LDL, thereby offering possible protection from heart disease. Moderate excesses of weight may be associated with increased levels of LDL in the blood and with high blood pressure and high blood sugar. The lack of physical activity that may be associated with excess weight has not been determined to be an independent cause of premature heart disease or stroke. Other risks for adults are stress, work, and genetic predisposition. Some drugs, such as oral contraceptives, may increase risks for these diseases.

The second most common disease in adults is cancer. Risk factors for cancer include consumption of alcohol and some diet-related components. Higher rates of head, neck, and liver cancers occur among people consuming large amounts of alcohol. Contaminants in the alcohol from the manufacturing process may prove to be carcinogenic rather than the alcohol itself. Some methods of food preparation, such as pickling, preserving, and charcoal broiling, have been proposed as producing certain carcinogens. Much of our information on dietary causes of cancer comes from animal studies and may have limited relevance to humans. Some data, however, come from comparison of human cancer rates in other cultures and among migrants from one country to another who exhibit distinctive food intake behavior. But the precise relationship between diet and various cancers is not yet known.

Other problems of adults with some relationship to nutrition are alcohol and drug abuse, mental illness, and periodontal disease (see Chapters 10 and

11). Many adults with mental illness accentuate the debilitating effects of the disease by significantly limiting total food intake or narrowing food choices to the point of nutrient deficiency. In addition, medications taken to alleviate the symptoms of illness may decrease interest in food and eating, as well as interact with foods to make some nutrients unavailable.

SUMMARY

The adult period extends from approximately 19 to 50 years. Individual psychological factors often result in a variety of activity, work, and eating patterns. The adult phase is the most stable physiologically. Nutritional requirements for adults are based on the observation of intakes by healthy adults, studies conducted with adults, rates of recovery from deficiency diseases, and assumptions made from animal studies. There are requirements for energy based on weight and activity and for protein and selected vitamins and minerals. Pregnancy increases the requirements for some nutrients much more than others and causes a number of physiological changes that affect nutritional status.

The higher incidence of chronic diseases in adults may also be related to nutritional status, although more research is needed. Some risk factors, such as obesity, high serum cholesterol, high blood pressure, and diabetes, have been identified.

references

1. CASSEL, J. "Social and Cultural Implications of Food and Food Habits." *American Journal of Public Health* 47 (1957): 732.
2. MILLS, E. R. "Psychological Aspects of Food Habits." *Journal of Nutrition Education* 9 (1977): 67.
3. CASPER, B. A., and L. M. WAKEFIELD, "Food Choices of Women: Personal, Attitudinal, and Motivational Factors." *Journal of the American Dietetic Association* 69 (1976): 152.
4. GRANDE, F., and A. KEYS. "Body Weight, Body Composition and Calorie Status." In *Modern Nutrition in Health and Disease,* 6th ed., Eds. R. S. Goodhart and M. E. Shils. Philadelphia: Lea and Febiger, 1981.
5. MCCAY, C. M., M. F. CROWELL, and L. A. MAYNARD. "The Effects of Retarded Growth upon the Length of Lifespan and upon the Ultimate Baby Size." *Journal of Nutrition* 10 (1935): 63.
6. ROSS, N. H. "Nutrition and Longevity in Experimental Animals." In *Nutrition and Aging,* ed. M. Winick. New York: Wiley, 1976.
7. GARROW, J. S. *Energy Balance and Obesity in Man,* 2nd ed. New York: Elsevier/North-Holland Biomedical Press, 1978.
8. FORBES, G. B., and J. D. REINA. "Adult Lean Body Mass Declines with Age: Some Longitudinal Observations." *Metabolism* 19 (1970): 653.
9. OHLSON, M. A., and L. J. HARPER. "Longitudinal Studies of Food Intake and Weight of Women from Ages 18 to 56." *Journal of the American Dietetic Association* 69 (1976): 629.
10. "Symposium on Role of Dietary Fiber in Health. Proceedings of a Workshop Sponsored by the Nutrition Coordinating Commitee, NIH." *American Journal of Clinical Nutrition* 31 (supp.) (1978): S1.
11. YOUNG, V. R., W. P. STEFFEE, P. B. PENCHARZ, J. C. WINTERER, and N. S. SCRIMSHAW. "Total Human Body Protein Requirements at Various Ages." *Nature* 253 (1975): 192.
12. SAUBERLICH, H. E., R. E. HODGES, D. C. WALLACE, H. KOLDER, J. E. CANHAM, J. HOOD, N. RAICA, JR., and L. K. LOWRY. "Vitamin A Metabolism and Requirements in the Human Studied with the Use of Labelled Retinol." *Vitamins and Hormones* 32 (1974): 251.
13. Food and Nutrition Board, National Research Council. *Recommended Dietary Allowances, 9th ed.* Washington, D. C.: National Academy of Sciences, 1980.
14. RAICA, N., JR., J. SCOTT, L. K. LOWRY, and H. E. SAUBERLICH. "Vitamin A Concentra-

tion in Human Tissues Collected from Five areas in the United States." *American Journal of Clinical Nutrition* 25 (1972): 291.

15. MITCHELL, G. V., M. YOUNG, and C. R. SEWARD. "Vitamin A and Carotene Levels of a Selected Population in Metropolitan Washington, D. C." *American Journal of Clinical Nutrition* 26 (1973): 992.
16. LOOMIS, W. F. "Skin-Pigment Regulation of Vitamin D Biosynthesis in Man." *Science* 157 (1967): 501.
17. BINDER, H. J., D. C. HERTIG., V. HURST, S. C. FINCH, and H. M. SPIRO. "Tocopherol Deficiency in Man." *New England Journal of Medicine* 273 (1965): 1289.
18. WITTING, L. A., and L. LEE. "Dietary Levels of Vitamin E and Polyunsaturated Fatty Acids and Plasma Vitamin E." *American Journal of Clinical Nutrition* 28 (1975): 571.
19. BIERI, J. G., and R. P. EVARTS. "Tocopherols and Fatty Acids in American Diets. The Recommended Allowance for Vitamin E." *Journal of the American Dietetic Association* 62 (1973): 147.
20. DAM, H. "Interrelations between Vitamin E and Polyunsaturated Fatty Acids in Animals." *Vitamins and Hormones* 20 (1962): 527.
21. HODGES, R. E., J. HOOD, J. E. CANHAM, H. E. SAUBERLICH, and E. M. BAKER. "Clinical Manifestations of Ascorbic Acid Deficiency in Man." *American Journal of Clinical Nutrition* 24 (1971): 432.
22. LEEVY, C. M., and H. BAKER. "Vitamins and Alcoholism." *American Journal of Clinical Nutrition* 21 (1968): 1325.
23. ROSKIN, N. H., and R. A. FISHMAN. "Neurologic Disorders in Renal Failure." *New England Journal of Medicine* 294 (1976): 204.
24. NADEL, A. M., and P. C. BURGER. "Wernicke Encephalopathy Following Prolonged Intravenous Therapy." *Journal of the American Medical Association* 235 (1976): 2403.
25. VIMOKESANT, S. L., S. NAKORNCHI, S. DHANAMITTA, and D. M. HILKER. "Effect of Tea Consumption on Thiamin Status in Man." *Nutrition Reports International* 9 (1974): 371.
26. PLATT, S. "Thiamin Deficiency in Human Beriberi and in Wernicke's Encephalopathy." in *Thiamin Deficiency,* eds. G. E. W. Wolstenholme and M. O'Connor. Boston: Little, Brown, 1967.
27. SAUBERLICH, H. E., Y. F. HERMAN, and C. O. STEVENS. "Thiamin Requirement of the Adult Human." *American Journal of Clinical Nutrition* 23 (1970): 671.
28. CONSOLAZIO, C. F., H. C. JOHNSON, H. J. KRZYWICKI, T. A. DAVIS, and R. A. BARNHORT. "Thiamin, Riboflavin, and Pyridoxine Excretion during Acute Starvation and Calorie Restriction." *American Journal of Clinical Nutrition* 24 (1971): 1060.
29. SEBRELL, W. H., JR., and R. E. BUTLER. *Riboflavin Deficiency in Man: Preliminary Note.* U. S. Public Health Report 53, 1938.
30. HORWITT, M. K., O. W. HILLS, C. C. HARVEY, E. LIEBERT, and D. L. STEINBERG. "Effects of Dietary Depletion of Riboflavin." *Journal of Nutrition* 39 (1949): 357.
31. DARBY, W. J., K. W. MCNUTT, and F. N. TODHUNTER. "Niacin." *Nutrition Reviews* 33 (1975): 289.

32. HORWITT, M. K., C. C. HARVEY, W. S. ROTHWELL, J. L. CUTLER, and D. HAFFRON. "Tryptophan-niacin Relationships in Man." *Journal of Nutrition* 60 (supp. 1) (1956): 1.

33. GOLDSMITH, G. A., O. N. MILLER, and W. G. UNGLAUB. "Efficiency of Tryptophan as a Niacin Precursor in Man." *Journal of Nutrition* 73 (1961): 172.

34. VIVIAN, V. M. "Relationship between Tryptophan-Niacin Metabolism and Change in Nitrogen Balance." *Journal of Nutrition* 82 (1964): 395.

35. HAWKINS, W. W., and J. BARSKY. "An Experiment on Human Vitamin B_6 Deprivation." *Science* 108 (1948): 284.

36. CANHAM, J. E., W. T. NUNES, and E. W. EBERLIN. "Electroencephalographic and Central Nervous System Manifestations of B_6 Deficiency and Induced B_6 Dependency in Normal Human Adults." In *Proceedings VI International Congress on Nutrition.* Edinburgh: E. and S. Livingstone, Ltd., 1964.

37. SAUBERLICH. H. E. "Human Requirements for Vitamin B_6." *Vitamins and Hormones* 22 (1964): 807.

38. LINKSWILER, H. M. "Vitamin B_6 Requirement of Men." In *Human Vitamin B_6 Requirements.* Washington, D. C.: National Academy of Sciences, 1978.

39. HERBERT, V., N. CUNEEN, L. JASKIELL, and C. KAPFF. "Minimal Daily Adult Folate Requirement." *Archives of Internal Medicine* 110 (1962): 649.

40. WILKINSON, R. "Absorption of Calcium, Phosphorus and Magnesium." In *Calcium, Phosphate and Magnesium Metabolism,* ed. B. E. C. Nordin. New York: Churchill Livingstone, 1976.

41. LOTZ, M., E. ZISMAN, and F. C. BARTTER. "Evidence for a Phosphorus Depletion Syndrome in Man." *New England Journal of Medicine* 278 (1968): 409.

42. GOODMAN, L. S., and A. Z. GILMAN. *The Pharmacological Basis of Therapeutics,* 3rd ed. New York: MacMillan, 1965.

43. WACKER, W. E. C., and A. F. PARISI. "Magnesium Metabolism." *New England Journal of Medicine* 278 (1968): 658.

44. HALLBERG, L., A. M. HOGDAHL, L. MILSSON, and G. RYBO. "Menstrual Blood Loss—A Population Study. Variation at Different Ages and Attempts to Define Normality." *Acta Obstetricia et Gynecologica Scandinavia* 45 (1966): 320.

45. GREEN, R., R. W. CHARLTON, H. SEFTEL, T. H. BOTHWELL, F. MAYET, E. B. ADAMS, C. A. FINCH, and M. LAYRISSE. "Body Iron Excretion in Man: A Collaborative Study." *American Journal of Medicine* 45 (1968): 336.

46. LAYRISSE, M., C. MARTINEZ-TORRES, and M. ROCHE. "Effects of Interaction of Various Foods on Iron Absorption." *American Journal of Clinical Nutrition* 21 (1968): 1175.

47. MONSEN, E. R., L. HOLLENBERG, M. LAYRISSE, D. M. HEGSTED, J. D. COOK, W. MERTZ, and C. A. FINCH. "Estimation of Available Dietary Iron." *American Journal of Clinical Nutrition* 31 (1978): 134.

48. SPENCER, H., D. OSIS, L. KREMER, and C. NORRIS. "Intake, Excretion, and Retention of Zinc in Man." In *Trace Elements in Human Health and Disease,* ed. A. S. Prasad. New York: Academic Press, 1976.

49. SANDSTEAD, H. H. "Zinc Nutrition in the United States." *American Journal of Clinical Nutrition* 26 (1973): 1251.

50. Food and Nutrition Board, National Research Council. *Iodine Nutriture in the United States.* Washington, D. C.: National Academy of Sciences, 1970.

51. ROBINSON, M. F., J. M. MCKENZIE, C. D. THOMSON, and A. L. VAN RIJ. "Metabolic Balance of Zinc, Copper, Cadmium, Iron, Molybdenum and Selenium in Young New Zealand Women." *British Journal of Nutrition* 30 (1973): 195.

52. SANDSTEAD, H. H., L. M. KLEVAY, R. A. JACOB, J. M. MUNOZ, G. M. LOGAN, JR., J. REEK, R. R. DINTZIS, G. E. INGLETT, and W. C. SHUEY. "Effect of Dietary Fiber and Protein Level on Mineral Element Metabolism." *Dietary Fibers: Chemistry and Nutrition,* eds. G. E. Inglett and S. I. Falkehag. New York: Academic Press, 1979.

53. KLEVAY, L. M., S. J. REEK, R. A. JACOB, G. M. LOGAN, JR., J. M. MUNOZ, and H. H. SANDSTEAD. "The Human Requirement for Copper." *American Journal of Clinical Nutrition* 33 (1980): 45.

54. MCCARRISON, R. "Nutritional Needs in Pregnancy." *British Medical Journal* 2 (1937): 256.

55. MELLANBY, E. "Nutrition and Childbearing." *Lancet* 2 (1933): 1131.

56. THOMSON, A. M. "Maternal Stature and Reproductive Efficiency." *Eugenic Review* 51 (1959): 157.

57. THOMSON, A. M., and W. Z. BILLEWIEZ. "Nutritional Status, Maternal Physique and Reproductive Efficiency." *Proceedings of the Nutrition Society* 22 (1963): 55.

58. VALADIAN, I., C. BERKEY, and R. B. REED. "Adolescent Nutrition as It Relates to Cardiovascular Disease and Reproductive Capacity Later in Life." *Nutrition Reviews* 39 (1981): 107.

59. "Workshop on Nutrition of the Child: Maternal Nutritional Status and Fetal Outcome." *American Journal of Clinical Nutrition* 34 (1981): 653–817.

60. FRISCH, R. E., and J. W. MCARTHUR. "Menstrual Cycles: Fatness as a Determinant of Minimum Weight for Height Necessary for Their Maintenance or Onset." *Science* 185 (1974): 949.

61. FRISCH, R. E., "Demographic Implications of the Biological Determinants of Female Fecundity." *Social Studies of Biology* 22 (1975): 17.

62. JOHNSTON, F. E., R. M. MALINA, and M. A. GALBRAITH. "Height, Weight and Age at Menarche and the 'Critical Weight' Hypothesis." *Science* 174 (1971): 1148.

63. STEIN, Z., and M. SUSSER. "Fertility, Fecundity, Famine: Food Rations in the Dutch Famine 1944–45 Have a Causal Relationship to Fertility and Probably Fecundity." *Human Biology* 47 (1975): 131.

64. TANNER, J. M. "Growth and Maturation during Adolescence." *Nutrition Reviews* 39 (1981): 43.

65. Task Force on Nutrition, The American College of Obstetricians and Gynecologists and The American Dietetic Association. *Assessment of Maternal Nutrition.* 1978.

66. Committee on Adolescence, The Academy of Pediatrics. "Statement on Teenage Pregnancy." *Pediatrics* 63 (1979): 5.

67. KULIN, J. E., M. M. GRUMBACK, and S. L. KAPLAN. "Gonadalhypothalamic Interaction

in Prepubertal and Pubertal Man: Effect of Clomiphene Citrate on Urinary Follicle-Stimulating Hormone and Luteinizing Hormone and Testosterone." *Pediatric Research* 6 (1972): 162.

68. MILLEN, J. W. *The Nutritional Basis of Reproduction.* Springfield, Ill.: Charles C Thomas, 1962.

69. RICHARDSON, S. A. "The Background Histories of School Children Severely Malnourished in Infancy." *Advances in Pediatrics* 21 (1975): 167.

70. PRASAD, A. S., A. MIALE, F. FACID, H. H. SANDSTEAD, and W. J. DARBY. "Biochemical Studies on Dwarfism, Hypogonadism and Anemia." *Archives of Internal Medicine* 111 (1963): 407.

71. RONAGHY, H. A., J. G. REINHOLD, M. MAHLOUDJI, P. GHAVAMI, M. R. SPIVEY FOX, and J. A. HALSTEAD. "Zinc Supplementation of Malnourished Schoolboys in Iran: Increased Growth and Other Effects." *American Journal of Clinical Nutrition* 27 (1974): 112.

72. MOUSTGAARD, J. "Nutritive Influences on Reproduction." In *Reproduction in Domestic Animals,* 2nd ed., eds. H. H. Cole and P. T. Cupps. New York: Academic Press, 1969.

73. KLATSKIN, G., W. T. SALTER, and F. D. HUMM. "Gynecomastia due to Malnutrition: Clinical Studies." *American Journal of Medical Science* 213 (1947): 19.

74. KEYS, A., J. BROZEK, A. HENSCHEL, O. MICKELSEN, and H. L. TAYLOR. "Growth and Development." In *The Biology of Human Starvation,* vol. 2. Minneapolis: University of Minneapolis Press, 1950.

75. MANN, T. "Biochemical Aspects of Sperm Maturation and Survival." In *Male Fertility and Sterility,* vol. 5. London: Academic Press, 1975.

76. RAMSEY, D. K. "Seven Years in Captivity." *Nutrition Today* 8 (1973): 14.

77. *Population Report: Effects of Child Bearing on Maternal Health.* Series J, No. 8, Department of Medicine and Public Affairs. Washington, D. C.: George Washington University Medical Center, 1975.

78. WRAY, J. D. "Population Pressures on Families: Family Size and Child Spacing." *Reports on Population and Family Planning* 9 (1971): 404.

79. *Population Report: Oral Contraceptives—Fifty Million Users.* Series A., No. 1, Department of Medicine and Public Affairs. Washington, D. C.: George Washington University Medical Center, 1974.

80. SAUNDERS, F. J. "Endocrine properties and mechanism of action of oral contraceptives." *Federation Proceedings* 29 (1970): 1211.

81. ROE, D. A. *Drug-induced Nutritional Deficiencies.* Westport, Conn.: AVI Publishing, 1976.

82. THEUER, R. C. "Effect of Oral Contraceptive Agents on Vitamin and Mineral Needs: A Review." *Journal of Reproductive Medicine* 8 (1972): 13.

83. PRASAD, A. S., K. S. MOGHISSI, K. Y. LEI, D. OBERLEAS, and J. C. STRYKER. "Effects of Oral Contraceptives on Micronutrients and Changes in Trace Elements due to Pregnancy." In *Nutritional Impacts on Women Throughout Life with Emphasis on Reproduction,* eds. K. S. Moghissi and T. N. Evans. Hagerstown, Md.: Harper and Row Publishers, 1977.

84. Rose, D. P. "The Influence of Estrogens on Tryptophan Metabolism in Man." *Clinical Science* 31 (1966): 265.

85. Adams, P. W., D. P. Rose, J. Folkard, V. Wynn, M. Sneed, and R. Strong. "Effects of Pyridoxine Hydrochloride (Vitamin B_6) upon Depression Associated with Oral Contraception." *Lancet* 1 (1973): 897.

86. Musa, B. V., R. P. Doe, and V. S. Seal. "Serum Protein Alterations Produced in Women Taking Synthetic Estrogens." *Journal of Clinical Endocrinology* 27 (1967): 1463.

87. Miale, J. B., and J. W. Kent. "The Effects of Oral Contraceptives on the Results of Laboratory Tests." *American Journal of Obstetrics and Gynecology* 120 (1974): 264.

88. Mann, J. I., M. P. Vessey, M. Thorogood, and R. Doll. "Myocardial Infarction in Young Women with Special Reference to Oral Contraceptive Practice." *British Medical Journal* 2 (1975): 241.

89. Hudiburgh, N. K., and A. N. Milner. "Influence of Oral Contraceptives on Ascorbic Acid and Triglyceride Status." *Journal of the American Dietetic Association* 75 (1979): 19.

90. Runner, M., and J. Miller. "Congenital Deformity in the Mouse as a Consequence of Fasting." *Anatomical Record* 124 (1956): 437.

91. Margen, S., and J. C. King. "Effects of Oral Contraceptive Agents on the Metabolism of Some Trace Minerals." *American Journal of Clinical Nutrition* 28 (1975): 392.

92. Simpson, G. R., and E. Dale. "Serum Levels of Phosphorus, Magnesium, and Calcium in Women Utilizing Combination Oral or Long-acting Injectable Progestational Contraceptives." *Fertility and Sterility* 23 (1972): 326.

93. Larsson, B., L. Hamberger, and G. Rybo. "Influence of Copper Intrauterine Contraceptive Devices (Cu-7 IUD) on the Menstrual Blood Loss." *Acta Obstetricia et Gynecologica Scandinavia* 54 (1975): 315.

94. Winick, M. *Nutrition: Pre- and Postnatal Development.* New York: Plenum Press, 1979.

95. Committee on Maternal Nutrition, Food and Nutrition Board, National Research Council, *Maternal Nutrition and the Course of Pregnancy.* Washington, D. C.: National Academy of Sciences, 1970.

96. Pitkin, R. M., H. A. Kaminetzky, M. Newton, and J. A. Pritchard. "Maternal Nutrition: A Selective Review of Clinical Topics." *Obstetrics and Gynecology* 40 (1972): 773.

97. Gold, E. M. "Interconceptional Nutrition." *Journal of the American Dietetic Association* 35 (1969): 27.

98. Stearns, G. "Nutritional State of the Mother prior to Conception." *Journal of the American Medical Association* 168 (1958): 1655.

99. Simpson, J. W., R. W. Lawless, and A. C. Mitchell. "Responsibility of the Obstetrician to the Fetus. II. Influence of Prepregnancy Weight and Pregnancy Weight Gain on Birth Weight." *Obstetrics and Gynecology* 45 (1975): 481.

100. Burke, B. S., V. A. Beal, S. B. Kirkwood, and H. C. Stuart. "The Influence of Nutrition during Pregnancy upon the Condition of the Infant at Birth." *Journal of Nutrition* 25 (1943): 569.

101. Burke, B. S., V. V. Harding, and H. C. Stuart. "Nutrition Studies during Pregnancy. IV. Relation of Protein Content of Mother's Diet during Pregnancy to Birth Length, Birth Weight and Condition of Infant at Birth." *Journal of Pediatrics* 23 (1943): 506.

102. Singer, J. E., M. Westphal, and K. Niswander. "Relationship of Weight Gain during Pregnancy to Birth Weight and Infant Growth and Development in First Year of Life. A Report from the Collaborative Study of Cerebral Palsy." *Obstetrics and Gynecology* 31 (1968): 417.

103. Smith, C. A. "Effects of Maternal Undernutrition upon Newborn Infants in Holland." *Journal of Pediatrics* 30 (1947): 229.

104. Stein, Z., M. Susser, G. Saenger, and F. Marolla. *Famine and Human Development: The Dutch Hunger Winter of 1944–1945.* New York: Oxford University Press, 1975.

105. Antonov, A. "Children Born during the Siege of Leningrad." *Journal of Pediatrics* 30 (1947): 250.

106. Gopalan, C., and A. N. Naidu. "Nutrition and Fertility." *Lancet* 2 (1972): 1077.

107. Habicht, J. P., C. Yarbrough, A. Lechtig, and R. E. Klein. "Relation of Maternal Supplementary Feeding during Pregnancy to Birth Weight and Other Socio-biological Factors." In *Nutrition and Fetal Development,* ed. M. Winick. New York: Wiley, 1974.

108. Tompkins, W. T., D. G. Wiehl, and R. Mitchell. "The Underweight Patient as an Increased Obstetric Hazard." *American Journal of Obstetrics and Gynecology* 69 (1955): 114.

109. Higgins, A. C. "Nutritional Status and the Outcome of Pregnancy." *Journal of the Canadian Dietetic Association* 37 (1976): 17.

110. Miller, H. C., and K. Hassanein. "Maternal Smoking and Fetal Growth of Full Term Infants." *Pediatric Research* 8 (1974): 960.

111. Roe, D. A. *Alcohol and the Diet.* Westport, Conn.: AVI Publishing, 1979.

112. Editorial. "Eclampsia Rare on War Diet in Germany." *Journal of the American Medical Association* 68 (1917): 732.

113. National Research Council. *Laboratory Indices of Nutritional Status in Pregnancy. Washington, D. C.: National Academy of Sciences, 1978.*

114. Calloway, D. H. "Nitrogen Balance during Pregnancy." In *Nutrition and Fetal Development, ed., M. Winick. New York: Wiley, 1974.*

115. King, J. C., D. H. Calloway, and S. Margen. "Nitrogen Nutrition, Total Body 40K and Weight Gain in Teenage Pregnant Girls." *Journal of Nutrition* 103 (1973): 772.

116. King, J. "Protein Metabolism during Pregnancy." *Clinical Perinatalogy* 2 (1975): 243.

117. Pike, R., and H. Smiciklas. "A Reappraisal of Sodium Restriction during Pregnancy." *International Journal of Gynecology and Obstetrics* 10 (1972): 1.

118. Robinson, M. "Salt in Pregnancy." *Lancet* 1 (1958): 178.

119. Sims, E., and K. Krantz. "Serial Studies of Renal Function during Pregnancy and the Puerperium in Normal Women." *Journal of Clinical Investigation* 37 (1958): 1764.

120. California Department of Public Health, MCH Unit. *Nutrition during Pregnancy and Lactation.* Sacramento, 1975.

121. WORTHINGTON, B., J. VERMEESCH, and S. WILLIAMS. *Nutrition in Pregnancy and Lactation.* St. Louis: C. V. Mosby, 1977.

122. *Healthy People, The Surgeon General's Report on Health Promotion and Disease Prevention.* DHEW (PHS), Publication No. 79–55071, 1979.

123. "Symposium, The Evidence Relating Six Dietary Factors to the Nation's Health." *American Journal of Clinical Nutrition* 32 (1979): 2621.

CHAPTER 6

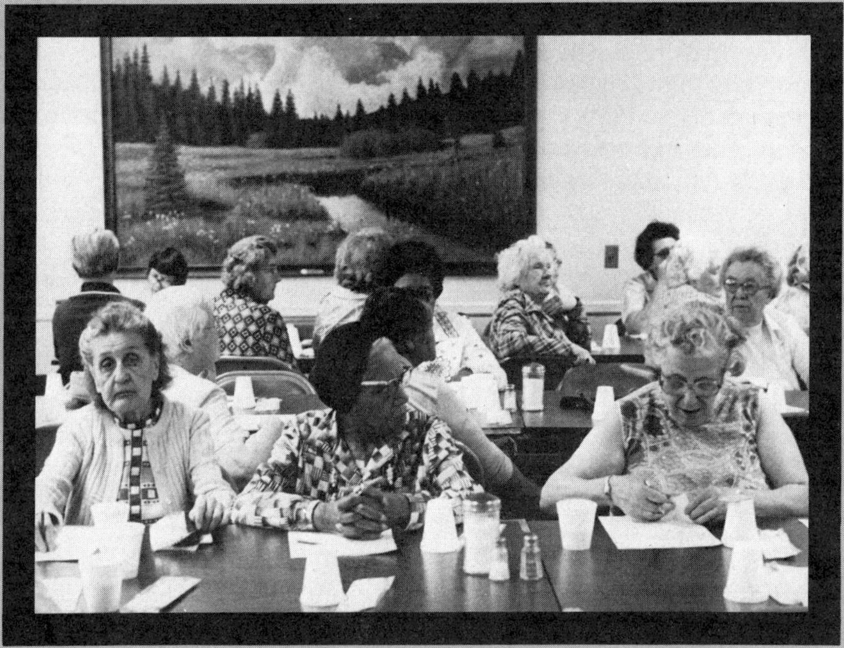

Photo by Irene Springer

nutrition during the later years

THE MOVEMENT FROM MIDDLE AGE INTO THE LATER YEARS has no clearly defined biological point of reference. By age 50, all humans show some physiological changes that can be related to aging, such as gray hair or skin wrinkles. The number of people with one or more chronic conditions increases greatly, and a large number of people die between 65 and 75. Figure 6–1 shows the increase in chronic conditions with an aging population.

In Germany in the 1880s, Chancellor Otto von Bismarck selected the age of 70 (it was lowered to 65) for retirement eligibility for benefits from social insurance legislation. In the United States today, although 65 is the common retirement age, the definition of who is aged varies. The National Academy of Sciences in the Recommended Dietary Allowances (appendix) begins the older age group at 51. Under Section 202 of the National Housing Act of 1959, benefits begin at 62. In the 1972 Nutrition Program for the Elderly Act, older people are those 60 years and older. The Social Security System uses age 65 for retirement benefits, with 62 for women at reduced benefits.

The elderly are our fastest growing population subgroup. In 1980 there were estimated to be 25 million elderly (aged 65 and over), or about 11 percent of the population (1). Population and mortality changes are shown in Figures 6–2 and 6–3. The children of the post-World War II baby boom will be over 65 in 2030, more than doubling the number of elderly living today, while the current birth rate is low. The great increase in the number and proportion of older people is the most startling demographic characteristic of the twentieth century. In 1900 individuals over 65 comprised 4 percent of the population; the projection is as high as 23 percent in 2030. At that point, one out of five Americans may be over 65.

Abolition of many fatal childhood diseases, drugs such as penicillin to cure pneumonia, and other improvements in health care have given Americans a greater opportunity to live longer. The leading causes of death in 1977 are shown in Table 6–1.

The elderly are often thought of as living in group care facilities, although statistics demonstrate only about 5 percent of America's older people live in institutions. Who are the aged? Definition is not an easy task. Terminology is important in studying nutrition and aging. Aging is a lifelong process; the aged are those who are near the end of this process. They are those who are close to death simply because of years and/or physical condition. By this definition the

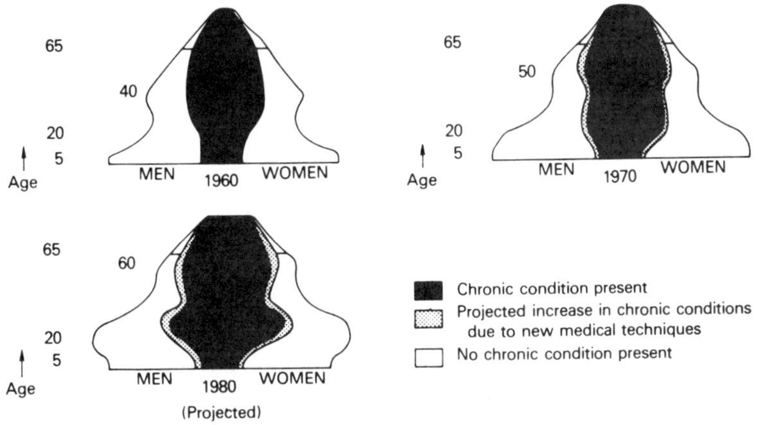

FIG. 6–1. Population pyramids for 1960, 1970, and 1980 showing that a larger proportion of the population has one or more chronic conditions as age increases. The 1970 and 1980 pyramids show how those who were age 40 in 1960 demonstrate the increased frequency of chronic conditions. *Source:* E. M. Gruenberg, *Patterns of Disease Among the Aged.* U.S. Department of Health, Education and Welfare Public Health Services, National Institutes of Aging, NIH Publication No. 79–1407 (rev. July, 1979).

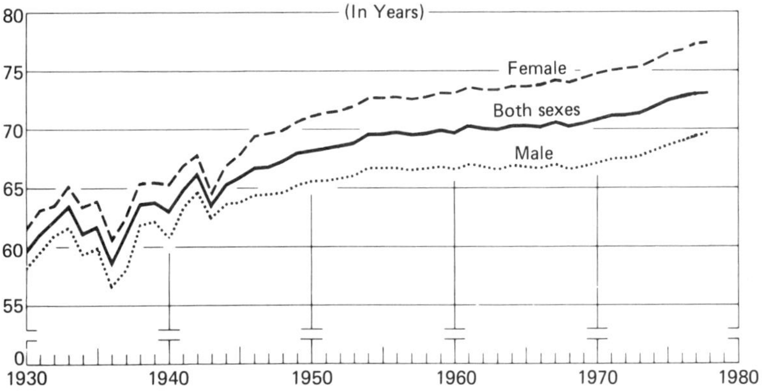

FIG. 6–2. Life expectancy by sex, 1930–1978. *Source: Vital Statistics Report, Final Mortality Statistics 1978,* DHHS Pub. No. (PHS) 80–1120, 29: (6) Suppt 2, 3, 1980. National Center for Health Statistics, Hyattsville, Md.

chronologically young person with a terminal disease would be aged because of the short distance from death. Biomedically, aging may be defined as the deteriorative changes that occur in the postreproductive period when the human organism has completed the task of perpetuation of the species. Senescence means to grow old. Senile means old; however, current usage implies negative connotations. Gerontology is the study of aging, including the processes and phenomena

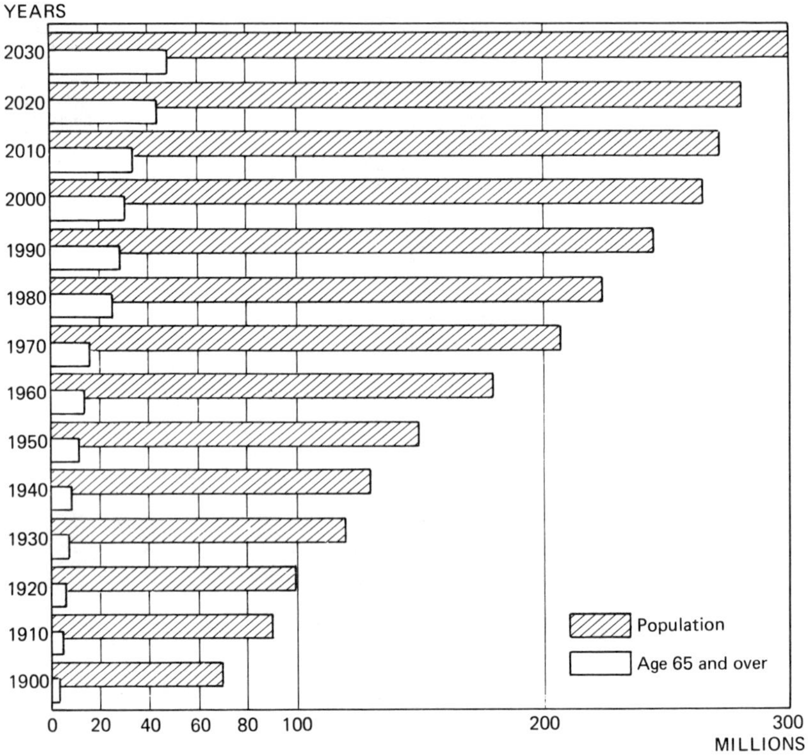

FIG. 6–3. Growth chart. Bars show the number of persons aged 65 and older, compared with the total population from 1900. The chart extends to the year 2030.

of aging; geriatrics is the study of the diseases of the aged and their treatment. We begin our examination of both the process and the people with an evaluation of the social and psychological aspects of this stage of the life cycle.

Social and Psychological Aspects of Aging

For older people who are well-integrated, the later years mean a new state of mind. There is the conviction that there is order and meaning in life, and that the life they have lived has been fully acceptable and necessary. The outcome is wisdom. Conversely, the older person without ego integrity feels despair, disgust, bitterness, and fear. Old age is partly a state of mind. Some people of advanced years are energetic and optimistic and have little concern for age. Everyone knows someone they consider "younger" than the person's chronological age. The satisfactions and quality of life in old age are determined more by success at social adaptation than by physical limitations.

Successful adaptation takes various routes. For some, a more contemplative mood represents successful coping; for others, an active social life is best. In the

TABLE 6–1. Death Rates for the 15 Leading Causes of Death: United States, 1978

rank[a]	cause of death	death rate (per 100,000 population)	percent of total deaths
	All causes	883.4	100.0
1	Diseases of heart	334.3	37.8
2	Malignant neoplasms, including neoplasms of lymphatic and hematopoietic tissues	181.9	20.6
3	Cerebrovascular diseases	80.5	9.1
4	Accidents	48.4	5.5
	Motor vehicle accidents	24.0	—
	All other accidents	24.4	—
5	Influenza and pneumonia	26.7	3.0
6	Diabetes mellitus	15.5	1.8
7	Cirrhosis of liver	13.8	1.6
8	Arteriosclerosis	13.3	1.5
9	Suicide	12.5	1.4
10	Certain causes of mortality in early infancy	10.1	1.1
11	Bronchitis, emphysema, and asthma	10.0	1.1
12	Homicide	9.4	1.1
13	Congenital anomalies	5.9	0.7
14	Nephritis and nephrosis	4.1	0.5
15	Septicemia	3.6	0.4
	All other causes	113.5	12.8

[a] Rank based on number of deaths.

SOURCE: Vital Statistics Report, Final Mortality Statistics, 1978 DHHS Pub. No. (PHS) 80–1120, 29: (2) Supplt. 2, 6, 1980, National Center for Health Statistics, Hyattsville, Md.

later years the person's role is often undefined or ambiguous. Retirement, death of a spouse, or a move into a group care facility or home of a relative alters the function of the individual in society. And retirement in a work-oriented society can be difficult. Many people view mandatory retirement with fear and misgiving. The first year of retirement especially is associated with mortality. Social and economic position may change. If most of the person's social contacts were related to work, retirement can result in social isolation and loss of self-esteem. Loss of income is a serious problem for many older adults. Among some middle-class families there is a refusal to accept available financial assistance because they consider this to be charity. The elderly are now one of the poorest segments of the population.

The mobility of young families and the death of a spouse and friends result in a large number of elderly who live alone and in isolation. Many of these people do not have the personal skills or the physical means to contact others. Friendships developed over a lifetime that have been lost through death cannot be replaced quickly, if at all. Fear of theft or molestation causes many elderly people to lock themselves in their apartments or homes. Many live in the center city or other high-crime areas where fear of violence or purse-snatching prevents them from leaving home often (2). Others may limit their activities to midday when they feel safe and avoid evening socials or meetings, which is a very different pattern from that of young adults who work during the day and socialize at night.

Physical changes may reduce mobility. The ability to drive a car or use public transportation may decline. If a car must be given up because of physical or economic reasons, there may be no public transportation available, especially in small towns and rural areas. Institutionalization may markedly affect an older person. Adjustment is difficult for some who must now depend on others. Others will feel abandoned and develop severe depression. An independent individual may resent the regimentation and lack of privacy.

In addition to coping with social and economic problems, the older person also has to cope with and accept many physiological changes.

The Physiology of Aging

The onset of aging occurs at an indeterminate point following maturity and has no objective landmarks in the early stages. The most consistent factor is a reduced compensation for physiological stress. In humans, vigor declines and susceptibility to disease multiplies with increasing age. Human tissue is of three kinds: cells that multiply throughout life (white corpuscles, epithelial cells), cells incapable of division or renewal (neurons), and noncellular material that may have much or little turnover (collagen, intercellular substance). All are subject to physiological control.

general changes

Separating normal age changes from changes associated with disease is difficult. Few longitudinal studies demonstrate the age changes in an individual over many years from youth to death. The work begun by Shock at the National Institutes of Health is providing the best information, but this research has only followed men for about 20 years (3). Other data are based on cross-sectional studies comparing 30-year-olds and 70-year-olds. But no one knows what characteristics the 70-year-olds had at 30. In addition, the 70-year-olds have achieved longevity while many of their cohorts died at an earlier age; thus, the older subjects in a cross-sectional study have been naturally selected for longevity.

Physiology is regarded as the study of functioning homeostasis. Homeostasis for the child is different from that for the young adult, and that of the young adult is different from that of the old person. This variation has been demonstrated in responses to the glucose tolerance test. The glucose tolerance test nomogram (Figure 6–4) is a realistic standard for the elderly because it takes into account the normal changes that occur with age. An individual's performance on the glucose test can be compared with that of others in the same age group by using the percentile ranking. By extending a line drawn from the subject's age through the blood glucose concentration, percentile rank can be determined. This schematic approach is also an imperfect yet useful guide to diabetes detection in the elderly. Older subjects retain a marked ability to maintain the chemical and physical composition of the blood under resting conditions.

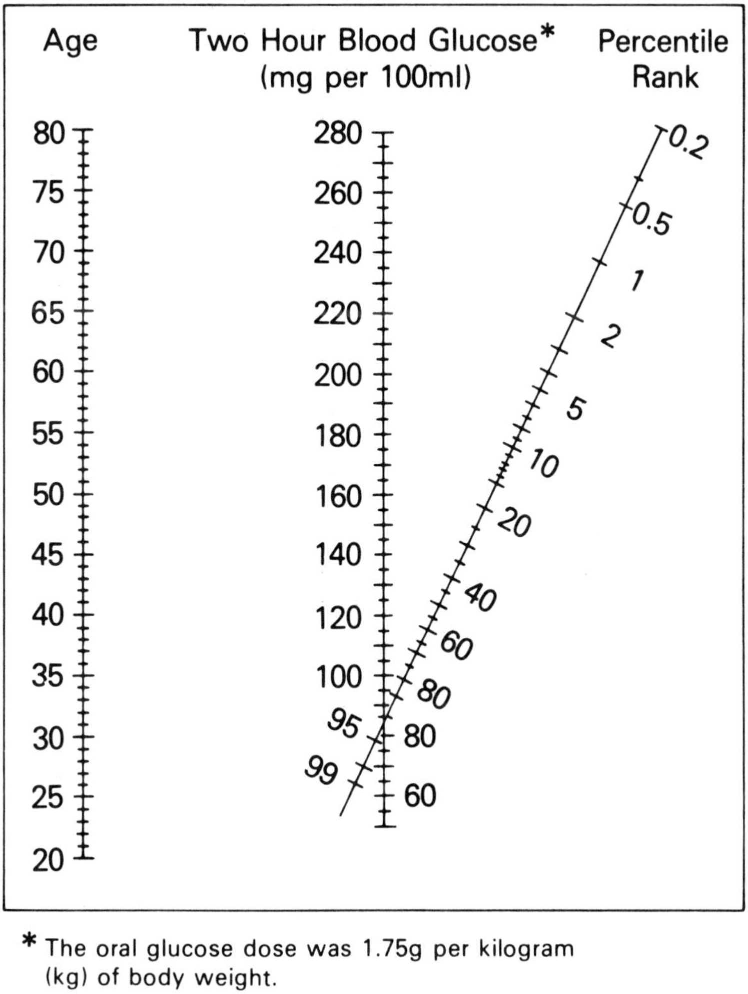

FIG. 6–4. Nomogram for glucose tolerance tests based on Baltimore Longitudinal Study Data. *Source:* J. Tobin and R. Andres, *Diabetes and Aging* (1978). DHEW Publication No. (NIH) 78–1408.

TABLE 6-2. Physiological Changes in Aging

declines or decreases

BODY COMPOSITION AND STRUCTURE

- Total body water and intracellular water
- Protoplasmic mass (by whole body ^{40}K counting)
- Stature and stem length
- Bone mass and skeleton
- Diameter and circumference of head, trunk, and limbs
- Muscle mass
- Grip strength in hands
- Skin elasticity
- Blood components
  - Ascorbic acid

FUNCTIONS

- Circulatory and respiratory Basal metabolic rate
  - Respirations per minute
  - Vital capacity: forced and one second
  - Diffusing capacity of the lungs
  - Cardiorespiratory performance during and after exercise
- Renal
  - Renal blood flow
  - Glomerular filtration rate
  - Functioning nephron units
- Endocrine
  - Glucose tolerance
  - Estrogens and other steroid hormones
  - Thyroid hormones
- Sensory
  - Visual acuity and amplitude of accommodations
  - Auditory acuity
  - Taste threshold
  - Evoked responses

increases

BODY COMPOSITION AND STRUCTURE

- Total body lipids
- Intracellular fat
- Body weight
- Skinfold thickness in some sites
- Blood components
  - Leucocyte count
  - Urea nitrogen
  - Creatinine
  - Cholesterol and cholesterol esters (until 60)
  - Triglyceride
  - Alkaline phosphate
  - Globulin
  - Autoantibody titers

FUNCTIONS

- Circulatory and respiratory
  - Systolic blood pressure (to age 70)
  - Diastolic blood pressure (or no change)
  - Residual capacity of the lungs

The physiological functioning of the aged differs widely. The only other stage of the life cycle that demonstrates such great variation is found in the male in the immediate prepubertal phase. Differences among the elderly are due to individual genetic and environmental influences, as well as to the consequences of deterioration in various systems and compensation for the deterioration. Eventually there is partial and irregular failure of homeostasis, and finally the deterioration that precedes death. At no other stage in life is the variation in individual pattern so marked or the complexity so great (4).

As the person ages, the system becomes increasingly unstable. The variations requiring response become larger, and the capacity to respond becomes less. At first compensatory mechanisms cover certain failures but eventually the failures multiply and the system collapses.

A description of the physiology of aging is a report of the variety of the observed changes, their sequence, and their interrelationships. It is a study of the mechanism of failing feedback systems. Intercellular physiology is concerned with chemical sources of damage, repair processes, and compensatory mechanisms. Intracellular physiology is concerned with normal or optimal feedback systems, sources of drift in these, secondary mechanisms of compensation, and the feedback between adjacent systems.

Disease and adaptive mechanisms affect each other. For example, degenerative changes in the heart affect the function of the kidneys. These modified kidney functions in turn alter the action of the heart and result in increased damage to the heart. The damaged heart results in retaining fluids in the lungs. Another example of the system's approach are changes in the cardiovascular system, such as plaque on the walls of the blood vessels. The decreased permeability of the vessel walls means that fewer nutrients move into the cells of the kidney and brain and less waste materials are removed than in a wall without disease. Identifying the sequences in the life cycle that control the stabilization of homeostasis in healthy, long-lived older persons is one way to discover the optimum way to live for healthy, productive old age (4).

With advancing age there is a loss of lean body tissues and an increase in the proportion of body weight that is fat. A reduction in total body water is a result of the lean tissue loss (see Figure 6–5). Body potassium decreases indicate a loss in lean body mass. Connective tissue increases in most organs. The collagen of older people has greater insolubility and increased rigidity. These changes play an important role in the age changes in blood vessels, lungs, and skin.

protein synthesis and basal metabolism

When total body protein synthesis was studied, older females exhibited lower rates of body protein synthesis than younger women, and males had rates similar to those of younger men (5). Different results are found when protein synthesis is related to lean body or cell mass instead of total body weight. By using urinary creatinine as an index of muscle mass and potassium for body cell mass, the

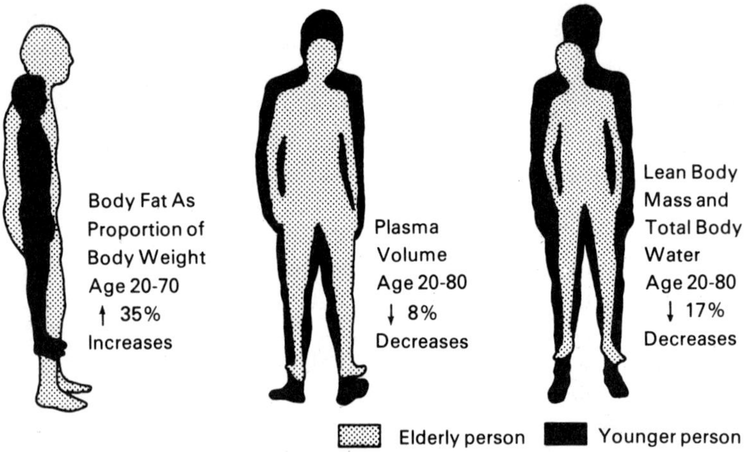

FIG. 6–5. Changes in the body with aging. *Source:* R. E. Vestal, *Drugs and the Elderly* (1979). NIH Publication No. 79–1449, U.S. Department of Health, Education and Welfare, Washington, D.C.

protein synthesis data show a relationship to body composition. Protein breakdown was significantly higher in elderly men than in young men. This relationship was also apparent for females. Because of decreased muscle mass in the elderly, more of the turnover comes from visceral organs than muscle protein. In general, muscle protein synthesis declines with advancing age.

Basal metabolism, when calculated as calories per square meter per hour, shows a gradual decline with age. The marked reduction in basal metabolism is a reflection of tissue loss rather than a reduction in the rate of cellular metabolism.

menopause

Menopause is the time of life for the human female when natural secretion of the sex hormones decreases (6). Estrogen is an anabolic agent for protein, producing strong bones and tissues. Estrogen aids in maintaining the moistness and pliability of the vagina and bladder. The hormone is also important in the balance of body chemistry. When the supply of estrogen declines, menopausal symptoms may develop: these include hot flashes, night sweats, chills, joint pains, backache, fatigue, insomnia, and depression. The severity varies; 50 percent of women go through menopause without any symptoms. This may be explained by individual variation of estrogen binding sites or other factors.

Physical changes include thinning of mucous membranes, development of dowager's hump, thinning of the hair, and hirsutism. Skeletal changes are decreased bone mass, increased bone porosity, and bone fragility. The incidence of osteoporosis of the spine is four times more common in women than in men. The cardiovascular system is affected, and cholesterol levels may increase. Atrophy occurs in the genital tract and the breasts.

Other hormones are affected by the decline in estrogen. The supply of thyroid and of adrenocortical hormones decreases somewhat. Pituitary gonadotropin increases. Vasomotor instability may be related to hormone decline.

neuroendocrine mechanisms

The effects of aging on the endocrine system vary from slight in some glands to marked in others. The most dramatic changes occur in the sex glands, leading to menopause in women and a decrease in testosterone secretion in men. There is a gradual decrease in the function of the thyroid and adrenal glands.

Age changes in noncentral nervous system tissues can markedly change the central nervous system mechanism. Changes in liver or kidney metabolism could alter steroid levels and influence the steroid-sensitive function of the nervous system. Future studies on the interaction of the brain and endocrine system should tell us exactly what happens where.

Brain failure may result from vascular disease of the brain or from conditions outside the brain, such as significant disease of the cardiovascular, renal, hepatic or endocrine systems. Brain disease may lead to behaviors that affect personal hygiene, feeding, impairment of domestic skills, and other patterns that adversely affect nutritional status. Reduced nutrient intake, especially of iron and certain vitamins, may hasten cognitive decline.

system changes

THE RENAL SYSTEM. At age 80, the glomerular filtration rate is about 50 percent of that at age 30 and is associated with a decrease in renal plasma flow. After age 40, the body's ability to regenerate nephrons seems to cease, and the number of nephrons gradually declines. On comparable diets the solute load excreted is similar for young and older adults; however, in older persons the solute load per nephron is greater due to fewer nephrons. The remaining nephrons show physiological impairment. The ability of the older kidney to form either a concentrated or dilute urine is decreased (7).

In the resting state, the older kidney can maintain fluid and electrolyte balance. During stress, the response of the kidney declines. The kidney changes in both structure and function. After reaching maximal size at maturation, the organ loses mass with age, primarily in the cortical area. Diminished regulatory mechanisms such as hormonal controls are the primary factors in the limited response to stress.

Impaired kidney function affects removal of waste products from the plasma and the maintenance of normal blood levels for some substances. Higher blood concentrations of urea may develop on high-protein diets.

THE DIGESTIVE SYSTEM. Poor eating and bowel habits lead to functional complaints of the digestive system that are not related to organic disorders. In the stomach the mucosal thickness decreases and atrophic gastritis occurs. There is an increase in leukocytes and lymphoid aggregates in the wall. The total volume of acid secreted declines in men and women, and the incidence of achlorhydria increases. Motor activity of the stomach decreases. But a hormone produced in the gut, gastric inhibitory polypeptide, may maintain blood sugar at healthy levels (1).

THE PULMONARY SYSTEM. Aging produces a primary change in the elastic properties of the lungs. There is an increase in fixed lung space (residual volume) which reduces the mobile lung space (vital capacity). Diffusing capacity of the lung decreases, but there are wide individual variations. Pulmonary capacity declines about 40 percent throughout life. Capability for energetic exercise may be limited. The extent to which environmental and disease factors modify aging in lungs is unclear (8).

THE CARDIOVASCULAR SYSTEM. The thickness of the wall of the left ventricle of the heart increases with age in the normal adult man. During maximal exercise, the cardiovascular response diminishes by about 20 percent at age 75. Decreased response to catecholamines may explain a limitation in maximal heart rate response. There is slowed myocardial relaxation in the hearts of aged men, although contractility does not necessarily decline. Interrelated factors regulate cardiac response to stress (9). One factor that regulates contraction duration and relaxation time is the length of time that calcium activates the myofibrils. The slower relaxation of advanced age may be related to a decrease in the rate at which the relaxing system can accumulate calcium.

In part, the body's ability to nourish cells depends on distribution by the vascular system. Removal of waste products depends on this system transporting substances to the kidney. In healthy elderly people, systolic blood pressure rises slightly with age and mean diastolic pressure remains fairly stable (10). Hypertension is any persistent level of systolic pressure above 160 mm Hg or of diastolic pressure above 100 mm Hg or both. An elderly man with a pressure below 110/70 or a woman with one below 105/65 is often considered hypotensive.

THE IMMUNE RESPONSE. From the early years the immune function increases rapidly; it peaks in adolescence and declines progressively in old age. Reduced immunological competence increases susceptibility to infections. A weakened immune system is probably one of the major sources of health problems in the elderly. The decline in immune function is involved in the development of a variety of age-related disease such as cardiovascular disease, kidney disease, and rheumatoid arthritis.

performance

Reaction times become progressively longer with age. Changes are small with simple tasks, but greater for complex jobs. Most sensorimotor performance in old people is limited by mechanisms of the central nervous system rather than impairments of the peripheral sense organs.

Sensory defects in vision and hearing increase. These are caused in part by central nervous system factors as well as organ changes. Taste sensitivity to sweet, sour, salty, and bitter substances declines. Odor response lowers.

Impaired performance in complex behavior is related to the breakdown in neural and endocrine regulatory mechanisms. The capacity of many hormone-producing organs declines. Reserve capacities are reduced, resulting in a lessened ability to meet daily environmental stresses. This loss in reserve capacity is caused by a gradual loss of functional units or by impairments of remaining units or by a combination of the two.

the rate of human aging

The study of aging and the testing of theories should benefit from the recent increase in information from longitudinal and cross-sectional sample studies, the availability of computers and of automated clinical chemistry, and the application of routine screening tests to many individuals (4).

Some currently used indices of aging are shown in Table 6–3. Currently, no uniformly applicable measure of the rate of aging is available. Figure 6–6 shows that the biological age profile may prove useful in gerontology. Visual assessment of age may reflect subconscious perception of physical and physiological status. The functional importance of the biological age test battery is shown by a comparison of deceased versus surviving subjects. Some of the parameters show no relation to mortality, but do show individual variation in aging. The rare syndrome of premature aging known as *progeria* is studied as a model for aging. The change in a single gene results in rapid aging beginning in infancy. Death occurs by the second decade, with signs of advanced age.

THEORIES OF AGING

Taken separately, there are more than 100 hypotheses about aging with enough research data to classify them as theories. Many of these, however, can be grouped into the major theories of aging (11, 12).

The **death gene theory** suggests an inherited mechanism that ultimately results in the cells of the organism dying. This theory is supported by an expected life span for various species. This species-specific life span seems to remain relatively constant. Among humans who survive to grow old, the life span seems

TABLE 6–3. Variables Used in Functional Age Prediction in Four Studies

WEBSTER AND LOGIE	FURUKAWA ET AL.	DIRKEN	BORKAN AND NORRIS
Plasma urea nitrogen	Glomerular filtration rate	Resting EKG	Forced expiratory volume (1 sec)
Log_{10} alkaline phosphatase	Renal plasma flow	Exercise EKG	Vital capacity
Erythrocyte sedimentation rate	Systolic blood pressure	Maximum energetic load	Maximum breathing capacity
Plasma triglycerides	Diastolic blood pressure	Maximum pulse frequency	Systolic blood pressure
Plasma cholesterol	Cholesterol	Maximum system blood pressure	Diastolic blood pressure
Systolic blood pressure	Red blood cells	VC_1	Hemoglobin
FEV_1	White blood cells	FEV_1	Serum albumin
	Hemoglobin concentration	Maximum breathing rate	Serum globulin
	Icterus index	Urinary 17-oxogenic	Creatinine clearance
	Total protein	17-oxosteroids	Plasma glucose (OGT test)
	Height	Creatinine	Auditory threshold (4000 cps)
	Weight	Psychomotor positioning	Visual acuity
	Vital capacity	Tapping rate	Visual depth perception
	Ocular accommodation	Hand dynamometry	Basal metabolic rate
	Vibratory sensation	Speech audiometry	Cortical bone percentage
	Grasping power	Pitch ceiling	Creatinine excretion
	Tapping rate	Presbycusis	Hand grip strength
	Body flexibility	Visual acuity	Maximum work rate
	Heart rate recovery	Picture completion	Benton visual memory test (errors)
		Reaction time	Tapping time (medium targets)
		Concentration	Tapping time (close targets)
			Reaction time (choice)
			Foot reaction time

SOURCES: I. W. Webster and A. R. Logie, "A Relationship between Functional Age and Health Status in Female Subjects, *Journal of Gerontology* 31 (1976): 546–550. T. Furukawa, M. Inoue, F. Kajiya, H. Inada, S. Takasugi, S. Fukui, H. Takeda, and H. Abe, "Assessment of Biological Age by Multiple Regression Analysis," *Journal of Gerontology* 30 (1975): 422–434. J. M. Dirken, *Functional Age of Industrial Workers* (Groningen: Netherlands Institute for Preventive Medicine TNO, Walter-Noordhoff Publishing, 1972). G. A. Borkan and A. H. Norris, "Assessment of Biological Age Using a Profile of Physical Parameters," *Journal of Gerontology* 35 (1980): 177–184.

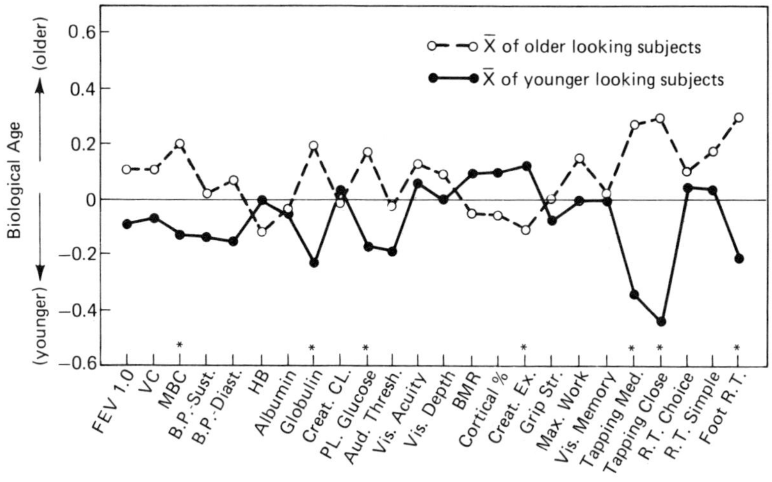

FIG. 6–6A. Biological age profile based on subjectively estimated age. Dotted line represents mean biological age scores of subpopulation which appeared most "old for their age" (top 15% of distribution). Solid line represents mean scores of subpopulation which appeared most "young for their age" (botton 15% of distribution). Starred parameters represent significantly different mean scores by *t*-test ($p < .05$).

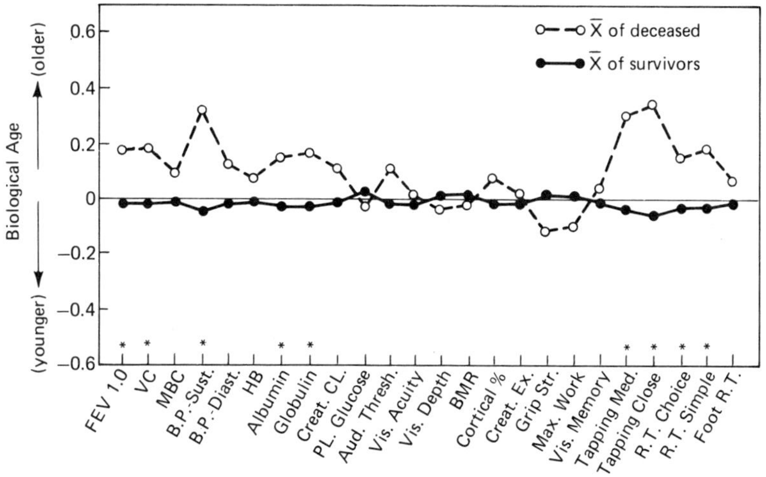

FIG. 6–6B. Biological age profile comparison of deceased with surviving study participants. Dotted line represents mean biological age scores of 166 men who have died since they were measured in the Baltimore Aging Study. Solid line represents mean scores for all other participants (N = 922) who remained alive in 1977. Starred parameters represent significantly different mean scores by *t*-test (*p*18 *fi* .05). *Source:* G. A. Borkan and A. H. Norris, "Assessment of Biological Aging Using a Profile of Physical Parameters," *Journal of Gerontology* 35 (1980): 177–184. Used with permission.

to have an upper limit of about 120 years, which is the oldest documented human age.

The **somatic mutation theory** considers aging to be a result of changes within the somatic cells of the body. These changes could be from DNA, deoxyribose nucleic acid; or RNA, ribose nucleic acid; or other cellular changes. These changes ultimately result in cell death randomly throughout the body. When enough cells die, the vigor of the organism declines and its ability to function ultimately ceases.

The **free radical theory** supports the idea that free hydroxyl groups are created as a result of lipid peroxidation or ionizing radiation. These free radicals damage subcellular membranes and ultimately result in cell death. The **cross-linking theory** indicates that aging is due to cross linkages of protein. Proteins are linked by tertiary bonds that make them more rigid. Collagen and elastin are the two proteins that show the most cross linkage, for these proteins have a long biological half-life. Cross linkage occurs in proteins that have a very low turnover rate in the body. The **genetic theory** of aging relates DNA deterioration to the aging process. The DNA either cross links or is damaged in some other way and can no longer replicate. Damage to the DNA can lead to defective protein synthesis, which could include faulty enzymes. In addition, damage could occur to the RNA templates, which could result in altered synthesis of amino acids or enzymes. Another theory of aging is related to the **autoimmune system** of the body. The autoimmune system may synthesize defective antibodies that not only attack foreign substances, but also could attack the body itself.

The **cell loss theory** implies that vigor declines through change or mutation in the properties of multiplying cells or loss and injury to nonmultiplying cells. Another theory holds that **dietary restriction** reduces the rate of aging. This has been shown in animal studies. Restrictions are accomplished by underfeeding the animals on a daily basis, by feeding every other day, and by feeding reduced amounts of protein to reduce growth rate. In a study using rats, total food intake was restricted either 33 or 46 percent. Nutritional restriction short of malnutrition seems to result in a prolonged life (13). At the Gerontology Research Center it was found that the increase in life span seems to be a result of protein restriction rather than simple caloric restriction. There is also a reduction in certain diseases through dietary restriction: either the onset of the disease is delayed, or an actual reduction in incidence occurs.

Other theories relate to the failure of mechanisms. Faulty copying of cellular signals can produce marked changes. Primary changes in the inert material of the body, such as collagen, produce mechanochemical failure. The tissues remain in the body, but in an altered form that affects either mechanical or chemical body functioning. Loss of physiological program would affect the timing of aging. This program determines aging by positive mechanisms or runs out of program when it passes beyond the reach of evolutionary selection. Studies of identical twins show that 60 to 80 percent of an individual's longevity is inherited.

Human aging is a very complex process. Although we may die sooner from single causes between 70 and 90 years of age, homeostasis declines across the board, causes of sickness accumulate, and possible causes of death multiply.

Nutrient Needs

Guidelines for the nutritional needs of the older adult are provided by the RDA (see Appendix). Many of these data are extrapolated from those for younger adults. But adults who are 50 years old are very different from those over 75 years, and little research has been conducted on those past 75. Another method of identifying needs is to survey the intake of healthy elderly adults and use these data estimates. Observation has been demonstrated to be more useful than interviews with institutionalized elderly (14). Madden et al. found that the 24-hour dietary recall is statistically conservative for calories and protein, with small intakes overreported and large intakes underreported (15). Recall data would not indicate a difference where no difference exists, but could yield a false negative or no significant difference where a difference does exist.

A number of dietary surveys have been conducted with older Americans. O'Hanlon and Kohrs have summarized 28 that were published between 1950 and 1978 (16). Data were collected by using food records, 24-hour recalls, or dietary histories. Most studies used the RDA as the standard for adequacy, although some established their own standards. An analysis of selected dietary records is shown in Table 6–4.

energy

Decreased physiological and physical activity result in a decline in the energy sources required by the aged. Loss of functioning cellular mass reduces the energy required in the resting state. The RDA for energy intake is 1800 kcal for females 51 to 75 and 2400 kcal for males; the range for females is 1400 to 2200 kcal and for males 2000 to 2800 kcal. For adults past 75, the recommendation is 1600 kcal (range 1200 to 2000 kcal) for females and 2050 kcal (1650 to 2450 kcal) for males.

Dietary surveys indicate that the mean energy intake of elderly people varies from 1000 to 1800 kcal per day. Most subjects are closer to 1500 or lower (17). In the HANES I survey, 74 percent of all persons consumed less than 90 percent of the established standard for calories, which was 34 kcal/kg body weight for males and 29 kcal/kg for females, or 1600 kcal/55 kg woman and 2400 kcal/70 kg man (18). About 32 percent consumed less than 60 percent of the standard, and about 11 percent consumed 110 percent or more of the standard for energy intake. When percentage of standard was used as the basis of comparison, there was little difference in males and females in the elderly age ranges. In order to

TABLE 6–4. Selected Dietary Studies on Older Americans

reference	number studied	state	standards and criteria used	mean nutrient intake less than standard	mean nutrient intake one-third below standard
HANES I (18)	1938	34 & D.C.	Own standards	Iron: low-income groups. Calories: all groups.	Calcium, iron, vitamin A, ascorbic acid.
Guthrie et al. (19)	109	PA	Two-thirds RDA (1968)	Calcium: females. Vitamin A: males and females.	Calories, calcium, vitamin A, thiamine, riboflavin, vitamin C.
Joering (20)	165	OH	Two-thirds RDA (1968)	Day including program meal: none below standard. Day with no program meal: calories; thiamin; males; calcium; females.	Not given.
Ten-State (21)	2076	Ten	Own standards	Calories: males and females. Iron: all black females, low-income white and high-income Spanish American females. Vitamin A: Spanish-Americans. Protein: low-income black males and white females, all black females, and high-income Spanish American females.	Calories and eight nutrients except vitamin C; intake of high-income black females and calcium intake of white males and high-income Spanish American males.
USDA (12)	1643	All	Own standards	65–74: Calories, calcium: both sexes; vitamin A, thiamin, riboflavin: females. 75+: Calories, vitamin C: males; calcium, riboflavin, vitamin A: both sexes.	Not given.
Davidson (22)	104	MA	100% RDA (1958)	Calories: both sexes.	Iron, thiamin, riboflavin.

TABLE 6–4. (Continued)

reference	number studied	state	standards and criteria used	mean nutrient intake less than standard	mean nutrient intake one-third below standard
				Food records (1–4 days)	
Kohrs (23)	466	MO	100% RDA (1974)	Calories: all groups; calcium: female participants, both nonparticipant groups; niacin: male participants, one nonparticipant group.	Not given.
Greger (24)	44	IN	100% RDA (1974)	Zinc, calcium: both sexes, calories: males.	Zinc.
Steinkamp (25)	229	CA	Two-thirds RDA (1964)	1962: Calories. niacin: males Calcium, niacin: females	1948, 1952, 1954, 1962: calcium: females; niacin: both sexes.
				Food records (over 4 days)	
Justice (26)	44	IN	100% RDA (1974)	Calories, calcium and niacin: both sexes; iron, thiamin: females only.	Calcium, protein, iron.
Dibble (27)	100	NY	Two-thirds RDA (1964)	None.	Calories: males; vitamin A, vitamin C: both sexes.
				Dietary histories	
Clarke (28)	197	KS	100% RDA (1968)	Calcium: both sexes; calories: males.	One-third had scores of 6 or lower (< 67% RDA for two or more nutrients)
Lyons (29)	100	MA	100% RDA (1953)	Calories: males; thiamin, iron: females.	< 75% RDA: iron: females; calories: males.

SOURCE: P. O. O'Hanlon and M. B. Kohrs, "Dietary Studies of Older Americans," *American Journal of Clinical Nutrition* 31 (1978): 1257.

obtain adequate nutrients on a lower caloric intake, food choices must be made carefully. At 1200 kcal or less, high nutrient density foods must be emphasized to obtain adequate intake. This eliminates many of the desserts so popular with the elderly. For some people, poor-quality diets are a result of low energy intakes of less than 1000 calories, with too little total food consumed to provide the necessary nutrients.

protein

Because the body is in a dynamic state, proteins and other constituents are being continuously synthesized and degraded. Protein intake provides essential amino acids and nitrogen replacement for the elderly. For people 51 and over, the allowance for protein from a mixed diet listed in the RDA is 0.8 g/kg body weight. Thus, the allowances are 56 g for the 70 kg male and 44 g for the 55 kg female reference persons. The FAO safe levels of protein intake based on values obtained using eggs and milk are 0.57 g and 0.52 g/kg for the reference man (65 kg) and woman (55 kg) (19). This is 39 g/day for the man and 29 g/day for the woman. Young has applied the factorial method and computed a "safe" level of intake of 0.42 g for egg and milk protein per kg of body weight per day, but found in balance studies that this amount was not adequate to maintain nitrogen balance for the elderly (5). A decrease in efficiency of utilization was suggested by the data. Only one elderly woman could maintain positive balance at the 0.52 g/kg of body weight per day. Zanni et al. found the safe level of intake to be 0.59 g protein per kg of ideal body weight (20). Thus, the difference in protein requirement for men aged 60 to 67 from that for younger men was quite small. As aging progresses, digestive system factors may decrease absorption from proteins.

For example, obligatory urinary N losses in 11 elderly women were similar to those for young women when expressed as unit of body weight, but higher when expressed per unit of creatinine excretion per lean body cell mass (21). In a review of kidney function, Parsons noted that protein intakes must be adjusted downward with emphasis on high-quality proteins for elderly patients who have residual kidney functions of 20 percent or less (22). The elderly do not have the reserve kidney function to handle dehydration, salt, or acid loading. A suggested protein intake is three times the urea output in grams.

Clinical conditions of severe infections, fever, and surgery will lead to increased protein requirements. In the elderly, recovery from an illness resulting in protein depletion may increase the requirement to that of a growth period until recovery is completed. Data from metabolic balance studies demonstrate that acute infectious illnesses are accompanied by negative body nitrogen balances which begin after the start of the febrile response. Body losses of nitrogen can usually be lessened by normal or increased dietary energy and protein intake (23).

Since balance studies cannot be performed on all people, one of the problems in determining protein needs rests in not having a simple and reliable tool to assess protein status. Serum protein and albumin have been widely used, with varying results. MacLennan found a significant positive correlation between albumin levels and protein intake in women, but not in men residents of a long-stay geriatric ward (24). Jordan found that protein did not correlate with serum albumin; however, protein content of hair root significantly correlated with dietary protein (25). In most studies there is a better relationship between serum albumin and protein intake when dietary protein is low.

The protein intake of the healthy elderly is also used as an indicator of needs. Numerous studies provide this information (16, 26, 27, 28). From studies of people living independently with adequate incomes, mean daily protein intake varies from 56 to 98 g. When calculated as g/kg/day, protein intake ranges from 0.9 to 1.2. From data collected by the recall method in HANES I, the mean protein intake of those 65 and over was 68.4 g/day. People below the poverty level consumed 57.7 g; above the poverty level, 69.4 g. When intake was calculated as a percentage of the standard for protein intake, which was 1 g/kg of body weight, about 45 percent of those over 65 consumed less than 90 percent of the standard, and about 14 percent consumed less than 60 percent (18). Note that this is more generous than the RDA, which is 0.8g/kg.

In nursing home diets, Justice found one-third of the subjects had individual intakes below the RDA (29). Of the four subjects who consumed less than 40 g of protein a day, four consumed no milk and one refused meat. Many could not eat meat because of mechanical difficulties associated with chewing and swallowing. In institutional care, alternate protein sources can be provided for those who have these problems—vegetable protein concentrate, pureed meats, or prepared protein supplements. Clark and Wakefield found no significant differences in nutritional intake between people living in a nursing home and independently (26). Nursing home residents had more changes in eating habits, and these changes correlated negatively with nutrition scores.

fats

The essential fatty acid, linoleic acid, is required by the elderly. Linoleic acid can be obtained by a small intake of polyunsaturated fats. Once this need is met, reduction of caloric intake can be accomplished using a lowered fat diet. For the elderly, usually not more than 35 percent of the energy should be provided by fat. Dietary fat serves as a carrier for fat-soluble vitamin absorption and as a satiety factor. Many elderly require dietary modification in type or amount of lipids due to atherosclerotic disease. Limitation in the amount of dietary cholesterol is also common. Increased use of polyunsaturated fats found in most vegetable oils instead of saturated fat found in animal foods, coconut and olive oil, may have beneficial effects on reducing elevated blood lipids.

vitamins

Vitamins are important components of the diet throughout the life cycle. Functioning mainly as coenzymes, vitamins are very important in metabolic processes. An adequate intake of vitamins is essential for mental, emotional, and physical health, but there is only limited research on vitamin requirements for the elderly. The RDAs indicate that most of the information for the elderly is based on the assumption that the requirements remain stable throughout the entire adult life span. The ability to absorb and utilize vitamins may decline with aging. In addition, some vitamins must be converted to an active form, and this ability may decline. Vitamin needs and requirements are based on the amount of energy, protein, and other nutrients consumed, absorbed, and metabolized. When dietary restrictions are medically or self imposed, certain vitamins may be eliminated or reduced along with the foods that are restricted. Because of the important balance with other nutrients, a varied food supply is preferable to supplements as a source of vitamins. Often supplements are not chosen correctly and replace the wrong vitamins unless they are prescribed after laboratory tests for nutrient status. Most vitamin deficiencies found in the elderly involve several vitamins. The vitamins are often associated with the perishable fruits and vegatables, meat, milk, and eggs, which are sometimes eliminated from the diet when there is inadequate income or storage facilities. In addition, storage of food for long periods of time under improper conditions may destroy the vitamins that are available. Long-term poor habits and inadequate vitamin intake may not manifest itself until old age. The water-soluble vitamins are excreted more readily in urine and sweat, but the fat-soluble vitamin stores are reduced through utilization. It takes many months to deplete stores of vitamin A.

B-VITAMINS. Only a small pool of most water-soluble vitamins is maintained by either young or old. In the elderly, long-standing marginal intake may eventually result in deficiency symptoms. Thiamin, riboflavin, and niacin changes in food intake may result in decreased thiamin and riboflavin blood levels. Although the smaller energy requirement may mean that less thiamin is required, thiamin is one vitamin frequently demonstrated to be deficient in the diets of the elderly (30, 31). The RDA is 1.2 mg for men and 1.0 mg for women. Altered intestinal flora and decreased gastric hydrochloric acid may inactivate thiamin. Requirements increase during fever, malignancy, increased carbohydrate intake, or increased excretion with diuretic therapy. Women with high dietary thiamin intakes have been shown to have a lower rate of death from cardiovascular disease.

Decreased riboflavin intake usually accompanies decreased amounts of other B-vitamins. Several studies noted reduced intakes of riboflavin. Increased protein intake, surgery, or trauma will affect riboflavin needs (32). Reduced riboflavin intake has been associated with diseases of the nervous and circulatory systems (11). The RDA is 1.3 mg for men over 51, and 1.2 mg for women.

Niacin tissue levels may decrease in the elderly, but true deficiency of niacin is rare. The RDA is 15 mg of niacin equivalents for men and 13 mg for women in the older age ranges.

FOLATE. Folate has been indicated as a nutritional problem in the United States. Intake may be reduced. In addition, the conversion of folate to folinic acid, the active form of the vitamin, may be reduced due to lower vitamin C levels in the blood of the elderly. Interference with absorption and utilization of folate may occur even when intake is adequate, and the requirement may increase due to metabolic changes or excessive excretion. Chronic loss of blood, hyperthyroidism, or malignancy can increase the requirements.

In the elderly, dementia due to folate deficiency should be considered. Early signs are lassitude, apathy, and weakness, in addition to megaloblastic red blood cells. Low serum folate correlates with organic brain disease in many elderly people. Megaloblastic anemia, which is the usual result of folate deficiency, is less common in older persons even when folate reserves are low. Enzyme deficiencies such as those that occur with liver disease may result in inadequate utilization of folate. The RDA for folate is 400 μg.

VITAMIN B_{12}. Absorption of this vitamin is reduced in some elderly due to lack of an intrinsic factor or consumption of drugs that reduce absorption of B_{12}. In the elderly, low serum levels of vitamin B_{12} are associated with confusion and psychiatric disorders (11). Hypotensive drugs require B_{12} for metabolism. Vegan diets that omit all animal products may affect the store of B_{12}, for this vitamin is found in foods of animal origin.

The classic B_{12} deficiency state known as pernicious anemia is not common in the elderly. The combined reduced intake of folate and B_{12} which leads to confusion and psychiatric disorders is a greater problem. In cases of dementia and confusion, B_{12} status should be considered. The RDA is 3 μg.

VITAMIN C. The requirement for this vitamin increases with aging. As with protein, it is difficult to determine whether the increased needs are because of tissue resistance, associated infections, or other problems. In addition, dietary habits may reduce the intake of vitamin C by elderly men and women. Physiological stress from burns or surgery increases vitamin C loss and reduces tissue levels. Anti-inflammatory drugs may inhibit metabolism. The RDA for vitamin C is 60 mg. Several surveys have reported low intakes of vitamin C (see Table 6–5).

In a study of 830 persons over 65, plasma and leucocyte vitamin C declined significantly with age (33). The mean plasma level at age 75 was 0.24 mg/100 ml for men and 0.37 mg/100 ml for women. In young adults, 1.0 mg/100 ml is the optimum level. Plasma levels and fruit intake were positively correlated, although higher fruit consumption did not account entirely for the higher blood levels. There seems to be a physiological difference between males and females in the

TABLE 6-5. Mean Intake of Calories and Selected Nutrients as Percentage of Standard for Persons over 65

	male			female		
	ALL INCOME	BELOW POVERTY INCOME	ABOVE POVERTY INCOME	ALL INCOME	BELOW POVERTY INCOME	ABOVE POVERTY INCOME
Calories	74%	70%	75%	77%	71%	78%
Protein	99%	91%	102%	90%	84%	92%
Calcium	179%	152%	184%	95%	88%	97%
Iron	121%	113%	123%	92%	80%	96%

NOTE: No one below standard for vitamin A, C, thiamin, or riboflavin.

SOURCE: *Preliminary Findings of the First Health and Nutrition Examination Survey, United States, 1971–1972, Dietary Intake and Biochemical Findings.* DHEW (HRA) 76–1219.

metabolism or retention of viatmin C. To maintain the plasma level at 1.0 mg requires a daily intake of more than 100 mg in men and 90 mg in women.

There is little agreement on the role of vitamin C in the aging process. Vitamin C plays a role in tissue repair and collagen formation; however, its place in the prevention of aging changes in connective and other tissue is unclear. The initial changes in blood vessels developing atherosclerosis resemble the lesions of vitamin C deficiency states in other tissues, but an actual relationship is undocumented. With acute and chronic stress there is increased liberation of adrenocorticotropin hormone (ACTH) and a reduction of the vitamin C available in the adrenals. Increased intake of vitamin C is useful in maintaining tissue levels during stress. Vitamin C requirements are increased during wound healing, such as following fractures or surgery, and during serious illness.

VITAMIN A. Although low intakes of vitamin A have been noted in some older adults who participated in nutrition surveys, the plasma level of vitamin A seems to rise with aging. Since vitamin A can be stored for long periods, there is difficulty in relating intake records with current blood status.

In older adults, low intakes of vitamin A were correlated with increased incidences of nervous, circulatory, and respiratory diseases. Skin and eye lesions that are frequently accepted as normal with aging are improved by vitamin A administration for adults with low serum levels. The RDA is 800 RE (retinol equivalents) or 4000 IU. One RE is equal to one μg of vitamin A alcohol (retinol) or 6 μg of B-carotene.

VITAMINS D AND E. The RDA for vitamin D is 5 μg as cholecalciferol (Vitamin D_3) or 200 IU. In the kidney and the liver, vitamin D must be converted to the metabolically active forms 25-hydroxy or 1,25-hydroxy cholecalciferol. The decline in kidney function may affect this activation.

Vitamin E functions as an antioxidant in biological systems and may reduce the formation of free radicals that damage cell membranes. Supplementation with vitamin E is popular, although there are no conclusive studies relating vitamin E to reduction of heart disease, reduced sterility, or improved sexual or athletic performance. The RDA is 8 mg α tocopherol equivalents (α TE) or 12 IU for females, and 10 mg α TE or 15 IU for males. If large amounts of polyunsaturated fats are consumed, the requirement increases.

minerals

In nutrition surveys, iron and calcium are the minerals most likely to be consumed in less than adequate amounts. Mineral nutrition is especially important in the later years because potassium, sodium, and chloride are important in the electrolyte balance in the body. Diuretic and other drugs may deplete the body of potassium. When normally active elderly people become weak and tired, electrolyte balance should be investigated.

CALCIUM. The RDA for calcium is 800 mg/day for men and women over 50. The amount of calcium required is related to phosphorus intake and vitamin D status. The calcium to phosphorus ratio should be from 1:2 to 1:1. The major portion of body calcium is in the bones; however, the bone can serve as a storage reservoir and be depleted to meet the cellular requirement for calcium when dietary calcium is not adequate. A number of studies have suggested that osteoporosis does not develop as readily in subjects with a high calcium intake (more than 1 g daily), so many experts recommend 1 g daily.

Calcium balance studies demonstrate that negative balance can result from inadequate intake, malabsorption, or excessive excretion (34). The efficiency of calcium absorption declines with age, and a high-fat diet may also reduce calcium absorption. Activation of vitamin D results in synthesis of a protein that enhances calcium absorption. Lactose forms a soluble complex with calcium, enhancing absorption. Phytate and oxalate interfere with absorption. Excessive excretion has been noted on very high-protein diets.

Serum calcium is quite stable in elderly adults at a mean of 10 mg/100 ml. This is under the control of the parathyroid hormone, which raises the blood level by mobilizing calcium from the bone, and calcitonin, which lowers the blood calcium level by decreasing the mobilization.

MAGNESIUM. The RDA for magnesium is 300 mg for women and 350 mg for men. No evidence exists for an increased need with aging. A severe loss of body fluid, malabsorption, or liver disease are the conditions that may lead to a deficiency. Dehydration is the most likely factor in the elderly. But because magnesium is so widely available from the food supply, deficiency is rare.

PHOSPHORUS. The RDA for phosphorus is 800 mg for men and women. Phosphorus is very available from a variety of foods, and deficient intakes are unlikely. Those taking antacids may have increased excretion of phosphates resulting in a deficiency.

POTASSIUM. In a study of 100 men and women over 65, grip strength declined with decreasing potassium intake although serum potassium levels were normal (35). A minimum daily intake of 2.3 g per day of potassium is recommended. Increased urinary excretion of potassium can result from injury, trauma, and diuretic drug therapy. Depletion of potassium may also occur with excessive loss of intestinal fluids. Depletion signs are impairment of muscular activity, weakness, and lassitude. Other disturbances in electrolytes usually accompany potassium deficiency.

SODIUM. The status of the kidney influences the sodium requirement. With aging, heart failure may result in sodium retention; kidney damage or adrenal insufficiency may result in sodium loss. Sodium loss can also occur from excessive vomiting or diarrhea. Although a lifetime pattern of a high consumption of sodium in some people may lead to high blood pressure, all people are not so affected. Sodium intake must be adjusted for the individual. There is no benefit for the healthy person in consuming excessive salt, and a possibility of harm.

IRON. Iron deficiency is relatively common in elderly people due to decreased intake and/or absorption. Lack of iron can lead to fatigue, behavioral changes, and anemia. The RDA for men and women over 50 is 10 mg/day. Iron deficiency anemia was indicated in the Ten-State Nutrition Survey by the high prevalence of low hemoglobin and hematocrit values found (36). The findings of the HANES survey indicated that iron was the nutrient most often found below standard for both blacks and whites aged 50 or over (18). In the lower-income brackets, 65 percent had intakes below the RDA; in the upper-income group the figure was 56 percent. However, serum iron and transferrin saturation levels were normal. Black adults in the lower-income group had the highest prevalence of low hemoglobin values, with a total of 29.6 percent. A larger percentage of 41.9 had low hematocrit values. All groups had more than 10 percent with low hemoglobin values. The incidence of low hemoglobin was 51 percent for men (below 13.5 g/dl) and 41 percent for women (below 12 g/dl) in geriatric hospital admissions in an English hospital (36). Grades of gastric mucosal change were not correlated with the presence or absence of anemia. However, Bird concluded that a small group had iron deficiency anemia as a result of gastric mucosal change, due to autoimmune mechanisms (37). In a study of iron fortification of foods for the elderly, Gershoff et al. found marked increases in hemoglobin levels in both fortified and unfortified groups (38). Thus, the undefined effects of intervention were as important as fortification.

ZINC. This trace mineral plays an important role in taste acuity for the elderly. Zinc is also required for wound healing and tissue repair. The RDA remains at 15 mg during the entire adult life span. Although zinc is available from many foods, decreased absorption occurs with aging; studies indicate low intakes and blood levels (39, 40).

fluids

In the elderly it is important to provide for adequate fluid intake because fluid reserves are low in older people. Both intracellular and extracellular water are reduced. Normally thirst will ensure sufficient intake of liquids; however, among the elderly chronic illness or habitual training may deemphasize the drinking of water. Sufficient intake of water not only provides for adequate body water, but maintains adequate kidney function.

Nutrition-Related Problems

The nutrition-related problems of aging require consideration on an individual basis. There are, however, certain problems common to many people (40).

hospital malnutrition

A substantial portion of hospitalized elderly patients suffer from protein calorie malnutrition. Most are malnourished due to illness-induced anorexia, catabolic response to disease or infection, or iatrogenic effects of multiple treatments including drugs. Some become malnourished after hospital admission for surgery, infection, or routine semi-starvation regimes. A preliminary survey of 67 adults, nonselected patients admitted to two teaching hospitals, demonstrated that 91 percent had overt or potential nutritional problems (41). Nutrition was neglected in the diagnosis and care of the patients.

The increased surgical risk associated with malnutrition in the elderly has often been emphasized (32, 42). Nutritional therapy appropriate to the individual patient will allow the person to undergo surgery with fewer risks and improved results.

bone loss

One of the major problems encountered by the elderly is bone loss. It seems to be a universal disease in aging humans. Optimum mineralization is reached by age 40 and decreases thereafter. All bone loss does not progress to the state of osteoporosis, although osteoporosis is a major health problem in women (34). Figure 6–7 shows the effect of the collapse of the vertebrae on height. In normal adults arm span is equal to height, but in osteoporotic adults arm span is greater than height; thus, the difference between arm span and height can be used as a means of estimating vertebral bone loss. Approximately 25 to 30 percent of women and 15 to 20 percent of men over age 50 have osteoporosis severe enough to involve vertebral compression. Osteoporosis is more common than arthritis and three times more prevalent than diabetes.

Sufficient calcium intake, adequate protein intake and other nutrients are important measures for preventing osteoporosis. Therapy with fluoride, calcium, and vitamin D, and its active forms, has increased the mineral content of bones. As with other problems, nutrition, heredity, and physical activity are factors. Bone demineralization in the elderly is also related to low calcium intakes over prolonged periods. Bone loss in the jaw leads to periodontal disease and tooth loss. Recent studies indicate increasing calcium requirements as high as 1000 to 1500 mg with aging. High protein intakes require increased calcium intakes to compensate for the increased urinary calcium loss, especially if phosphorus intakes are also high, as in meat and cereal consumption. Although inactivity hastens bone loss, there is little evidence that increasing activity such as jogging in normally active people prevents bone loss. This remains to be investigated.

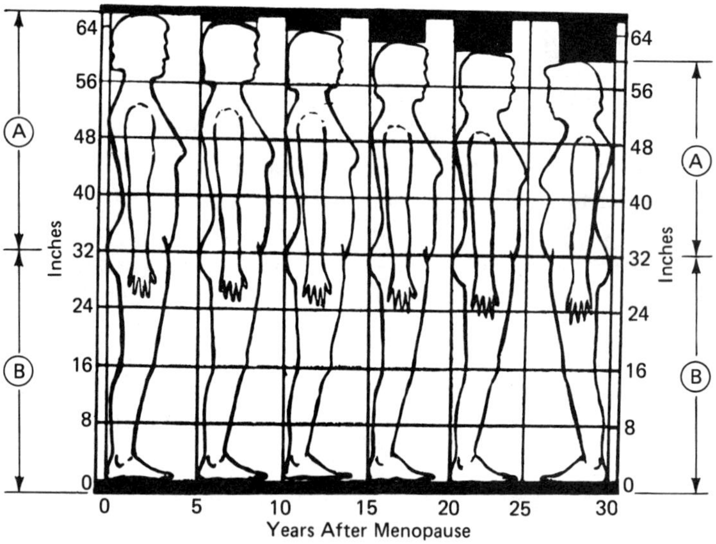

FIG. 6–7. Effect of postmenopausal osteoporosis on height of women. Decrease in distance from hip to top of head (A) with little or no change in distance from hip to heel of foot (B). *Source:* Anthony A. Albanese, "Bone Loss: Causes, Detection and Therapy," *Current Topics in Nutrition and Disease* (New York: Alan R. Liss, Inc., 1977). Used by permission.

constipation

This is a concern for many elderly people. Foods high in water or fiber content are suggested. By preventing excess absorption of water from the bowel, fiber increases passage of bulky, soft fecal material. Increased intracolonic pressures may cause diverticulosis. Emphasis should be on consumption of minimally processed cereal foods plus fruits and vegetables for the treatment of constipation (43). Deficiencies in fat-soluble vitamins such as A, D, and E in the aged are frequently due to habitual use of the common laxative mineral oils, which interfere with absorption.

changes in food patterns

A long life results from a combination of genetic endowment and environmental factors. Changing biological and physical status and the different social environment that accompany aging may affect food patterns and intake (see Table 6–6).

PERCEPTUAL CHANGES. Perceptual changes in hearing, vision, taste, and smell are important to eating and drinking patterns.

Hearing is more important than vision in maintaining integration of personality and adaptation psychologically. Elderly with impaired hearing may be reluctant to eat in public places because of the difficulty of conversation with others. Vision is reduced by the loss of ability of the lens to accommodate to a near point and can be corrected by an appropriate lens. Slowed adaptation to darkness and increased need for light is noted in advanced age. Many older people object to eating in dimly lighted areas and are bothered by flickering candlelight. Taste declines with age due to the aging process or as a result of disease and smoking habits. The overall number of papillae decreases with age. Old people demonstrate a decline in taste buds per papilla which beings at middle life with the taste buds on the anterior part of the tongue and progresses to the posterior taste buds. The taste buds that detect sweet and salt deteriorate first. This may explain the complaint by some elderly that food tastes bitter or sour (44). The ability to identify foods by taste while blindfolded declines significantly in the aged.

The loss of ability to detect odors by the elderly is well documented. In one study, at least 11 times the concentration of odor was required for smelling by the elderly when compared to young adults. Dissatisfaction with both taste and smell by the elderly has been reported by Cohen and Gitman (45). The most frequent complaint is related to a sour or bitter taste or dryness of the mouth. Some vegetables have a pleasant odor, but a bitter taste. If detection of the pleasant odor is lost, only the bitter taste is perceived.

PREFERENCES. Preferences may revert to foods associated with previous pleasant life experiences or security foods. These memories are not confined to childhood.

TABLE 6-6. Conditions Implicating Nutrition for the Later Years

condition	effect	nutritional or clinical implications
SOCIOECONOMIC		
Reduced income retirement or inflation	Reduction in food expenditure—meat, milk and fresh vegetables.	Reduced intake of protein, vitamins and calcium.
Changes in family size Institutionalization Changes in environment	Changed availability of food and altered intake.	Weight loss or gain, malnutrition.
Lack of storage or preparation facilities	Excessive ingestion of processed foods, snacks.	
PSYCHOLOGICAL		
Changes in dietary habits	Overeating, erratic diets; reduced food intake.	Obesity; undernutrition, deficiency.
Depression Loneliness Confusion	Overeating or no interest in food.	Obesity; undernutrition, deficiency.
PHYSIOLOGICAL		
Reduced BMR	Less energy, but same amount of other nutrients required.	Obesity or deficiency.
Loss of teeth, atrophy of jaws	Difficulty chewing, changed food intake.	Digestive disorders, constipation, deficiencies.
Reduced secretion of HCl and digestive enzymes	Altered digestion.	Dietary deficiencies, i.e. calcium, iron.
Hepatic and biliary insufficiency	Reduced absorption of lipids.	Fat-soluble vitamin deficiency, weight loss, flatulence.
Atrophy of intestinal mucosa and muscles	Poor absorption; slower movement of food through intestine.	Vitamin and mineral deficiencies; constipation.
Decreased secretion of intestinal mucus	Decreased lubrication of intestine.	Constipation.
Diverticulosis	Entrapment of hard food particles in diverticula.	Diverticulitis.
Altered glucose metabolism	Decreased glucose tolerance.	Hyperglycemia or hypoglycemia.
Decreased renal function	Reduced ability to handle renal solute loads.	Elevated blood urea, alkalosis.
Altered bone metabolism	Reduced bone formation, increased bone destruction.	Bone loss, osteoporosis.

Food has symbolic value and provides rewarding experiences that may assist in maintaining self-esteem. Cultural attitudes toward food are established early in life and are difficult to change.

In a study of cohort influences, Garcia et al. found that food patterns do not change significantly from early middle age to old age (28). Habitual eating patterns of individuals are important in the nutritional care and group feeding of the elderly. Some foods have deep significance and emotional meaning to older people (46). Although food patterns are relatively stable throughout the life cycle, with education, changes are made even by the elderly. The concern of the older population for their health improves the response to education. Nutrition counseling is needed especially when modification must be made in energy, sodium, fat, or other nutrient content (47).

Physical changes in the body that require alteration in the characteristics or consistency of food may force alteration in preferences. Loss of teeth or ill-fitting dentures may require alteration in the consistency and form of food before it can be eaten. Physical disabilities interfere with cutting or peeling foods. Fatigue prevents some elderly people from preparing food or eating sufficient amounts or variety to maintain nutritional status. There is a need to produce nutritious, inexpensive, single-serving, easily opened foods that require minimal effort in preparation for all age groups, but especially for the elderly. Their use of baby and junior foods indicates this need. In addition, culturally acceptable formulations and recipes that are high in micronutrient density proportionate to calories must be produced (48). However, no food should be specifically designed or recommended for the aged. Any food a person has been able to eat for a number of years and continues to tolerate should be allowed.

FOOD SERVICE. The manner of serving food varies from culture to culture. Appropriate temperature and method of preparation affect acceptance. A person may eat a fried oyster but not a raw one. Some prefer baked fish; others eat only fried fish.

Since many elderly use the side of the plate to push food onto the fork or spoon, a deep plate is a wise choice. Heavy mugs and glasses or those wide in diameter may be difficult to handle, especially for those with arthritic problems or other disabilities.

KNOWLEDGE. The aged are bombarded by nutrition information, much of it incorrect or unsubstantiated. This leads to expensive, wasteful, and often harmful nutritional regimens. The informational assault comes not only from outright faddists, but also from the persistent use of the mass media by self-serving sponsors who influence dietary practices to the detriment of the consumer (49).

Most elderly today were born before the discovery of vitamins. In their youth, the valued foods were bread, potatoes, and meat. Most fruits and vegetables were special treats or seasonal pleasures. Their period of formal education was completed before many major nutrients were discovered. Many of our elderly still carry the idea that the most important foods are meat, potatoes, and bread.

The greater percentage of rural families produced their own food supply which dictated the variety of foods available. Now the urbanized elderly are unable to produce their own foods. It is important to recognize these concepts in encouraging new food patterns.

SOCIAL SITUATIONS. Loss of self-esteem, isolation, and frustration may lead to refusal of food or to overeating and obesity. Many people who live alone have little interest in food preparation and eat snack foods or other convenience items. Some individuals do not know how to cook in small amounts.

Food also has social functions. Food and eating can be sources of esthetic and creative satisfaction. Religious observances and holiday traditions are often combined with food. In institutions for the elderly, residents often focus much of their interest and activity around meals. Food is important to basic feelings of security.

With no public or private transportation available, many elderly people must shop near home or rely on family or friends for assistance in shopping. Lack of transportation is common in rural areas. In cities, transportation systems may be too complex or fast moving for the elderly. Perishable foods may not be purchased because of reduced shopping trips.

INCOME. Large numbers of the elderly have incomes below the poverty level; in some studies, as many as 75 percent of the respondents. Limited income restricts the dietary choices. Poverty, disease, and malnutrition are an inseparable trio. Nutrition and health may be the most compressible items in a limited budget (49).

EXERCISE. Lack of physical activity may affect appetite. Exercise benefits pulmonary and circulatory function, helps preserve bones, maintains body weight, relieves depression and anxiety, and enhances self-esteem.

STATE OF HEALTH AND FOOD PROGRAMS. Illness and chronic disease can alter food patterns. Fatigue from illness or lack of an adequate diet can intensify the cycle of malnutrition. Poor health or poor nutrient intake may lead to irritability, moodiness, depression, and inability to make decisions.

Chronic brain syndrome and Alzheimer's disease may result in undesirable behavior that can affect nutritional status (50). Lapses in feeding behavior can result in refusal of food, objectionable eating habits, or consumption of inappropriate materials. Domestic skills may be impaired so that meals are not prepared, food spoils, or insufficient food is purchased. Lack of personal hygiene can result in contamination of food and digestive disturbances.

There are some federally funded programs designed to improve the nutritional status of the elderly. The Food Stamp Program is available to low-income persons. Food stamps are issued according to income and are redeemed for food at participating grocery stores. Feeding programs are provided under the Older Americans Act. A hot noon meal is served on weekdays, and the food must provide at least one-third of the RDA. Nutrition education and socialization are part of the program goals. Local communities operate home delivery programs using volunteers to deliver the food. Many churches, service clubs, and other groups have meal programs for older adults.

A Summary Note on Nutrition, Aging, and Health

Research on aging has demonstrated that aging and disease are not the same. The old are not necessarily diseased, and many illnesses in the elderly are treatable.

Good nutrition aids older people to be active and productive. The incidence of physical and emotional disability and need for medical attention increases with poor nutrition. Adequate diet is an effective means to maintain good health and minimize degenerative changes in old age.

In nutrition for the elderly we must consider the long-term effect of infant and childhood feeding. Level of nutrition in early postnatal or in post-weaning life affects rate of growth, maximum body size, development of age-associated changes, and the time of death in a variety of species of laboratory animals (51, 52, 53). Nutrition for a healthy old age must begin early in life.

Summary

The number of people who live to be old has increased in the United States. Aging is accompanied by a greater incidence of chronic diseases. Many social and psychological factors influence the ability of an individual to age well. Successful adaptation takes various routes; only a small part of the elderly population is institutionalized. The major problems are physical changes and isolation from others. The physiological changes that accompany age influence the ability to eat and to assimilate food. Included are general changes and changes in body composition; neuroendocrinisms; menopause; changes in the renal system, the digestive system, the pulmonary system, and the cardiovascular system; changes in the immune response; and changes in the ability to perform.

There are a number of theories on aging, but our information is still scanty. There are, however, data on nutritional needs for protein, energy, and vitamins and minerals in the later years.

references

1. *Special Report on Aging 1980.* U.S. Department of Health and Human Services, National Institutes of Health, National Institute of Aging, NIH Pub. No. 80-2135, 1980.
2. SHERWOOD, S. "Sociology of Food and Eating." *American Journal of Clincal Nutrition* 26 (1973): 1108.
3. SHOCK, N. W. "Physiologic Aspects of Aging." *Journal of the American Dietetic Association* 56 (1970): 491.
4. COMFORT, ALEX. *The Biology of Senescence,* 3rd ed. New York: Elsevier, 1979.
5. YOUNG, V. R., W. D. PEREA, J. C. WINTERER, and N. S. SCRIMSHAW. "Protein and Amino Acid Requirements of the Elderly." In *Nutrition and Aging,* ed. M. Winick. New York: Wiley, 1976.
6. BANNER, EDWARD A. "The Menopause and Thereafter." *Postgraduate Medicine* 59 (1976): 174.
7. GOLDMAN, R., and M. ROCKSTEIN. *The Physiology and Pathology of Human Aging.* New York: Academic Press, 1975.
8. MANDERLY, J. L. "Effect of Age on Pulmonary Structure and Function." *Federation Proceedings* 38 (1979): 173.
9. LAKATTA, E. G. "Alterations in the Cardiovascular System That Occur in Advanced Age." *Federation Proceedings* 38: 163, 1979.
10. BABU, T. N., F. NAZIR, D. B. RAO, and A. A. LUISADA. "What Is 'Normal' Blood Pressure in the Aged?" *Geriatrics* 32 (1977): 73.
11. WEG, RUTH. *Nutrition and the Later Years.* Andrus Gerontology Center, University of Southern California Press, 1978.
12. TIMIRAS, P. S. *Developmental Physiology and Aging.* New York: Macmillan, 1972.
13. HAYNES, S. G., and M. FEINLEIB. *Second Conference on the Epidemiology of Aging.* U. S. Department of Health and Human Services, Public Health Service, National Institutes of Health, National Institute on Aging, National Heart, Lung, and Blood Institute. NIH Publication No. 80-969, July 1980.
14. BROGDON, H. G., and B. B. ALFORD. "Food Preferences in Relation to Dietary Intake and Adequacy in Nursing Home Population." *Gerontologist* 13 (1973): 354.
15. MADDEN, J. P., S. J. GOODMAN, and H. A. GUTHRIE. "Validity of the 24-hour Recall. Analysis of Data Obtained from Elderly Subjects." *Journal of the American Dietetic Association* 68 (1976): 143.
16. O'HANLON, P. O., and M. B. KOHRS. "Dietary Studies of Older Americans." *American Journal of Clinical Nutrition* 31 (1978): 1257.

17. HOWEL, S. C., and M. B. LEOB. "Nutrition and Aging: A Monograph for Practitioners." *Gerontologist* 9 (1969): 1.

18. *Preliminary Findings of the First Health and Nutrition Examination Survey, United States, 1971–1972, Dietary Intake and Biochemical Findings.* DHEW (HRA) 76-1219.

19. PASSMORE, R., B. M. NICHOL, and N. RAO. *Handbook of Human Nutritional Requirements.* No. 28-61, Food and Agricultural Organization of the United Nations, Rome, 1974.

20. ZANNI, E., D. H. CALLOWAY, and A. Y. ZEZULLA. "Protein Requirements of Elderly Men." *Journal of Nutrition* 109 (1979): 513.

21. SCRIMSHAW, N. S., W. D. PEREA, and V. R. YOUNG. "Protein Requirements of Man: Obligatory Urinary and Fecal Nitrogen Losses in Elderly Women." *Journal of Nutrition* 106 (1976): 665.

22. PARSONS, V. "What Decreasing Renal Function Means to Aging Patients." *Geriatrics* 32 (1977): 93.

23. BEISEL, W. R. "Magnitude of the Host Nutritional Response to Infection." *American Journal of Clinical Nutrition* 30 (1977): 1236.

24. MACLENNAN, W. J., P. MARTIN, and B. J. MASON. "Protein Intake and Serum Albumin Levels in the Elderly." *Gerontology* 23 (1977): 360.

25. JORDAN, V. E. "Protein Status of the Elderly as Measured by Dietary Intake, Hair Tissue, and Serum Albumin." *American Journal of Clinical Nutrition* 29 (1976): 522.

26. CLARKE, M., and L. M. WAKEFIELD. "Food Choices of Institutionalized vs. Independent-Living Elderly." *Journal of the American Dietetic Association* 66 (1975): 600.

27. BROWN, E. L. "Factors Influencing Food Choices and Intake." *Geriatrics.* 31 (1976): 89.

28. GARCIA, P. A., G. E. BATTESE, and W. D. BREWER. "Longitudinal Study of Age and Cohort Influences on Dietary Patterns." *Journal of Gerontology* 30 (1975): 349.

29. JUSTICE, C. L., J. M. HOWE, and H. E. CLARK. "Dietary Intakes and Nutritional Status of Elderly Patients: Study in a Private Nursing Home." *Journal of the American Dietetic Association* 65 (1974): 639.

30. GUTHRIE, H. A., K. BLACK, and J. P. MADDEN. "Nutritional Practices of Elderly Citizens in Rural Pennsylvania." *Gerontology* 12 (1972): 380.

31. JOERING, E. "Nutrient Contribution of a Meals Program for Senior Citizens." *Journal of the American Dietetic Association.* 59 (1971): 129.

32. *Ten-State Nutrition Survey 1968 to 1970.* DHEW Publication No. 72-8130-34, Washington, D.C., 1972.

33. BURR, M. L., P. C. ELWOOD, D. J. HALE, R. J. JURLEY, and R. E. HUGHES. "Plasma and Leukocyte Ascorbic Acid Levels in the Elderly." *American Journal of Clinical Nutrition* 27 (1974): 144.

34. ALBANESE, A. A. "Calcium Nutrition in the Elderly: Maintaining Bone Health to Minimize Fracture Risk." *Postgraduate Medicine* 63 (1978): 167.

35. JUDGE, T. G., and N. R. COWAN. "Dietary Potassium Intake and Grip Strength in Older People." *Gerontologia Clinica* 13 (1971): 221.

36. Bistrian, B. R. "Interaction of Nutrition and Infection in the Hospital Setting." *American Journal of Clinical Nutrition* 30 (1977): 1223.

37. Bird, T., M. R. P. Hall, and R. O. K. Schade. "Gastric Histology and Its Relation to Anemia in the Elderly." *Gerontology* 23 (1977): 309.

38. Gershoff, S. N., O. A. Brusis, H. V. Nino, and A. M. Huber. "Studies of the Elderly in Boston. 1. The Effects of Iron Fortification on Moderately Anemic People." *American Journal of Clinical Nutrition* 30 (1977): 226.

39. Gregor, J. L. "Dietary Intake and Nutritional Status in Regard to Zinc of Institutionalized Aged." *Journal of Gerontology* 32 (1977): 549.

40. Barrows, C. H. "Nutrition and Aging: The Time Has Come to Move from Laboratory Research to Clinical Studies." *Geriatrics* 32 (1977): 39.

41. Tobias, A. L., and T. B. Vanitallie. "Nutritional Problems of Hospitalized Patients." *Journal of the American Dietetic Association* 71 (1977): 253.

42. Harken, D. E. "Malnutrition: A Poorly Understood Surgical Risk Factor in Aged Cardiac Patients." *Geriatrics* 32 (1977): 83.

43. Burkitt, D. P., and P. Meisner. "How To Manage Constipation with a High Fiber Diet." *Geriatrics* 34 (1979): 33.

44. Schiffman, S. S. "Changes in Taste and Smell in Old Persons." *Advances in Research,* vol. 2. Durham, N. C.: Duke University, 1978.

45. Cohen, T., and L. Gitman. "Oral Complaints and Taste Perception in the Aged." *Journal of Gerontology* 14 (1959): 294.

46. Boykin, L. S. "Soul Foods for Some Older Americans." *Journal of the American Geriatric Society* 22 (1975): 380.

47. Young, C. M. "Nutritional Counseling for Better Health." *Geriatrics* 29 (1974): 83.

48. Mann, G. V. "Relationship of Age to Nutrient Requirements." *American Journal of Clinical Nutrition* 26 (1973): 1096.

49. Watkin, D. M., and G. V. Mann. "Nutrition for the Aged: A Summation." *American Journal of Clinical Nutrition* 26 (1973): 1159.

50. Isaacs, B. "The Evaluation of Drugs in Alzheimer's Disease." *Age and Aging* 9 (1979): 137.

51. Leto, S., G. C. Kokkonen, and C. H. Barrows, Jr. "Dietary Protein, Life-Span and Biochemical Variables in Female Mice." *Journal of Gerontology* 31 (1976): 144.

52. Ross, M. H. "Protein, Calories and Life Expectancy." *Federation Proceedings* 18 (1959): 1190.

53. McCay, C. M., M. F. Cromwell, and L. A. Maynard. "The Effect of Retarded Growth upon the Length of Life Span and upon the Ultimate Body Size." *Journal of Nutrition* 10 (1935): 63.

SECTION 11

IMPORTANT NUTRITIONAL CONCERNS DURING THE LIFE CYCLE

CHAPTER 7

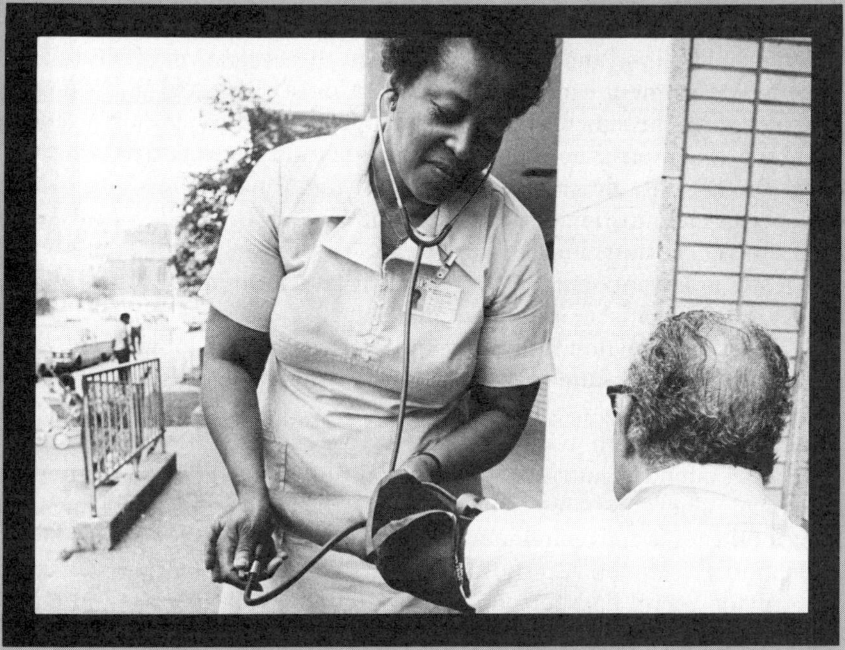

Photo courtesy of the New York Heart Association

assessing nutritional status

Assessment of the nutritional status of an individual should be part of all routine health examinations and should be used in the evaluation of all data collected. Nutrition assessment can confirm or reject most suspected nutritional deficiencies, including the subclinical ones when proper techniques are selected. Nutritional status demonstrates the relationship of food consumed to utilization by the body. Dietary data describe eating patterns and may or may not coincide with evidence of malnutrition; biochemical, anthropometric, and clinical data are necessary to reflect nutritional status. *Nutritional status* describes the body, not the diet. Only in advanced stages of malnutrition will there be a strong correlation between dietary intake and nutritional status.

Other information important in determining nutritional status includes a general evaluation of the social environment and health history of the individual or group, the availability of money for food and environmental sanitation, medical problems, and emotional factors.

Assessment of nutritional status can be conducted on a community or an individual. There are similarities and differences in both types of assessment. Some of the tools and techniques are the same, with differences in application and evaluation. For example, certain methods are too general for use with individuals, but provide useful data for populations. Some techniques are too costly to use with groups, but may add significant information for research or treatment of individuals with disease (1).

Nutritional assessment is part of the current effort to determine needs, evaluate feeding programs, and assess the state of health of groups and individuals. The basic goal of an assessment determines the techniques to be used. Other factors involved include time, available facilities and personnel, and money.

Community Assessment

Knowledge of the nutritional status of populations has been gained from over thirty national surveys in Asia, Africa, Europe, and the Americas conducted by the Interdepartmental Committee on Nutrition for National Defense of the United States (ICNND), which published a comprehensive manual for nutritional surveys. Community nutrition surveys have been conducted by the Food and Agriculture Organization (FAO), the World Health Organization (WHO), and the

United Nations Children's Emergency Fund (UNICEF), all United Nations organizations. The United States has obtained data through the Agency for International Development (AID) and the Interdepartmental Committee on Nutrition for National Defense. After the World War II, many new nations were established. Surveys were devoted to the unique nutritional problems of the country, the scarcity and abundance of food, and specific nutritional deficiencies in the general population and specific subgroups.

In the late 1960s children and some adults in low-income groups in various parts of the United States seemed to be hungry or malnourished. A national nutrition survey was organized using the guidelines for international studies. Regions of the country were selected for study, and the result was the TEN-State Nutrition Survey. Subsequently, the National Center for Health Statistics established a continuing national surveillance system to measure the nutritional status of the U.S. population and to monitor changes in the status over time. The Health and Nutrition Examination Survey (HANES) selected a population sample to represent the total population between ages 1 and 74 years (3). Included with the general population were certain groups at risk of malnutrition—the poor, preschool children, women of childbearing age, and the elderly. HANES used dietary intake (kind and quantity of food consumed and its nutritional value), biochemical tests of blood and urine for nutrients and related substances, clinical examinations by doctors and dentists, and various body measurements.

Conducting a successful nutrition survey requires fulfilling several conditions. These include a clear statement of objectives, which influences the choice of appropriate sampling; the utilization of valid methods for the assessment of nutritional status; and accurate analysis and utilization of the data collected. The larger the population group to be studied and the more intensively it is studied, the greater the cost. All nutrition surveys, of course, are subject to financial and technical constraints.

types of studies

Comprehensive epidemiological surveys are used when baseline data are needed for intervention programs. Where baseline data are assumed or known, surveys of a more limited scope may be conducted. Surveys can be limited by studying fewer members of the population or smaller age ranges, or by measuring only certain parameters. Some studies include only certain nutrients or anthropometric factors. A small survey can involve a particular sex, socioeconomic group, or geographic location.

Nutrition surveys can be a tool for evaluating the effectiveness of feeding or nutrition education programs. Another type of group assessment is called *nutrition surveillance.* It identifies changes in nutritional status or dietary intake (4). Inventories of food supply, food stock disappearance rates, consumption patterns, and anthropometric measurements are among the methods used in nutrition surveillance.

When studying the food intake of a population, it is important to determine more than the average intake, which usually fails to identify the proportion of the population with poor food intake. Percentile distributions are often a useful form of presenting data (see Figure 7–1) because they allow identification of those more likely to be malnourished. Another method of interpreting data is cross correlation of related measures. This procedure identifies the proportion of the population at risk according to dietary data, clinical signs, or biochemical measures alone, and those at risk according to a combination of factors.

Another important consideration in evaluating nutritional data on populations is the method of gathering age-related information. The two primary methods are: 1) cross-sectional studies, a one-time assessment of people of different ages; and 2) longitudinal assessments, repeated measurement of a group of individuals over an extended period of time. Most of the data we have currently are cross-sectional because they are much easier to collect. But they present a number of problems because ours is a rapidly changing society. Those who are elderly today, for example, had a very different food supply and environment in their early childhood years than the children of today; therefore, when today's children become elderly, they may exhibit very different nutritional problems and habits. Longitudinal studies offer the advantage of accuracy of ages, genetic homogeneity, and simultaneous correlation with history and background (diet, illnesses, previous socioeconomic circumstances). However, they require years of careful supervision and collection of data.

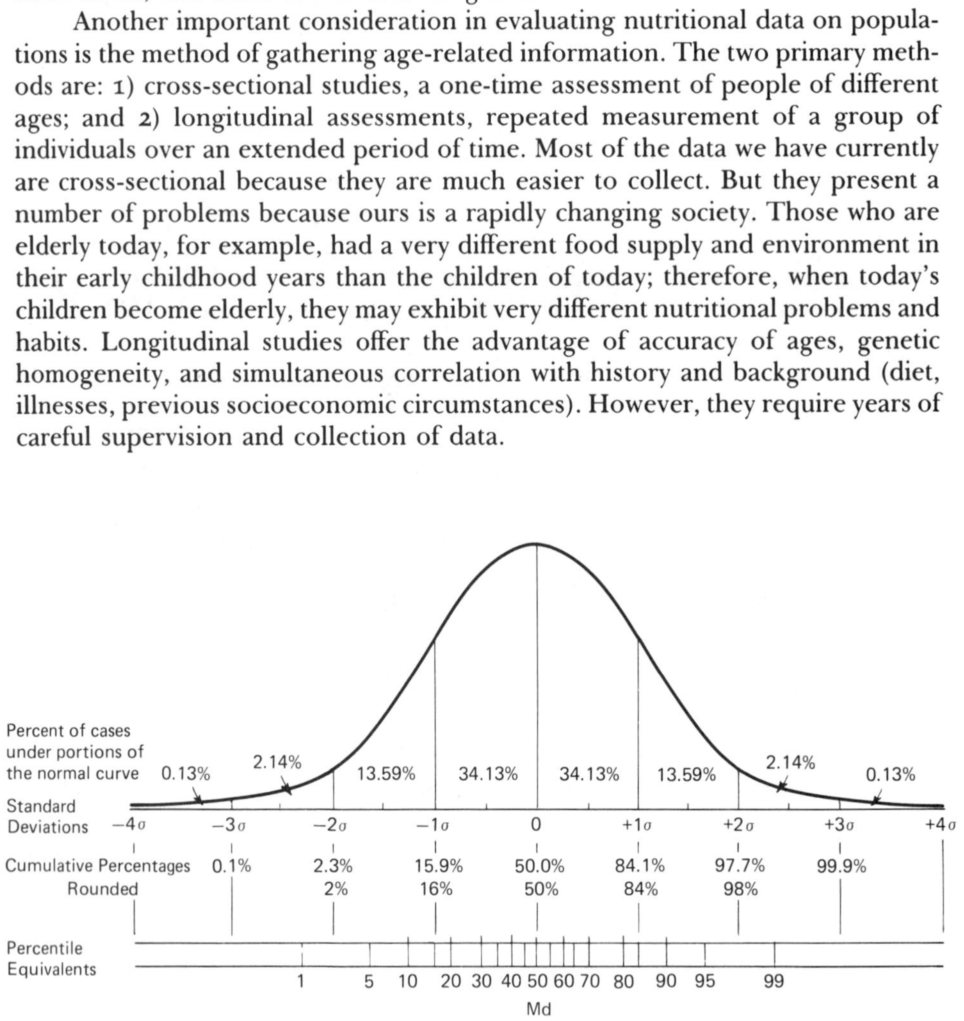

FIG. 7–1. Percentile and standard deviation show how a measurement deviates from the mean in a set of measurements. With a set of measurements, percentiles can be converted to standard or the reverse. The standard deviations and the percentage of measurements under each portion are shown for the normal curve.

Individual Assessment

In assessing individual nutritional status, available resources often dictate the methods used. The most standardized method available should be selected. Standardization increases the level of confidence of the data obtained and allows comparison with data on different populations or of an individual to norms.

The process of determining nutritional status should begin with the most simple procedures and move toward the more complex ones. The methods include clinical examination, anthropometric measurements, biochemical studies, and collection of dietary information (5). As an initial step in assessing nutritional status, current dietary intake should be determined. This current dietary intake should be related to lifetime habits and eating patterns through the use of historical methods such as the dietary history developed by Beal (6). Let us look first at how dietary assessment is done, and then at anthropometric measurements and clinical techniques.

dietary assessment

TWENTY-FOUR HOUR RECALL. A popular method of assessing current food intake is the 24-hour recall (7, 8, 9). This method involves asking the person what foods have been consumed during the last 24 hours. A structured form is usually used to record the information (10). One widely used form is divided by meals, with snacks grouped at the end or spaced between the meals. Because vocabulary for meals varies among localities and groups in a given community, sometimes the forms designate times of the day, such as morning, mid-morning, noon, afternoon, and night. The least structured forms give instructions but no meal divisions. Such forms are useful in determining if people eat meals in a traditional pattern or follow a small and frequent meal or snack plan. This form usually has a column for the time of consumption.

In collecting recall data, some interviewers begin with the last meal and work backward for the 24 hours; other interviewers begin at the other end and work forward to the last meal consumed. On all types of forms, additional information needs to be incorpoated: is this a typical or nontypical meal, recent significant changes in food patterns, and data on frequency.

The interviewing techniques and rapport established with the person affect the quality of the information obtained. Training and practice sessions are important in acquiring the necessary skills to obtain reliable data. An accepting, nonjudgmental attitude and skill in encouragement are important. The person being interviewed should understand the purpose of the history or dietary recall. The person must know that the reliability of the information depends on the individual.

The reliability of the serving size recorded on the 24-hour recall can be increased by use of food models. Moore et al. have reported an inexpensive system of making food models by using paraffin, rice, and beans(11). Models representing various portion sizes can be made to help people identify the serving sizes they usually eat. Research has shown this is vital because many people assume that the amount they consume is a "normal serving size." The typical example is a four-cup mixing bowl used for a serving of ice cream and reported as a normal serving, when the normal serving size is actually one-half cup. The reported amount is eight times what would be an average serving size in a food composition table.

There are some problems with the 24-hour recall technique. The recall can sometimes be a psychological test based on ability to remember. Some people tend to describe what they think they should have eaten. Many people do not accurately observe what they eat, or the amount of food consumed. Periods longer than 24 hours further reduce the accuracy of the recall and should not be used.

FOOD RECORDS. Food intake can also be determined by means of a written record of all food eaten maintained by an individual for a specified period of time. The length of the food record is determined by the purpose of the assessment. One-day diet records are more satisfactory for collecting information about groups than for individuals, because individuals fluctuate widely in daily food consumption patterns. On some days intakes are considerably less than the long-term average, and on other days intakes are more. The variability will be greater in one-day diet records than in three- to seven-day records. So periods of from three to seven days are needed to make an accurate evaluation. Three days that include a weekend day or one atypical day of the week is adequate. For long-term changes in food habits, food records may be maintained for weeks or even months. Once a person begins recording food eaten, the awareness of the quantity or quality of the diet often results in changed intake.

Detailed instructions for recording are necessary, and completed sample records may be helpful. Accuracy is improved by providing sets of measuring cups and spoons, as well as a ruler. The use of scales further increases accuracy. In addition, the food record should be reviewed with the individual to determine its completeness. A well-done food record is an accurate and economical assessment tool.

Forms for the records vary with the goals of the assessment, but should include as a minimum the food eaten, time consumed, amount eaten, and method of food preparation. A reminder to include all beverages, seasonings, condiments, and other items should be on every page. Failure to record fats, sugar, sauces, jellies, and so on will result in underestimation of caloric intake. Information on feeding, activity, or site of consumption is often collected as well.

The problem with correlating dietary intake to individual biochemical or clinical studies is that the dietary intake record may represent a short period of time, while clinical and biochemical studies show the results of long-term nutrient intake. Short-term studies of dietary intake for groups, however, show more correlation with biochemical and clinical observations than those for individuals.

INTAKE OBSERVATION. Observation assures the assessor that the intake data are accurate; but this one-to-one procedure is very expensive and time-consuming. Only a few people can be observed. The number can be increased slightly by premeasuring food and serving it on trays. The remains of the food can be measured to determine consumption as long as the trays are closely monitored. Subjects must be placed in a controlled environment. Often a parent or caretaker serves as the observer. But many adults and children change their consumption patterns when they are observed, and some foods may be eliminated or appetite lost when people pay close attention to their food intake. So observation may not yield accurate information.

EVALUATION OF INTAKE. Determining the adequacy of dietary intake is usually more successful for groups than for individuals. The purpose of evaluation is to identify problems that need further study or trends that need positive reinforcement. The simplest standard for comparison is with a food grouping, as shown in Appendix Table A–3. A checklist can be developed to rank the quality of food intake to the extent that it meets serving requirements. If dietary inadequacy is indicated by the checklist, then a more comprehensive form of evaluation may be needed.

A rating based on the Recommended Daily Allowances or the FAO standards (see Appendix) may be used. Both guides were developed for groups, and thus are limited for individual application. Usually, a healthy individual who meets two-thirds of the RDA for all nutrients except energy and possibly protein has an adequate intake. The RDA has a margin of safety and does not represent minimum needs or requirements; the FAO standards are closer to requirement or minimum needs. The standards used in the HANES (3) study are shown in Table 7–1.

anthropometric measures

Anthropometric measurements are noninvasive, relatively easy to perform, and inexpensive. The most common measures are height, weight, skinfold thickness, mid arm circumference, and head circumference. Guidelines are necessary for obtaining these measurements, since they are subject to error from poor technique, inaccurate instruments, and incorrect readings and recordings. The value of these measures depends entirely on the accuracy with which they are done and the standards to which they are compared. Except for height, weight, and head circumference, anthropometric measurements are not yet adequately standardized; much additional work needs to be done in this area.

GROWTH CHARTS. Anthropometry is an effective screening procedure for child health and nutrition, but the accuracy and reliability of physical growth data depend on the method of recording and interpretation (12). The National Center for Health Statistics (NCHS) growth charts can indicate potential nutritional problems and facilitate comparison of one group of children with another (13). These growth

TABLE 7-1. Standards for Evaluation of Daily Dietary Intake Used in the Health and Nutrition Examination Survey, United States, 1971–1972

AGE AND SEX	CALORIES (per kg)	PROTEIN (gm per kg)	CALCIUM (mg)	IRON (mg)	VITAMIN A (IU)[a]	VITAMIN C (mg)
1–5 years						
12–23 months, male and female	90	1.9	450	15	2,000	40
24–47 months, male and female	86	1.7	450	15	2,000	40
48–71 months, male and female	82	1.5	450	10	2,000	40
6–7 years, male and female	82	1.3	450	10	2,500	40
8–9 years, male and female	82	1.3	450	10	2,500	40
10–12 years						
Male	68	1.2	650	10	2,500	40
Female	64	1.2	650	18	2,500	40
13–16 years						
Male	60	1.2	650	18	3,500	50
Female	48	1.2	650	18	3,500	50
17–19 years						
Male	44	1.1	550	18	3,500	55
Female	35	1.1	550	18	3,500	50
20–29 years						
Male	40	1.0	400	10	3,500	60
Female	35	1.0	600	18	3,500	55
30–39 years						
Male	38	1.0	400	10	3,500	60
Female	33	1.0	600	18	3,500	55
40–49 years						
Male	37	1.0	400	10	3,500	60
Female	31	1.0	600	18	3,500	55
50–54 years						
Male	36	1.0	400	10	3,500	60
Female	30	1.0	600	18	3,500	55
55–59 years						
Male	36	1.0	400	10	3,500	60
Female	30	1.0	600	10	3,500	55
60–69 years						
Male	34	1.0	400	10	3,500	60
Female	29	1.0	600	10	3,500	55

TABLE 7-1. (Continued)

AGE AND SEX	CALORIES (per kg)	PROTEIN (gm per kg)	CALCIUM (mg)	IRON (mg)	VITAMIN A (IU)[a]	VITAMIN C (mg)
70 years and over						
Male	34	1.0	400	10	3,500	60
Female	29	1.0	600	10	3,500	55
Pregnancy (fifth month and beyond), add to basic standard	200	20	200		1,000	5[b]
Lactating, add to basic standard	1,000	25	500		1,000	5

[a]Assumed 70 percent carotene, 30 percent retinol.

[b]For all pregnant women.

SOURCE: U.S. Department of Health, Education and Welfare, National Center for Health Statistics, *Preliminary Findings of the First Health and Nutrition Examination Survey, United States, 1971–1972* (Washington, D.C.: Superintendent of Documents, 1979).

charts appear in the Appendix. Age of the child must be known for the height and weight charts, but not for the weight-length chart. Until the charts were prepared by the NCHS for assessing the physical growth of children in the United States, the only available data had been collected early in this century by Stuart in Boston and Meredith in Iowa from white, middle- and upper-class children of Northern European ancestry living in a limited geographic region. The NCHS growth curves represent percentile ranks for all contemporary American children of the same age and sex.

Racial, socioeconomic, and geographic variability have been documented in an extensive series of publications by NCHS that permit adjustment of normal limits for children from various segments of the population. The extreme percentiles ($<$ 5th and $>$ 95th) on the charts can be used as indicators to suspect health or nutritional problems sufficiently severe to impair growth. In nutrition screening programs, percentiles can be used to determine whether or not follow-ups should be undertaken. Growth is within normal limits by current standards when values follow the central or median percentile, between the 25th and 75th. Comparison of growth assessment of one population with another can be very precise when it is made using a common reference. For example, when a 4-year-old girl is found to be at the fifth NCHS percentile for body weight or stature, wherever she lives in the world, she is smaller than 95 percent of the 4-year-old girls in the United States. This kind of anthropometric classification is an essential early step in evaluating growth and nutritional status.

Standard growth charts show percentile curves for body weight and stature. The data are plotted to create a percentile distribution of weight for length or weight for stature, not a ratio of weight divided by length. The relationship is assumed to be independent of age until the marked change in body proportion that begins in early pubescence. Where birth date or age is unknown or unreliable, these curves may serve their most important applied use. Stature and chronological age are used in the construction of charts for older children because data were not available on the presence or absence of the clinical signs of pubescence for all sets of measurements in the population. The weight for stature charts are appropriate for plotting values for most prepubescent boys and girls regardless of chronological age, but not for a child showing signs of pubescence, such as breast enlargement, testicular development, or coarsening and pigmentation of axillary and pubic hair.

Normal growth is measured between the 25th and 75th percentiles. Crossing percentiles within this range is not unusual during growth. Measurements between the 10th and 25th and the 75th and 90th percentiles may or may not be normal depending on previous measurements and on genetic or environmental factors. Values above the 90th and below the 10th percentile should be carefully checked for measurement and recording accuracy. If accurate, these children need much more careful evaluations. Measurements above the 95th and below the 5th percentile should be given priority for further investigation. When height is above the 10th percentile but weight is below the 5th, nutritional deficiency may be suspected. Weight for height greater than the 95th percentile suggests obesity, although not necessarily. The weight can be due to good muscle development, especially in the athlete.

Growth charting is a screening and classifying procedure, not a diagnostic one (14). Small size may reflect impaired growth or undernutrition, or it can be related to small ancestors or slow but normal rate of maturation. This technique must be used in conjunction with other means of evaluating nutritional status.

HEIGHT AND WEIGHT. The basic measurement for all ages must include height and weight. For infants and children, techniques and standards are well established. For adults, height and weight charts have been developed by insurance companies (see Appendix). In addition, NCHS is preparing height and weight standards for adults.

Height is measured without shoes with the individual standing on a flat, stable surface with feet parallel and with heels, buttocks, shoulders, and back of head touching an upright surface such as a wall. Accuracy is increased by use of a wide board placed on the head and extending to a vertical scale (see Figure 7–2). The height measuring device on standard weight scales is too narrow and unsteady for accurate results. Infant length is measured in a recumbent position. Two people are required to position the infant to obtain accurate and reliable length measurement. Length data on the birth to 36-month charts developed by the NCHS represent recumbent (not upright) length without shoes. Standing height or stature should not be plotted on the birth to 36-month chart. This will result in a child appearing shorter than recumbent length by as much as 2 cm or more (see Figure 7–3).

Weight is measured on scales with a platform wide enough to be comfortable. For those unable to stand, there are chair or bed scales. Infants are weighed in a reclining position. Accurate scales are important and should be checked by standard weights frequently. Usually light clothing is worn, except for infants, who are weighed nude.

SKINFOLD MEASUREMENT. Subcutaneous fat is measured by using skinfold calipers such as the Lange or Harpenden.[1] The instrument exerts a constant pressure, has a standard contact surface, and is accurate to 0.1 mm. A double layer of skin and subcutaneous fat is included in the pinch, but no muscle. The usual sites are the back of the upper midarm (the triceps) and the base of the shoulder blade on the back (the subscapular). Measurements are made on the left side of the body. For undernutrition and obesity, the triceps skinfold is the most practical for all ages. To determine the midpoint, bend the arm at a right angle over the stomach. Measure from the point where the arm joins the shoulder to the elbow and work

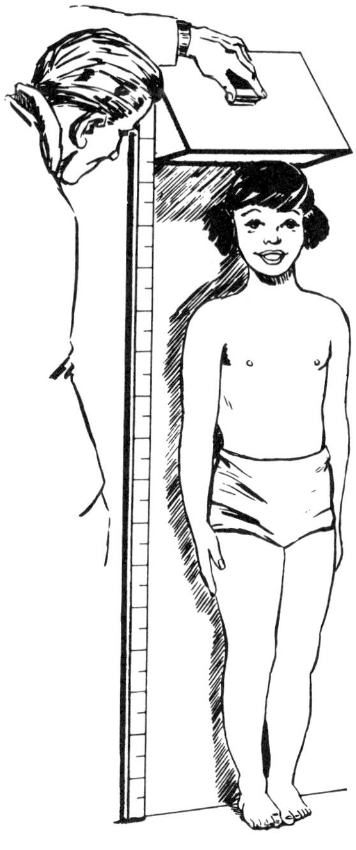

FIG. 7–2. Height measurement of schoolchild.

[1]Lange Skinfold Calipers, Cambridge Scientific Industries, Inc., Cambridge, Md.; Harpenden Skinfold Calipers, British Indicators, Ltd., St. Albans, Hertfordshire, England.

the midpoint for measurement at the back of the arm (see Figure 7–4). Then, a lengthwise skinfold is grasped firmly and lifted slightly between the index finger and thumb, avoiding the inclusion of underlying muscle (see Figure 7–5). Three measurements should be made and the results averaged. Training and practice are necessary for reliable results because of variability of pressure and grasp. Edema and softer fat increase compressibility and make measurement difficult.

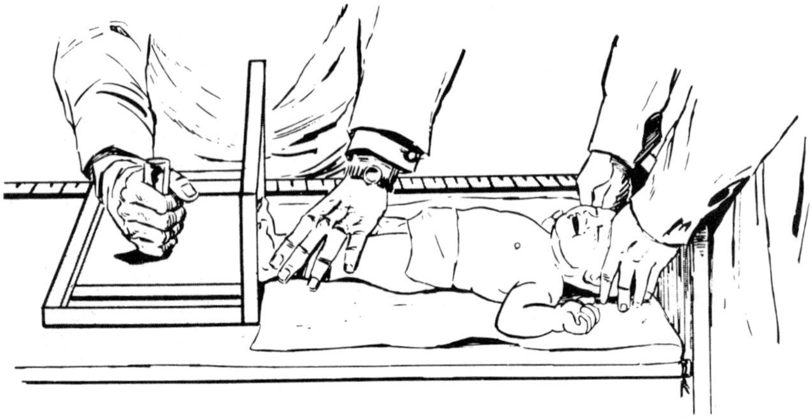

FIG. 7–3. Length measurement of infant.

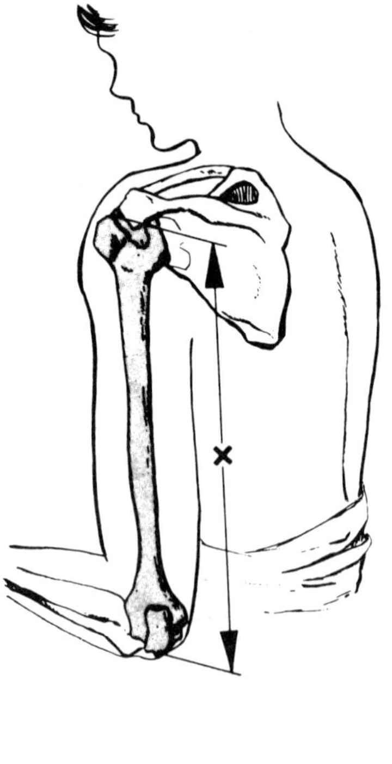

FIG. 7–4. Assessing midpoint of upper arm (halfway between the acromial process of the scapula and the olecranon process of the ulna).

Midarm circumference can indicate muscle mass and fatty tissue. With use of the skinfold measure, a reasonable estimation of the muscle is indicated. Measure with the arm hanging relaxed to the side. Use a flexible metal or non-stretch tape (see Figure 7–6). Measure to the nearest 0.1 cm, but avoid compression of soft tissue (15).

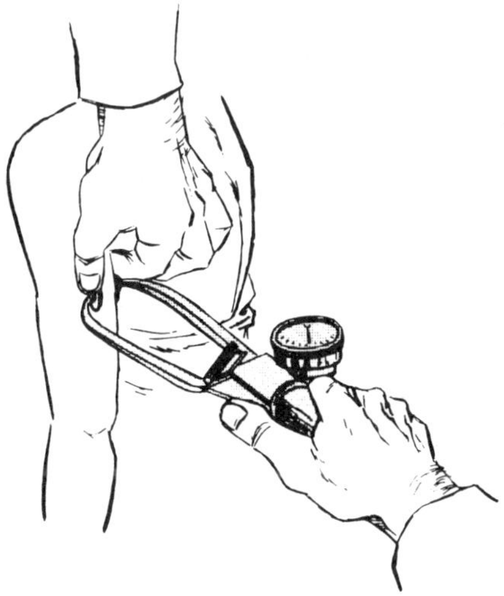

FIG. 7–5. Measurement of triceps skinfold with Harpenden Calipers.

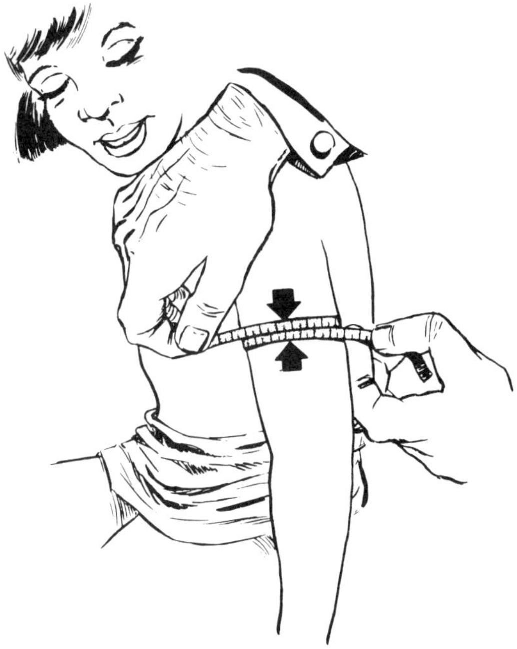

FIG. 7–6. Measurement of mid upper-arm circumference. *Source* (Figs. 7–2 – 7–6): D. B. Jelliffe, *The Assessment of the Nutritional Status of the Community* (Geneva: World Health Organization, 1966).

Measures of arm muscle are only estimates because of difference in bone thickness, bone shape, and compressibility of fat. Using the triceps skinfold and the arm circumference measurements, arm muscle circumference and arm muscle can be estimated. They may be derived mathematically or with the use of nomograms (see Figures 7–7, 7–8, and 7–9) (16). Some standards are available for both males and females of most ages, but additional work is needed in this area to establish standards for meaningful comparisons (17, 18) (see Tables 7–2, 7–3, and 7–4).

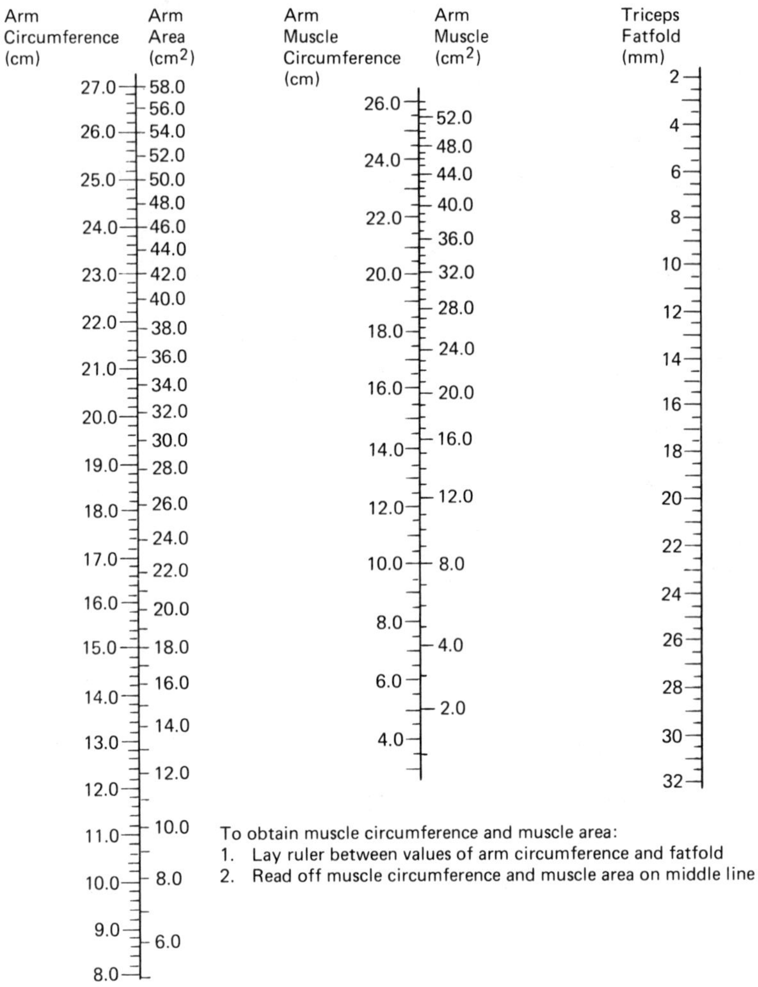

FIG. 7–7. Nomogram for the determination of arm muscle circumference and arm muscle area.

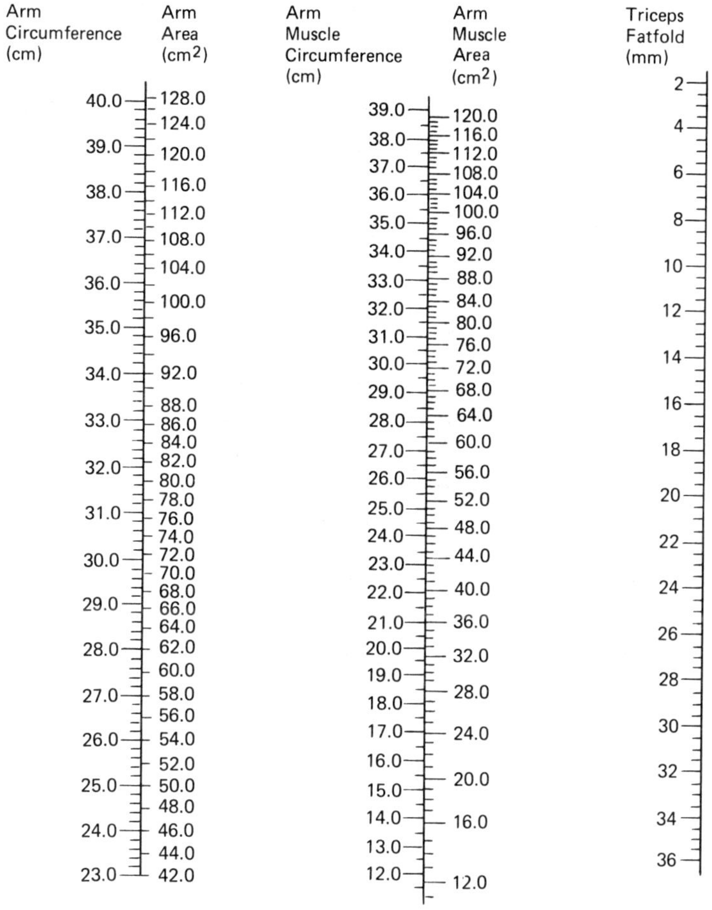

To obtain muscle circumference and muscle area:
1. Lay ruler between values of arm circumference and fatfold
2. Read off muscle circumference and muscle area on middle line

FIG. 7–8. Nomogram for determination of arm muscle circumference and arm muscle area. *Source* (Figs. 7–7 and 7–8): J. Gurney and D. Jelliffe, "Arm Anthropometry in Nutritional Assessment; Monogram for Rapid Calculation of Arm Muscle Circumference and Cross-sectional Muscle and Fat Areas," *American Journal of Clinical Nutrition* 26 (1973): 912. Reproduced with permission.

SKELETAL DEVELOPMENT. Greulich and Pyle have published a system of determining the maturation of the skeleton using X rays of the hand and wrist (19). From birth until growth is completed, minerals are deposited in the protein matrix. Stages of development can be assessed from the degree of development of ossification

Figure 7–9

example

triceps fatfold (from direct measurement) = 21 millimeters (mm)
arm circumference (from direct measurement) = 35 centimeters (cm)
arm muscle circumference (from nomogram) = 28.5 centimeters (cm)
arm muscle area (from nomogram) = 65 square centimeters (cm^2)

calculation of arm muscle circumference

Arm muscle circumference is derived mathematically using the following formula:

$C_m = C_a - \pi S$ where C_m = arm muscle circumference in centimeters

C_a = mid-upper arm circumference in centimeters

S = triceps fatfold in centimeters*

π = 3.14

*To use the formula, the fatfold value obtained with the calipers will need to be converted to centimeters (divide by 10).

example

C_a = 35 centimeters

S = 2.1 centimeters

$C_m = 35 - (3.14)(2.1)$

$= 35 - 6.59$

$= 28.4$ centimeters

calculation of arm muscle area

Arm muscle area can be calculated by the following formula:

$M = \frac{(C_a - \pi S)^2}{4\pi}$ where M = arm muscle area in square centimeters

C_a = mid-upper arm circumference in centimeters

S = triceps fatfold in centimeters

π = 3.14

centers (see Figures 7–10 and 7–11). All centers are mineralized when growth is completed. White middle-class children were the population for standard development. Tanner et al. developed a different standard for British children (20). These standards for skeletal mass and bone mineral are not appropriate for American blacks (21). The American black of largely African ancestry is of smaller size at birth, but of greater size from 2 to 14 years; has advanced skeletal development for bone age; and has advanced dental development. The skeletal mass and bone density of blacks is larger, and a lesser rate of adult bone loss is found in the black female after age 40.

Bone density measurements can indicate the degree of mineralization of bones. The common techniques for measuring bone density are X rays or the

TABLE 7–2. Percentiles for Upper Arm Circumference and Triceps Skinfolds for Whites of the Ten-State Nutrition Survey of 1968–1970

age group	age midpoint, years	No.	arm circumference percentiles, mm					triceps skinfold percentiles, mm				
			5th	15th	50th	85th	95th	5th	15th	50th	85th	95th
MALES												
0.0–0.4	0.3	41	113	120	134	147	153	4	5	8	12	15
0.5–1.4	1	140	128	137	152	168	175	5	7	9	13	15
1.5–2.4	2	177	141	147	157	170	180	5	7	10	13	14
2.5–3.4	3	210	144	150	161	175	182	6	7	9	12	14
3.5–4.4	4	208	143	150	165	180	190	5	6	9	12	14
4.5–5.4	5	262	146	155	169	185	199	5	6	8	12	16
5.5–6.4	6	264	151	159	172	188	198	5	6	8	11	15
6.5–7.4	7	309	154	162	176	194	212	4	6	8	11	14
7.5–8.4	8	301	161	168	185	205	233	5	6	8	12	17
8.5–9.4	9	287	165	174	190	217	262	5	6	9	14	19
9.5–10.4	10	315	170	180	200	228	255	5	6	10	16	22
10.5–11.4	11	294	177	186	208	240	276	6	7	10	17	25
11.5–12.4	12	294	184	194	216	253	291	5	7	11	19	26
12.5–13.4	13	266	186	198	230	270	297	5	6	10	18	25
13.5–14.4	14	207	198	211	243	279	321	5	6	10	17	22
14.5–15.4	15	179	202	220	253	302	320	4	6	9	19	26
15.5–16.4	16	166	217	232	262	300	335	4	5	9	20	27
16.5–17.4	17	142	230	238	275	306	326	4	5	8	14	20
17.5–24.4	21	545	250	264	292	330	354	4	5	10	18	25
24.5–34.4	30	679	260	280	310	344	366	4	6	11	21	28
34.5–44.4	40	616	259	280	312	345	371	4	6	12	22	28
FEMALES												
0.0–0.4	0.3	46	107	118	127	145	150	4	5	8	12	13
0.5–1.4	1	172	125	134	146	162	170	6	7	9	12	15
1.5–2.4	2	172	136	143	155	171	180	6	7	10	13	15
2.5–3.4	3	163	137	145	157	169	176	6	7	10	12	14
3.5–4.4	4	215	145	150	162	176	184	5	7	10	12	14
4.5–5.4	5	233	149	155	169	185	195	6	7	10	13	16
5.5–6.4	6	259	148	158	170	187	202	6	7	10	12	15
6.5–7.4	7	273	153	162	178	199	216	6	7	10	13	17
7.5–8.4	8	270	158	166	183	207	231	6	7	10	15	19
8.5–9.4	9	284	166	175	192	222	255	6	7	11	17	24
9.5–10.4	10	276	170	181	203	236	263	6	8	12	19	24
10.5–11.4	11	268	173	186	210	251	280	7	8	12	20	29
11.5–12.4	12	267	185	196	220	256	275	6	9	13	20	25
12.5–13.4	13	229	186	204	230	270	294	7	9	14	23	30
13.5–14.4	14	184	201	214	240	284	306	8	10	15	22	28
14.5–15.4	15	197	205	216	245	281	310	8	11	16	24	30
15.5–16.4	16	187	211	224	249	286	322	8	10	15	23	27
16.5–17.4	17	142	207	224	250	291	328	9	12	16	26	31
17.5–24.4	21	836	215	233	260	297	329	9	12	17	25	31
24.5–34.4	30	1153	230	243	275	324	361	9	12	19	29	36
34.5–44.4	40	933	232	250	286	340	374	10	14	22	32	39

SOURCE: A. R. Frisancho, "Triceps Skinfold and Upper Arm Muscle Size Norms for Assessment of Nutritional Status," *American Journal of Clinical Nutrition* 27 (1974): 1054.

TABLE 7-3. Percentiles for Upper Arm Diameter and Upper Arm Circumference for Whites of the Ten-State Nutrition Survey of 1968–1970

age midpoint, years[a]	arm muscle, diameter percentiles, mm					arm muscle, circumference percentiles, mm				
	5th	15th	50th	85th	95th	5th	15th	50th	85th	95th
					MALES					
0.3	26	30	34	40	42	81	94	106	125	133
1	32	34	39	44	46	100	108	123	137	146
2	35	37	40	44	46	111	117	127	138	146
3	36	38	42	46	48	114	121	132	145	152
4	38	39	43	48	50	118	124	135	151	157
5	39	41	45	50	53	121	130	141	156	166
6	40	43	47	51	53	127	134	146	159	167
7	41	43	48	52	55	130	137	151	164	173
8	44	46	50	55	59	138	144	158	174	185
9	44	46	51	58	64	138	143	161	182	200
10	45	48	53	59	64	142	152	168	186	202
11	48	50	55	62	67	150	158	174	194	211
12	49	52	58	66	70	153	163	181	207	221
13	51	54	62	71	77	159	169	195	224	242
14	53	58	67	74	84	167	182	211	234	265
15	55	59	70	80	86	173	185	220	252	271
16	59	65	73	83	89	186	205	229	260	281
17	66	69	78	86	92	206	217	245	271	290
21	69	74	82	91	97	217	232	258	286	305
30	70	77	86	94	100	220	241	270	295	315
40	71	76	86	96	101	222	239	270	300	318
					FEMALES					
0.3	27	29	33	37	40	86	92	104	115	126
1	31	32	37	41	43	97	102	117	128	135
2	34	36	40	44	46	105	112	125	140	146
3	34	37	41	44	46	108	116	128	138	143
4	36	38	42	46	48	114	120	132	146	152
5	38	40	44	48	51	119	124	138	151	160
6	38	41	45	49	53	121	129	140	155	165
7	39	42	47	52	56	123	132	146	162	175
8	41	44	48	53	59	129	138	151	168	186
9	43	45	50	56	62	136	143	157	176	193
10	44	47	52	58	62	139	147	163	182	196
11	44	48	55	62	67	140	152	171	195	209
12	48	51	57	64	68	150	161	179	200	212
13	49	53	59	66	71	155	165	185	206	225
14	53	56	61	70	74	166	175	193	221	234
15	52	55	62	70	74	163	173	195	220	232
16	54	57	64	72	83	171	178	200	227	260
17	54	56	62	71	77	171	177	196	223	241
21	54	58	65	73	80	170	183	205	229	253
30	56	60	68	78	87	177	189	213	245	272
40	57	61	69	80	89	180	192	216	250	279

[a] The age group and *n* are the same as in Table 7–2.

SOURCE: A. R. Frisancho, "Triceps Skinfold and Upper Arm Muscle Size Norms for Assessment of Nutritional Status," *American Journal of Clinical Nutrition* 27 (1974): 1054.

TABLE 7-4. Percentiles for Arm Muscle Area of Whites Derived from the Ten-State Nutrition Survey of 1968-1970

age midpoint, year[a]	male arm, muscle area percentiles, mm					female arm, muscle area percentiles, mm				
	5th	15th	50th	85th	95th	5th	15th	50th	85th	95th
0.3	522	703	892	1,244	1,414	591	670	866	1,058	1,272
1	791	928	1,201	1,500	1,690	756	821	1,084	1,304	1,460
2	978	1,082	1,284	1,525	1,686	885	991	1,241	1,551	1,693
3	1,027	1,163	1,384	1,670	1,842	928	1,068	1,298	1,516	1,628
4	1,106	1,224	1,451	1,805	1,973	1,040	1,143	1,390	1,693	1,828
5	1,171	1,342	1,579	1,930	2,193	1,119	1,227	1,516	1,825	2,045
6	1,275	1,435	1,700	2,019	2,220	1,163	1,333	1,563	1,902	2,174
7	1,342	1,485	1,815	2,152	2,386	1,213	1,384	1,700	2,096	2,433
8	1,506	1,647	1,987	2,398	2,729	1,322	1,513	1,818	2,239	2,758
9	1,522	1,637	2,074	2,645	3,188	1,473	1,625	1,955	2,477	2,978
10	1,608	1,832	2,239	2,753	3,239	1,528	1,727	2,115	2,637	3,066
11	1,801	1,987	2,406	3,000	3,544	1,551	1,842	2,335	3,018	3,486
12	1,874	2,126	2,603	3,401	3,902	1,781	2,052	2,558	3,183	3,582
13	2,012	2,273	3,013	3,998	4,661	1,905	2,178	2,711	3,382	4,014
14	2,231	2,645	3,544	4,358	5,601	2,186	2,430	2,952	3,883	4,358
15	2,375	2,729	3,867	5,060	5,826	2,126	2,387	3,031	3,838	4,279
16	2,741	3,331	4,184	5,363	6,266	2,316	2,510	3,198	4,096	5,386
17	3,373	3,743	4,771	5,826	6,713	2,316	2,502	3,058	3,968	4,612
21	3,748	4,273	5,315	6,529	7,411	2,289	2,679	3,341	4,164	5,089
30	3,837	4,634	5,802	6,912	7,918	2,486	2,856	3,606	4,772	5,889
40	3,938	4,563	5,820	7,183	8,041	2,566	2,926	3,724	4,991	6,195

[a] The age group and *n* are the same as in Table 7-2.

SOURCE: A. R. Frisancho, "Triceps Skinfold and Upper Arm Muscle Size Norms for Assessment of Nutritional Status," *American Journal of Clinical Nutrition* 27 (1974): 1054.

photon absorption method using a radioactive iodine source usually known as the Cameron method (22, 23). Degree of mineral loss can be shown by serial bone density measures. However, these are not part of routine screening because of the expense and the technical difficulty.

clinical evaluation of nutritional problems

Nutritional deficiencies are usually shown by changes in the skin, eyes, oral cavity, skeletal system, or neuromuscular system. Clinical signs usually appear after the deficiency has become severe (see Table 7-5). Severe deficiencies are rare in the United States, so the clinical examiner must look for subtle changes in size, color,

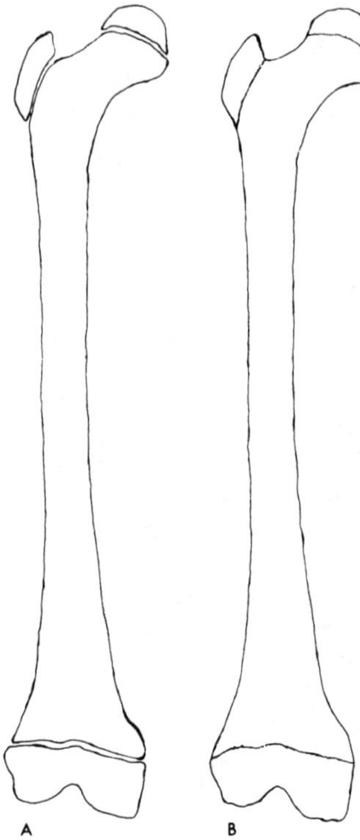

FIG. 7–10. Skeletal growth and maturation. Skeletal growth is the same for bones A and B; however, bone B is mature due to the fusion of the primary and secondary ossification centers which indicates the completion of growth. Growth and maturation are controlled by different hormones.

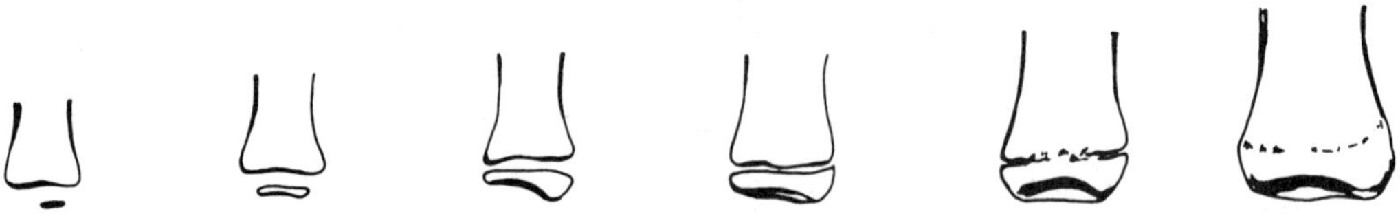

FIG. 7–11. Bone maturation. The stages from birth to maturity of bone maturation begin on the left with the appearance of the secondary ossification center and end with epiphyseal-diaphyseal fusion on the right.

or texture. Clinical screening should be performed by a physician or nurse practitioner who can distinguish between nutritional deficiencies and disease states that present symptoms similar to nutritional deficiencies. Subclinical deficiencies, those that cannot be seen by clinical examination, can be determined by laboratory assays.

biochemical assessment

Laboratory methods for assessment of nutritional status can provide more objective and precise approaches than dietary records or clinical assessment alone (24). Circulating levels of nutrients in the blood or urine may be measured, or

TABLE 7–5. Physical Signs Indicative or Suggestive of Malnutrition

body area	normal appearance	signs associated with malnutrition
Hair	Shiny; firm; not easily plucked	Lack of natural shine; hair dull and dry; thin and sparse; hair fine, silky and straight; color changes (flag sign); can be easily plucked
Face	Skin color uniform; smooth, pink, healthy appearance; not swollen	Skin color loss (depigmentation); skin dark over cheeks and under eyes (malar and supra-orbital pigmentation); lumpiness or flakiness of skin of nose and mouth; swollen face; enlarged parotid glands; scaling of skin around nostrils (nasolabial seborrhea)
Eyes	Bright, clear, shiny; no sores at corners or eyelids; membranes a healthy pink and are moist. No prominent blood vessels or mound of tissue or sclera	Eye membranes are pale (pale conjunctivae); redness of membranes (conjunctival injection); Bitot's spots; redness and fissuring of eyelid corners (angular palpebritis); dryness of eye membranes (conjunctival xerosis); cornea has dull appearance (corneal xerosis); cornea is soft (keratomalacia); scar on cornea; ring of fine blood vessels around corner (circumcorneal injection)
Lips	Smooth, not chapped or swollen	Redness and swelling of mouth or lips (cheilosis); especially at corners of mouth (angular fissures and scars)
Tongue	Deep red in appearance; not swollen or smooth	Swelling; scarlet and raw tongue; magenta (purplish color) of tongue; smooth tongue; swollen sores; hyperemic and hypertrophic papillae; and atrophic papillae
Teeth	No cavities; no pain; bright	May be missing or erupting abnormally; gray or black spots (fluorosis); cavities (caries)
Gums	Healthy; red; do not bleed; not swollen	"Spongy" and bleed easily; recession of gums
Glands	Face not swollen	Thyroid enlargement (front of neck); parotid enlargement (cheeks become swollen)
Skin	No signs of rashes, swellings; dark or light spots	Dryness of skin (xerosis); sandpaper feel of skin (follicular hyperkeratosis); flakiness of skin; skin swollen and dark; red swollen pigmentation of exposed areas (pellagrous dermatosis); excessive lightness or darkness of skin (dyspigmentation); black and blue marks due to skin bleeding (petechiae); lack of fat under skin
Nails	Firm, pink	Nails are spoon-shape (koilonychia); brittle, ridged nails

TABLE 7-5. (Continued)

body area	normal appearance	signs associated with malnutrition
Muscular and skeletal system	Good muscle tone; some fat under skin; can walk or run without pain	Muscles have "wasted" appearance; baby's skull bones are thin and soft (craniotabes); round swelling of front and side of head (frontal and parietal bossing); swelling of ends of bones (epiphyseal enlargement); small bumps on both sides of chest wall (on ribs)—beading of ribs; baby's soft spot on head does not harden at proper time (persistently open anterior fontanelle); knock-knees or bow-legs; bleeding into muscle (musculoskeletal hemorrhages); person cannot get up or walk properly
Internal Systems:		
Cardiovascular	Normal heart rate and rhythm; no murmurs or abnormal rhythms; normal blood pressure for age	Rapid heart rate (above 100 tachycardia); enlarged heart; abnormal rhythm; elevated blood pressure
Gastrointestinal	No palpable organs or masses (in children, however, liver edge may be palpable)	Liver enlargement; enlargement of spleen (usually indicates other associated diseases)
Nervous	Psychological stability; normal reflexes	Mental irritability and confusion; burning and tingling of hands and feet (paresthesia); loss of position and vibratory sense; weakness and tenderness of muscles (may result in inability to walk); decrease and loss of ankle and knee reflexes

SOURCE: G. Christakis, "Nutritional Assessment in Health Programs," *American Journal of Public Health* 63 (1973): part 2, supplement.

functional tests made. The third form of testing involves providing a measured dose of the test nutrient and then measuring blood or excretion levels. Measurement of circulating levels of a nutrient can identify nutritional problems. Loading tests can measure tissue saturation. Functional tests can indicate the severity of a nutritional problem. Functional tests measure effect or lack of effect, usually within an enzyme system requiring a nutrient. Selection of the method to be used in laboratory assessment is important, but the method of collecting and storing samples is critical. The personnel involved in such tests need special instructions on the assessment goals. The simplest, most reliable method available should be chosen. The range of reproducibility for the tests must be known in order to interpret results. In addition, the physiological significance of the test must be considered. Commonly performed laboratory tests should be used first.

In most clinical laboratories, some screening tests are routinely used. Many hospitals and clinics use automated equipment that provides total protein, albumin, globulin, cholesterol, triglycerides, calcium, phosphorus, sodium, potassium, glucose, hemoglobin, and hematocrit measures. If the diet and clinical examination indicate more information is needed, other tests can be added. Most common nutrients and related substances analyzed for nutritional status are serum protein, serum albumin, vitamin A, beta carotene (the precursor of vitamin A), transferrin saturation, and serum iron. A listing of normal values used in the HANES survey is shown in Table 7–6.

Vitamin C analysis is a simple and inexpensive laboratory procedure that reflects recent intake. Vitamin A analysis of the blood is a better indicator of long-term intake of the vitamin. There are a number of commercial kits for analysis of nutrient and blood fractions, such as those for folate analysis using a radio assay technique. A microbiological procedure may also be used for folate. Low hemoglobin and hematocrit may indicate deficiencies of protein, iron, folate, B_{12}, and/or B_6. Attitude, age, sex, and diseases not related to nutrition are also influential. For measurement of iron status, serum iron, total iron-binding capacity (TIBC), and percent saturation of transferrin are widely used. Iron deficiency is usually indicated by serum iron levels less than 50 mg/dl, elevated TIBC, and saturation less than 15 percent. Serum ferritin provides a sensitive assessment of iron stores except in the presence of liver disease and inflammation.

Plasma zinc is the most reliable measure of zinc status. Values between 80 and 115 mg/dl are normal. Zinc levels in hair are less reliable measures, but may be used in conjunction with serum levels. Thiamin and riboflavin may be measured in urine, although these are cumbersome techniques. A functional test of erythrocyte transketolase is a reliable and sensitive indicator of thiamin and erythrocyte glutathione for riboflavin. Other common substances to analyze for nutritional status are niacin, vitamin B_6 (pyridoxine), vitamin B_{12}, vitamin D, iodine, and selected trace minerals, such as zinc or copper, various enzymes, and selected hormones.

Nutritional Assessment over the Life Cycle

infancy and childhood

Assessment of infants and children requires close involvement of the parent and/or the caretaker. Diet records require observation by an adult until the children can read and write all food items consumed, describe the preparation, and understand the importance of cooperation. This is usually near the end of the elementary school years. In the very young child, who is generally under constant supervision, observation is much easier. As the child becomes more independent, it is difficult to determine food intake. When the child reaches

TABLE 7-6. Guidelines for Classification of Biochemical Determinations Used in the Health and Nutrition Examination Survey, United States, 1971–1972

biochemical determination, age, and sex	classification category LOW	ACCEPTABLE	HIGH
Hemoglobin (gm/100 ml)			
1–5 years	< 10.0	10.0–11.0	> 11.0
6–11 years	< 11.5	11.5–12.5	> 12.5
12–17 years, male	< 13.0	13.0–14.0	> 14.0
12–17 years, female	< 11.5	11.5–12.5	> 12.5
18 years and over, male	< 14.0	14.0–16.5	> 16.5
18 years and over, female	< 12.0	12.0–14.5	> 14.5
Hermatocrit (percent)			
1–5 years	< 31	31–34	> 34
6–11 years	< 35	35–39	> 39
12–17 years, male	< 40	40–44	> 44
12–17 years, female	< 36	36–38	> 38
18 years and over, male	< 44	44–52	> 52
18 years and over, female	< 38	38–48	> 48
Serum iron (μg/100 ml)			
1–5 years	< 40	40–49	> 49
6–11 years	< 50	50–59	> 59
12 years and over, male	< 60	60–149	>149
12 years and over, female	< 40	40–119	>119
Transferrin saturation (percent)			
1–5 years	< 15	15–29	> 30
6–11 years	< 20	20–29	> 30
12 years and over, male	< 20	20–29	> 30
12 years and over, female	< 15	15–29	> 30
Serum protein (gm/100 ml)			
1–5 years	< 5.0	5.0–6.0	> 6.0
6–17 years	< 6.0	6.0–8.0	> 8.0
Adult	< 6.5	6.5–8.5	> 8.5
Serum albumin (gm/100 ml)			
1–5 years	< 2.5	2.5–3.5	> 3.5
6–17 years	< 3.0	3.0–4.0	> 4.0
Adult	< 3.5	3.5–5.5	> 5.5
Serum vitamin A (μg/100 ml)			
All ages	< 20	20–80	> 80

SOURCE: U.S. Department of Health, Education and Welfare, National Center for Health Statistics, *Preliminary Findings of the First Health and Nutrition Examination Survey, United States, 1971–1972* (Washington, D.C.: Superintendent of Documents, 1979).

school age and food sources come from many places other than the home, dietary records become more and more inadequate in providing dietary information. Often children want to please and provide the interviewer with information they think the interviewer wants.

Children have difficulty giving the historical information that is necessary for a complete clinical examination. For biochemical and urinary studies, adequate sampling presents problems. The blood volume of the child is small; therefore, a limited amount can be taken. Micro methods help resolve this problem. Twenty-four-hour urine specimens are very difficult to get from children (2, 10). Special apparatus is necessary for infants and is successful only with male infants. Because of lack of bladder control, complete sampling is most difficult in young children. And as children become older, there is great resistance to urine sampling.

adolescence

Some of the same problems exist for the adolescent as for the young child. A particular problem of the adolescent is the great individual variety in stages of maturity (see Chapter 4). Sexual maturation and the growth spurt begin much earlier in girls than in boys. During adolescence, the proportion of body fat accumulates in girls and declines in boys. Muscle mass increases in both sexes, but at a greater rate in boys. Since it is often difficult to determine the stage of the growth cycle, skeletal measures may be the best way to determine how close the child is to maturity.

The eating patterns and places of adolescents may be irregular. With the greater use of snacks, diet histories are more complicated to obtain and recorded information is difficult to collect. Food intake may be highly variable. Consumption of alcoholic beverages may not be reported. The adolescent may find great humor in providing false information unless made to understand the importance and purposes of the data collected.

A private area must be established for the collection of urine samples from adolescents. Urine sampling may be accompanied by a great deal of embarrassment, and 24-hour samples may be difficult to obtain.

adulthood

The busy life styles of many adults may interfere with recordkeeping, recall, or sampling. During working hours adults are often unwilling to keep urine specimens for a 24-hour sampling. Circadian rhythms are clearly established for adults for many substances; however, there is great individual variation.

Assessment for the elderly adult again poses particular problems. If there is neurological disease, it may be difficult for adults to recall food consumed. There is a great desire to please the interviewer, which can result in false dietary information.

Height is especially difficult to obtain because of the stooped posture that some elderly people assume. Elderly who have difficulty balancing on platform scales need chair or under-bed scales for weight measurement.

Looking Ahead

The work on assessment of nutritional status (5, 25, 26) points to the need for simplified and inexpensive methods. Automated equipment and computers are providing data more rapidly. Home computers or telephone connections to large computers are available to program for data entry to determine the nutrient content of food eaten and compare it with appropriate standards. Small automated analytical equipment for analysis of blood or urine could be housed in vans or placed in shopping centers or apartment complexes. This would make assessment available to a large segment of the healthy population as well as the sick. Research in the area of behavioral aspects of food consumption is needed, and it is difficult to obtain and interpret.

Summary

Assessment of nutritional status is ordinarily conducted for communities of individuals. Community assessments have been made in many parts of the world. Data are collected in cross-sections of the population or over a period of time to give longitudinal data. Objectives and cost are factors in the methods used in assessment. Dietary intake is determined by recalls, food records, or observations. These data are then compared with a standard or measure of status. Laboratory analyses are used with physiological samples. Anthropometric measures of height, weight, skinfold thickness, and mid-arm circumference are also made. Certain physical signs are suggestive of malnutrition, and at each stage of the life cycle there are special considerations for assessment. Nutrition assessment is the foundation of any health program.

references

1. JELLIFFE, D. B. *The Assessment of the Nutritional Status of the Community.* Geneva: WHO Monograph Series No. 53, 1966.
2. Interdepartmental Committee on Nutrition for National Defense. *Manual for Nutrition Surveys,* 2nd ed. Washington, D.C.: U.S. Government Printing Office, 1963.
3. National Center for Health Statistics. *Plan and Operation of the Health and Nutrition Examination Surveys, United States, 1971–1973.* DHEW Pub., (PHS) 79-1310. Public Health Service, Washington, D.C., 1979.
4. BERRY, W. T. C. "Nutrition Surveillance in Affluent Nations." *Nutrition Reviews* 30 (1972): 127.
5. CHRISTAKIS, G. "Nutritional Assessment in Health Programs." *American Journal of Public Health* 63 (1973): part 2, supplement.
6. BEAL, V. A. "The Nutritional History in Longitudinal Research." *Journal of the American Dietetic Association* 51 (1967): 426.
7. GRAHAM, G. T. "Validity of 24-hour Diet Recalls." *American Journal of Clinical Nutrition* 30 (1977): 1939.
8. YOUNG, C. M., and M. F. TRULSON. "Methodology for Dietary Studies in Epidemiological Surveys. I. Strengths and Weaknesses for Existing Methods." *American Journal of Public Health* 50 (1960): 503.
9. MADDEN, J. P., J. GOODMAN, and H. A. GUTHRIE. "Validity of 24-hour Recall." *Journal of the American Dietetic Association* 68 (1976): 143.
10. *Screening Children for Nutritional Status: Suggestions for Child Health Programs.* U.S. DHEW, Public Health Service No. DHE (HSM) 72-5603, 1972.
11. MOORE, C. M., B. C. JUDLIN, and P. M. KENNEMUR. "Using Graduated Food Models in Taking Dietary Histories." *Journal of the American Dietetic Association* 51 (1967): 447–452.
12. ANDERSON, M. A. "Comparison of Anthropometric Measures of Nutritional Status in Preschool Children in Five Developing Countries." *American Journal of Clinical Nutrition* 32 (1979): 2339.
13. HAMMIL, P. V., et al. "Physical Growth: National Center for Health Statistics Percentiles." *American Journal of Clinical Nutrition* 32 (1979): 607–629.
14. OWEN, G. M. "The Assessment and Recording of Measurements of Growth of Children: Report of a Small Conference." *Pediatrics* 51 (1973): 461.
15. ZERFAS, A. J. "The Insertion Tape: A New Arm Circumference Tape for Use in Nutritional Assessment." *American Journal of Clinical Nutrition* 28 (1975): 782.

16. GURNEY, J. M., and D. B. JELLIFFE. "Arm Anthropometry in Nutritional Assessment; Nomogram for Rapid Calculation of Muscle Circumference and Cross-Sectional Muscle and Fat Areas." *American Journal of Clinical Nutrition* 26 (1973): 912.

17. FRISANCHO, A. R. "Triceps Skinfold and Upper Arm Muscle Size Norms for Assessment of Nutritional Status." *American Journal of Clinical Nutrition* 27 (1974): 1052.

18. TANNER, J. M., and R. H. WHITEHOUSE. "Revised Standards for Triceps and Subscapular Skinfolds in British Children." *Archives of Diseases of Children* 50 (1975): 142.

19. GREULICH, W. W., and S. I. PYLE. *Radiographic Atlas of Skeletal Development of the Hand and Wrist,* 2nd ed. Stanford, Calif.: Stanford University Press, 1959.

20. TANNER, J. M., R. H. WHITEHOUSE, W. A. MARSHALL, M. J. R. HEADY, and H. GOLDSTEIN. *Assessment of Skeletal Maturity and Prediction of Adult Height.* New York: Academic Press, 1975.

21. GARN, S. M., and D. C. CLARK. "Problems in the Nutritional Assessment of Black Individuals." *American Journal of Public Health* 66 (1976): 262.

22. GARN, S. M. "An Annotated Bibliography on Bone Densitometry." *American Journal of Clinical Nutrition* 10 (1962): 59.

23. CAMERON, J. R., and J. A. SORENSON. "Bone Mineral Measurement by Improved Photon Absorption Technique." In *Progress in Development of Methods in Bone Densitometry.* Eds. G. D. Whedon, et al. National Aeronautics and Space Administration, NASA SP-64, 1966, p. 87.

24. SAUBERLICH, H. E., R. P. DOWDY, and J. H. SKALA. *Laboratory Tests for the Assessment of Nutritional Status.* Cleveland: CRC Press, 1974.

25. SABRY, E. I. "Assessing the Nutritional Status of Populations." *Food and Nutrition* 3 (1977): 2.

26. HARKIN, J. H., and R. HUENEMAN. "A Short Study Method for Epidemiological Studies." *Journal of the American Dietetic Association* 50 (1967): 487.

CHAPTER 8

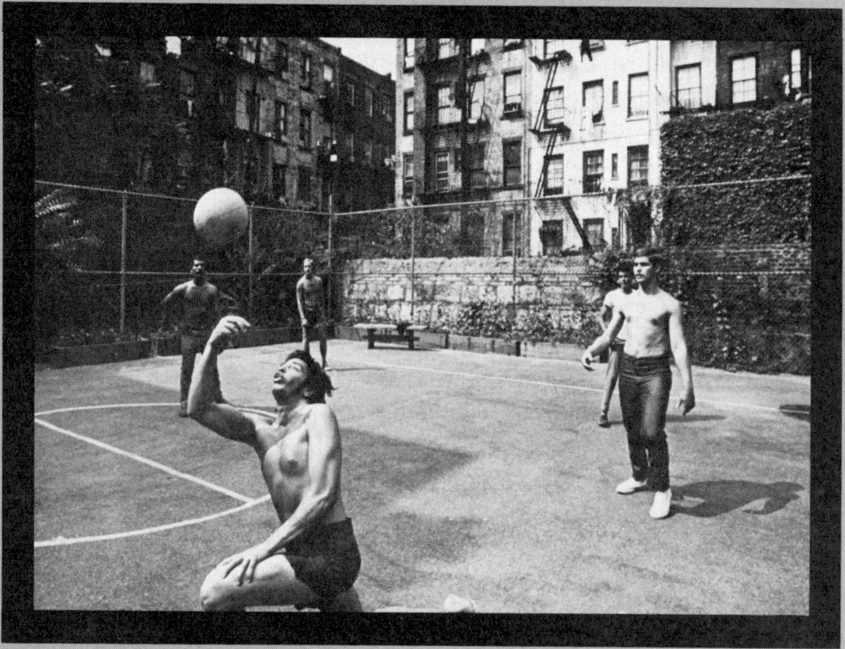

WHO photo by C. Blackwell

physical fitness, athletics, and nutritional needs

TODAY THERE IS MUCH INTEREST IN PHYSICAL FITNESS for health, prevention of disease, and sports. As more Americans become involved in exercise and physical activities, it is important to recognize certain physiological and nutritional interrelationships. Health and physical fitness are influenced by genetics, psychological states, life styles, and use of drugs, as well as by food intake and exercise.

The benefits of physical activity are many, including improved work capacity, improved muscular strength, increased endurance, better muscle tone, and usually reduced blood pressure and pulse rates. Exercise has important effects on metabolism, temperature regulation, salt and water balance, and endocrine response. In addition, the amount of body fat may be modified.

Improved or superior physical performance is the goal of many who participate in rigorous exercise programs—particularly athletes. The competition of sports and athletic events leads athlete and coach to seek every possible means of improving performance. Through the years, nutrition fads have become a way of life for athletes (1). The athlete is eager to manipulate food intake in an effort to increase output and improve performance. Unfortunately, the information available concerning nutrition and athletics is not well understood and is easily misinterpreted. Only in recent years has research been designed to look at the effects of specific foods and/or feeding regimens on the outcomes of physical performance (2).

Most of the current practices of both coaches and athletes are based on their own personal opinions and their past experiences, rather than on research data, although Werblow showed a positive correlation between nutritional knowledge and attitudes about sports nutrition in a group of female athletes she studied (3, 4). Another study reported by Cho indicated that physical education majors knew less about nutrition than college students who had completed a basic course in nutrition (5). Both groups recommended a multivitamin supplement for athletes. In addition, the physical education majors recommended such "magical" foods as honey, wheat germ, gelatin, lecithin, and sugar more often than did nutrition students.

It is no wonder that in the face of no knowledge, few scientific facts, and much faddism and tradition, many athletes do not know where to turn and what the best regimens to follow are (6). The difficulty in discounting many of the fads relates to their having been practiced for generations. People have always assumed that somewhere there is a food that will increase physical abilities and produce better athletes.

The Pregame Meal

Much of the faddism centers around the pregame meal. Most athletes and coaches have strong ideas about the specific timing and content of this meal. The ideas are not totally unfounded, for certain physiological concepts do apply to the pregame meal. For example, pregame tension is evident in most athletes. Emotional tension decreases gastric motility, thereby increasing digestion time and delaying gastric emptying. It may cause nausea, vomiting, or stomach cramps. So the stomach should be empty at the time of physical performance or competition. The foods that are eaten should be those that are well tolerated by the individual. There should be adequate time (three to four hours) for digestion prior to the actual physical exertion (7, 8). A large meal containing significant amounts of fat and protein is not recommended, as it may interfere with respiration and circulation. The digestion and absorption of food competes with muscle metabolism for the blood supply, resulting in reduced muscle work.

Some people recommend a high-carbohydrate meal because it is easily digested and absorbed. But carbohydrate supplements should relate to the energy expended and to the depletion and replenishment of glycogen stores (9). For "quick energy," some athletes consume candy or sweetened beverages just prior to competition. Costill has shown that this practice may in fact be detrimental because of the insulin-producing effect, which reduces the ability of the muscles to use fat (10). This places excessive demands on blood glucose and muscle glycogen for energy for the physical event. The onset of exercise causes a rapid intake of blood glucose by the muscles and could cause hypoglycemia (reduced glucose levels of blood). If sugar is taken after exercise has started, insulin is not increased, blood glucose is maintained, and the athlete does not become hypoglycemic. This also helps conserve liver glycogen stores (11, 12).

Another factor in discouraging "concentrated" sweets just prior to physical activity relates to the hyperosmolar load sugars give the gastrointestinal tract, which responds by drawing in water to dilute the sugar solutions. This may result in cramps, dehydration, delayed stomach emptying, and/or osmotic diarrhea. The carbohydrates taken during exercise should be in the form of chilled fluids, diluted, and taken in small amounts spread over the period of physical activity. Sugar content should not be in excess of 2.0 to 2.5 g per 100 ml of water. Chilled fluids leave the stomach faster than warm fluids.

Currently, the best recommendations for the pregame meal are foods that are familiar and well tolerated by the individual, including some protein, a small amount of fat, and generous amounts of complex carbohydrates (13).

Fats are generally restricted in the pregame meal of the athlete because of the delay in digestion; however, they should not be excluded from the athlete's daily intake. This is relevant in planning meals to meet the caloric needs of athletes because of the excessive energy expenditures associated with intense physical activity. Some athletes will need in excess of 4000 kcal per day, and it is difficult to eat the quantity of food needed when fat, a concentrated source of calories, is not used. This increased caloric need is related specifically to energy expended in physical activity and will vary considerably from one athlete to another.

Carbohydrate Loading

Carbohydrate loading has been suggested as a means of supplying sufficient energy to marathon athletes such as long-distance runners (14, 15, 16). The first step in loading involves depletion of glycogen stores by strenuous exercise and a carbohydrate intake of less than 100 g. In the week prior to the event, the athlete consumes large amounts of carbohydrates (250–500 g daily). Complex carbohydrates are preferred over concentrated sweets because they are good sources of vitamins and minerals as well. The carbohydrate provides a source of energy during intense exercise over a long period of time because the stored muscle and liver glycogen has been increased (17). Carbohydrate loading is not recommended for the preadolescent or adolescent athlete, nor for the short-time, high-intensity competitor (18, 19). It has been shown to be of benefit only in endurance-type competition.

Jette has described a study that compared the benefits of a protein and low-fat meal with a carbohydrate-rich meal (20). The results suggested the need for further study into the possibility of supplementing the carbohydrate meal with niacin. Niacin intakes were low in the study and could have accounted for the decreased performance level shown by those on the high-carbohydrate meal. Recommendations are difficult to make because the results of studies so far are inconclusive (21, 22).

Protein and Vitamin Recommendations

Large quantities of protein—even protein supplements—are advocated by some coaches and athletes (23, 24 25). During training, when muscle mass is increasing with growth, the need for increased protein is evident. Protein is necessary for synthesis of muscle tissue and for the increased blood volume required to oxygenate the additional muscle mass. The most common recommendation for adolescent athletes who are still growing is 2 grams of protein per kilogram of body weight per day. This represents approximately 15 to 20 percent of the total calories ingested. If the athlete is not growing rapidly, the recommendation for protein is only 1 gram per kilogram of body weight, or approximately 10 to 12 percent of total calories. These amounts can easily be obtained from a variety of foods without the necessity for protein supplements (26).

Various studies have looked at the possibility of vitamin supplementation for improvement of physical activity (27, 28, 29). The only need for increased amounts of vitamins is related to the increased calorie need and specifically those vitamins necessary for energy release—primarily thiamin, niacin, and riboflavin.

Consuming a variety of foods to get the increased calories will usually provide adequate vitamins without supplements.

Fluid and Mineral Replacement

Water and mineral replacement during and after strenuous exercise is of prime concern. It is not unusual for an athlete to lose several pounds in the course of a game, most of it water. Fluid loss is even more important in environmental areas where temperature is hot because water losses increase, thereby increasing need for both water and electrolytes (30, 31). Water losses of as little as 2 percent of body weight can cause circulatory problems during exercise.

Electrolyte and fluid imbalance does lead to decreased athletic performance and attitudinal changes of "not wanting to perform." If the physical activity is intense and prolonged and the environmental temperature is hot, the increase in body heat production and losses of water and electrolytes will be relative or proportional. The body attempts to maintain temperature equilibrium by removing body heat through sweating and subsequent evaporation. Rest periods and appropriate clothing aid in this process. If sweat is not replaced by water intake as physical activity progresses, the body becomes dehydrated and overheated and is unable to maintain thermal balance. A weight loss of greater than 5 percent may lead to heat exhaustion, which indicates defects in the heat regulation system and may occur quite suddenly if precautions to replace fluids are not taken (32). Renal failure and loss of consciousness are additional possibilities. See Table 8–1 for estimates of possible water losses compatible with survival and physiological changes with athletic performance and/or physical exertion.

Other researchers have shown that the maximum performance can be expected only when intake of water is equivalent to water losses in perspiration (33, 34). It is generally concluded that the fluid balance is best maintained with small amounts of water taken before and over the course of the physical performance, not in large amounts at intermissions or only at the end of the activity (35).

Water is the preferred fluid to quench thirst and prevent dehydration. Most prepared fluids have too much concentration of sugar, which may cause cramps and diarrhea (36).

If the weight loss is greater than 4 percent, it may take 24 to 36 hours before complete rehydration is affected. Adequate fluids must be provided to prevent dehydration and maintain appropriate body temperatures. Weight loss is the best indicator of water lost; therefore, athletes should weigh themselves before and after physical activities in order to determine amount of fluid that needs to be replaced.

The loss of weight from water loss and dehydration has been used by some coaches to get athletes into specific weight categories such as those required for wrestlers and boxers (37). This came to be such a detriment to the health of these

TABLE 8-1. Body Water Loss and Survival

water loss as a percentage of body weight	equivalent body water loss		symptoms
	70 kg MAN	80 kg MAN	
3	2.1	2.4	First signs of dehydration; decreased work performance. Some psychological upsets occur.
5–6	3.5–4.2	4.0–4.8	"Dehydration exhaustion syndrome" occurs (increased body temperature and heart rate).
6–10	4.2–7.0	4.8–8.0	Increased respiration rate, decreased blood volume, GI upsets, nausea, loss of appetite, numbness, emotional instability, and dangerous hallucinations.
11–15	7.7–10.5	8.8–12.0	Results in delirium, deafness, dimmed vision, swollen tongue, anuria, and possibly death. Heat stroke is likely to occur. Man is totally incapacitated.
15–20	10.5–14.0	12.0–16.0	This is the greatest water loss compatible with survival in acute dehydration.

SOURCE: Reprinted with permission from: C. F. Consolazio, "Physical Activity and Performance of the Adolescent." In *Nutrient Requirements in Adolescence*, eds. J. I. McKigney and H. N. Munro. (Cambridge, Mass.: MIT Press, 1976), p. 211.

athletes that the American College of Sports Medicine issued a position stand on weight loss in wrestlers (38). At no time should dehydration and/or water deprivation be considered an appropriate form of weight reduction in the growing adolescent athlete (see Chapters 4 and 9 for a discussion of weight control). The overfat adolescent needs to lose stored body fat, not water and lean body mass, which requires careful manipulation of caloric intake and energy expenditure (39).

The use of salt tablets to replace salt lost in perspiration has also been questioned. Most authorities agree that salt losses are best replaced with regular foods and liquids if weight loss is less than 6 pounds per day. A pound of weight loss equals approximately one pint of sweat. As salt is replaced water should be also, especially if salt tablets are used. A pint of water for each tablet (equivalent to 200 mg sodium) is recommended, but salty fluids are not recommended with salt tablets. Salt tablets are to be discouraged when they cause nausea and vomiting, because this will cause further dehydration. There is great individual variation in tolerance for salt replacement. Potassium may also need to be replaced if sweating is excessive, and it can be done easily with certain fruits and fruit juices.

Providing Energy

Some athletes and coaches will attempt severe caloric restriction (near starvation) of less than 1000 kcal/day to get within weight limits or to improve speed. This is an extremely unsafe practice, because it is usually accomplished by narrow food and beverage choices that are totally inadequate nutritionally (40). The current fad seems to be to include small amounts of protein with little or no other foods. Sometimes vitamin and mineral supplements will be given, but frequently they are ignored. Serious problems develop with electrolyte imbalances, especially sodium and potassium. These result in neuromuscular changes and decreases in blood volume, with resultant circulatory system changes, all of which greatly impair physical performance. Aside from debilitation, in the adolescent athlete these practices may be so nutritionally detrimental as to prevent growth.

No beneficial effects have been determined for honey, lecithin, wheat germ, vitamin E, alkaline salts, or protein supplements. They are expensive and can give false security to the athlete who believes they have special powers. Van Huss did not find evidence of any special beneficial effects on endurance (41). Some individuals may find that certain foods are gas forming and therefore should be restricted prior to physical activity because of discomfort and inconvenience. In addition, the consumption of foods high in fiber should be avoided in the pregame meal because gastrointestinal motility may be accelerated. These symptoms vary from individual to individual, so these suggestions are intended only as general recommendations.

The performance or work capacity for a muscle depends on the nature and availability of energy sources. The muscle uses several fuels and regenerates some itself. The direct source of muscle energy is adenosine triphosphate (ATP), which is synthesized continuously since little is stored in the muscle. Figure 8–1 outlines the relationships among the sources of muscular energy.

During moderate exercise, muscles do not produce lactic acid. Exercise maintained at a constant level of energy consumption results in a balance of splitting and resynthesis of the phosphagens. Under these conditions, net expenditure of energy can be calculated from the consumption of oxygen (5 kcal per ml of oxygen consumed). For strenuous exercise, energy cannot be provided in sufficient quantity through oxidation because of the limit on the rate of delivery of oxygenated blood to the tissues. The muscle supplements the energy through glycolysis, resulting in the production of lactic acid. The degree of training of the athlete and the amount of atmospheric oxygen will influence the level at which oxygen becomes depleted.

The best work performance can be obtained by avoiding lactic acid debt (see Figures 8–2 and 8–3). More than an hour is required to reduce lactic acid to the

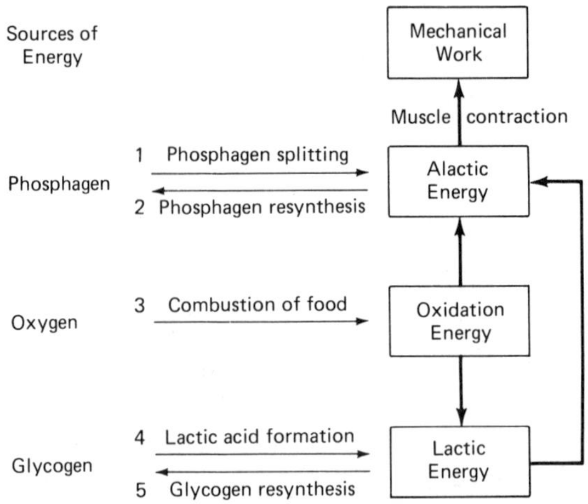

FIG. 8–1. Relations of sources of muscular energy are outlined. "Phosphagen," the direct source of energy, is a general term for the high-energy phosphates such as ATP and creatine phosphate (CP) that are found in cells. Energy is released by the splitting of phosphagen molecules. The split phosphagen is almost immediately resynthesized. Energy for the recombination is supplied by the two secondary energy sources: the combustion of food and the breakdown of glycogen, a carbohydrate stored in the muscle, into lactic acid. Glycogen in turn is resynthesized from lactic acid with energy from oxidation. The overall cycle consists fosfi of five reactions, three of which release energy and two of which absorb it. Source: R. Margaria, "Sources of Muscular Energy in Food." In J. E. Hoff and J. Janick (Eds.), *Readings from Scientific American* (San Francisco: W. H. Freeman, 1973).

point of acidosis that hampers muscle performance and causes discomfort. When the oxygen debt is only alactic, there is no acidosis and the return to a steady state is rapid, occurring in a few minutes. For the athlete or worker, proper spacing of work and intervals of rest can improve performance. More work can be produced with short bursts of strenuous activity and short rest periods than by driving relentlessly to exhaustion, which requires extremely long recovery periods.

Exercise and Insulin

Physical exercise can alter the level of plasma insulin and the binding of insulin to its receptors (42). Plasma insulin levels fall during acute exercise in proportion to the length of the exercise period. This stimulates glucose production by the liver and mobilization of lipids.

In sedentary subjects, submaximal exercise for 3 hours will result in a 30 to 35 percent increase in insulin binding. The same effect is produced in obese subjects, but at a smaller intensity. In well-trained athletes, insulin binding is 70 percent greater in the resting state than in nonathletes. The increment in insulin binding is proportional to the level of fitness of the athlete. During acute exercise, athletes use less carbohydrate and a larger amount of fat for fuel. This may be related to the fall in insulin binding observed during acute exercise by trained athletes.

Women in Sports

Recently there has been much interest in the differences in physical performance between males and females. Men seem to have an advantage over women in sports that require great strength, speed, and endurance. Women have an advantage in sports based on balance, flexibility, and buoyancy. We have little information on the female's true potential for sports performance. It remains unclear whether the differences are related to physical and physiological characteristics or cultural biases toward the activities promoted for girls and young women.

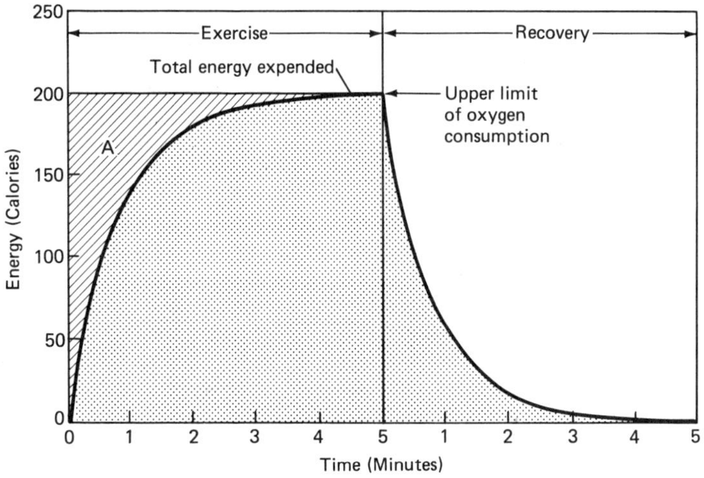

FIG. 8–2. Alactic oxygen debt is created by muscles drawing energy from phosphagen-splitting (area A) while the oxidation mechanism is being activated. In moderate exercise that does not lead to the formation of lactic acid, oxygen consumption quickly rises to its upper limit of about 40 milliliters (equivalent to 200 calories) per minute per kilogram of body weight and provides all of the energy required by the muscles. At the end of the exercise additional oxygen is consumed (gray area) to repay the alactic oxygen debt (A). The repayment energy is used to resynthesize the phosphagens that were split. Source: R. Margaria, "Sources of Muscular Energy in Food." In J. E. Hoff and J. Janick (Eds.), *Readings from Scientific American.* (San Francisco: W. H. Freeman, 1973).

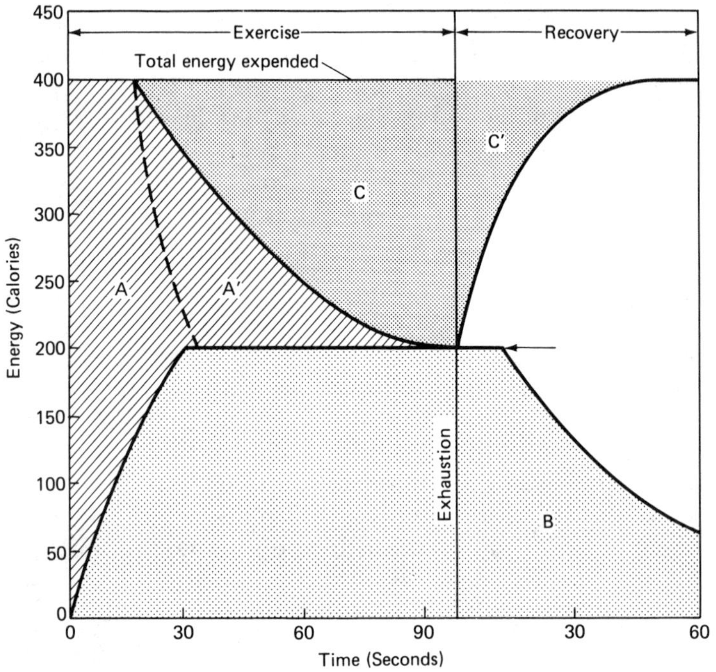

FIG 8–3. Alactic and lactacid debts are incurred when the exercise calls for superexertion to exhaustion. The alactic oxygen debt (areas A and A') is formed by the muscles obtaining energy from phosphagen-splitting while energy from oxygen consumption (area B) is rising to its upper limit (arrow). The lactacid oxygen debt (areas C and C′) is the result of energy obtained from the formation of lactic acid. During recovery from superexertion oxygen consumption remains at a high level for 15 to 20 seconds and then begins to drop. Energy from the delayed oxygen consumption (area B) pays the greater part (area A) of the alactic oxygen debt. Continued production of lactic acid (C') after the exercise is over provides energy to pay the fraction A' of the alactic debt. Source: R. Margaria, "Sources of Muscular Energy in Food." In J. E. Hoff and J. Janick (Eds.), *Readings from Scientific American* (San Francisco: W. H. Freeman, 1973).

Prior to puberty there is little difference in strength, endurance, or performance (44). Females reach their peak performance by 12 or before maturation. Male adults have more muscle mass as a result of the hormone testosterone, which increases rapidly at puberty. Females have very small amounts of testosterone and large amounts of estrogen, which may inhibit the development of muscle mass and increase the accumulation of fat (45, 46). From adolescence into adult life, men become more efficient in oxygen utilization for energy production. This is due in part to conditioning, but even more to differences in body composition.

It is apparent that with training and conditioning, women are competitive athletes (43). College women who participate in weight training programs can make strength improvements similar to men's when strength is expressed per pound of body weight. In women the improvement in strength is not accompanied by muscular enlargement. The testosterone level in males has an influence on the enlargement of the muscles.

SUMMARY

The priorities of an athlete's diet should be adequate calories for the increased energy expenditure; adequate intake of fluids and electrolytes to replace losses due to exertion and heat regulation; and increased protein only during training if muscle mass is increasing with growth (as in the adolescent). In addition, the diet should provide for body weight equilibrium without sudden fluctuations up or down. There is no significant improvement in performance with excessive protein intake, which becomes an expensive (both physiologically and economically) source of energy. A variety of foods is more likely to include the necessary nutrients than any one "special" food or food supplement, and at the same time be more palatable. Faddists' claims for "special powers" related to certain foods in improving athletic abilities must be discounted with facts. Adequate overall nutrition is necessary for optimum growth and performance. "Magical" claims are erroneous and some common practices, especially if they involve dehydration or extreme weight loss, are hazardous and may be fatal.

references

1. WILLIAMS, M. H. "Nutritional Faddism and Athletes." *Nutrition and the M.D.* 4 (1977): 1.
2. HANLEY, D. F. JR., "Athletic Training and How the Diet Affects It." *Nutrition Today* 14 (1979): 5.
3. CHO, M., and B. A. FRYER. "Nutrition Knowledge of Collegiate Physical Education Majors." *Journal of the American Dietetic Association* 65 (1974): 30.
4. WERBLOW, J. A., H. M. FOX, and A. HENNEMAN. "Nutritional Knowledge, Attitudes and Food Patterns of Women Athletes." *Journal of the American Dietetic Association* 73 (1978): 242.
5. CHO, M, and B. A. FRYER. "What Foods do Physical Education Majors and Basic Nutrition Students Recommend for Athletes?" *Journal of the American Dietetic Association* 65 (1974): 541.
6. VAN ITALLIE, T. B. "If Only We Knew." *Nutrition Today* 3 (1968): 3.
7. HIRATA, I. "Pre-game Meals: A Discussion." *Journal of School Health* 40 (1970): 409.
8. VAN ITALLIE, T. B., L. SINESTERRA, and F. J. STARE. "Nutrition and Athletic Performance." *Journal of the American Medical Association* 172 (1956): 1120.
9. BERGSTROM, J., and E. HULTMAN. "Nutrition for Maximal Sports Performance." *Journal of the American Medical Association* 221 (1972): 999.
10. COSTILL, D. L. "Sports Nutrition: The Role of Carbohydrates." *Nutrition News* 41 (1978): 1.
11. BERGSTROM J., and E. HULTMAN. "A Study of the Glycogen Metabolism during Exercise in Man." *Scandinavian Journal of Clinical and Laboratory Investigation* 19 (1967): 218.
12. COSTILL, D. L., A. BENNETT, G. BRANAM, and D. EDDY. "Glucose Ingestion at Rest and during Prolonged Exercise." *Journal of Applied Physiology* 34 (1973): 764.
13. The American Dietetic Association. "Nutrition and Physical Fitness." *Journal of the American Dietetic Association* 76 (1980): 437.
14. KARLSSON, J., and B. SALTIN. "Diet, Muscle Glycogen, and Endurance Performance." *Journal of Applied Physiology* 31 (1971): 203.
15. SLOVIC, P. "What Helps the Long Distance Runner." *Nutrition Today* 10 (1975): 18.
16. SPENCE, H. A. "Dietary Requirements of Ultra-Long Distance Runners." *Food and Nutrition* 34 (1977): 172.
17. FORGAC, N. T. "Carbohydrate Loading: A Review." *Journal of the American Dietetic Association* 75 (1979): 42.

18. SMITH, N. J. "Nutrition and the Athlete." in *Sports Medicine and Physiology*. Ed. R. H. Strauss. Philadelphia: Saunders, 1979.

19. MIRKIN, G. "Carbohydrate Loading: A Dangerous Practice." Letter. *Journal of the American Medical Association* 223 (1973): 1511.

20. JETTE, M., O. PELLETIER, L. PARKER, and J. THODEN. "The Nutritional and Metabolic Effects of a Carbohydrate-rich Diet in Glycogen Super Compensation Training Program." *American Journal of Clinical Nutrition* 31 (1978): 2140.

21. BERGSTROM, J., E. HULTMAN, B. PERNOW, L. JORFELDT, and J. WAHREN. "Effect of Nicotinic Acid on Physical Working Capacity and on Metabolism of Muscle Glycogen in Man." *Journal of Applied Physiology* 26 (1969): 170.

22. JENKINS, D. J. A. "Effects of Nicotinic Acid on Carbohydrates and Fat Metabolism during Exercise." *Lancet* 1 (1965): 207.

23. BULLEN, B., J. MAYER, and F. J. STARE. "Athletics and Nutrition." *American Journal of Surgery* 98 (1959): 343.

24. COOPER, D. L. "Nutrition and Athletes." *Journal of the American College Health Association* 14 (1966): 261.

25. MANN, G. "Nutritional Practices in Athletics Abroad." *Physician and Sports Medicine* 5 (1977): 33.

26. CONSOLAZIO, C. F. "Protein Metabolism during Intense Physical Training in the Young Adult." *American Journal of Clinical Nutrition* 28 (1975): 29.

27. SHARMAN, I. M., M. G. DOWN, and R. N. SEN. "The Effect of Vitamin E and Training on Physiological Function and Athletic Performance in Adolescent Swimmers." *British Journal of Nutrition* 26 (1971): 265.

28. LAWRENCE, J. D., R. C. BOWER, W. P. RIEHL, and J. L. SMITH. "Effects of α-tocopherol Acetate on the Swimming Endurance of Trained Swimmers." *American Journal of Clinical Nutrition* 28 (1975): 205.

29. GEY, G. O., K. N. COOPER, and R. A. BOTTENBERG. "Effect of Ascorbic Acid on Endurance Performance and Athletic Injury." *Journal of the American Medical Association* 211 (1970): 105.

30. ADOLPH, E. F. *Physiology of Man in the Desert.* New York: Interscience, 1947.

31. COSTILL, D. L., and K. SPARKS. "Rapid Fluid Replacement Following Thermal Dehydration." *Journal of Applied Physiology* 34 (1973): 299.

32. Committee on Nutritional Misinformation, Food and Nutrition Board. "Water Deprivation and Performance of Athletes." *Nutrition Review* 32 (1974): 314.

33. PITTS, G. C., R. E. JOHNSON, and C. F. CONSOLAZIO. "Work in the Heat as Affected by Intake of Water, Salt and Glucose." *American Journal of Physiology* 142 (1944): 253.

34. SMITH, J. H., S. ROBINSON, and M. PEARCY. "Renal Responses to Exertion, Heat and Dehydration." *Journal of Applied Physiology* 4 (1952): 659.

35. KENNEY, R. A. "The Effects of Drinking Pattern on the Water Economy in a Hot, Humid Environment." *British Journal of Industrial Medicine* 11 (1954): 38.

36. COSTILL, D. L., and B. SALTIN. "Factors Limiting Gastric Emptying during Rest and Exercise." *Journal of Applied Physiology* 37 (1974): 679.

37. SMITH, N. J. "Gaining and Losing Weight in Athletics." *Journal of the American Medical Association* 236 (1976): 149.

38. American College of Sports Medicine. "Position Stand on Weight Loss in Wrestlers." *Sports Medicine Bulletin* 11 (1976): 1.

39. SHAFFER, T. E. "The Adolescent Athlete." *Pediatric Clinics of North America* 20 (1973).

40. HENSCHEL, A., H. L. TAYLOR, and A. KEYS. "Performance Capacity in Acute Starvation with Hard Work." *Journal of Applied Physiology* 6 (1954): 624.

41. VAN HUSS, W. D., G. MICKLES, E. M. JONES, J. J. MONOTOYE, D. C. CEDERQUIST, and L. SMEDLEY. "Effect of Milk Consumption on Endurance Performance." *Research Quarterly* 33 (1962): 120.

42. KOIVISTO, V., V SOMAN, E. NADEL, W. V. TAMBORLANE, and P. FELIG. "Exercise and Insulin: Insulin Binding, Insulin Mobilization and Counterregulatory Hormone Secretion." *Federation Proceedings* 39 (1980): 1481.

43. ASTRAND, P. O. "Human Physical Fitness with Special Reference to Sex and Age." *Physiological Review* 36 (1956): 307.

44. Committee on Pediatric Aspects of Physical Fitness, Recreation and Sports. "Participation in Sports by Girls." In *Food for Sport.* Ed. N. J. Smith. Palo Alto, Calif.: Bull Publishing, 1976.

45. ERDELYI, G. J. "Women in Athletics." *Proceedings of the Second National Conference on Medical Aspects of Sports.* Chicago: The American Medical Association, 1961.

46. MOREHOUSE, L. E., and D. J. RAND. "Age and Sex Factors in Athletics." in *Scientific Basis of Athletic Training,* eds. L E. Morehouse and P. J. Rasch. Philadelphia: Saunders, 1958.

CHAPTER 9

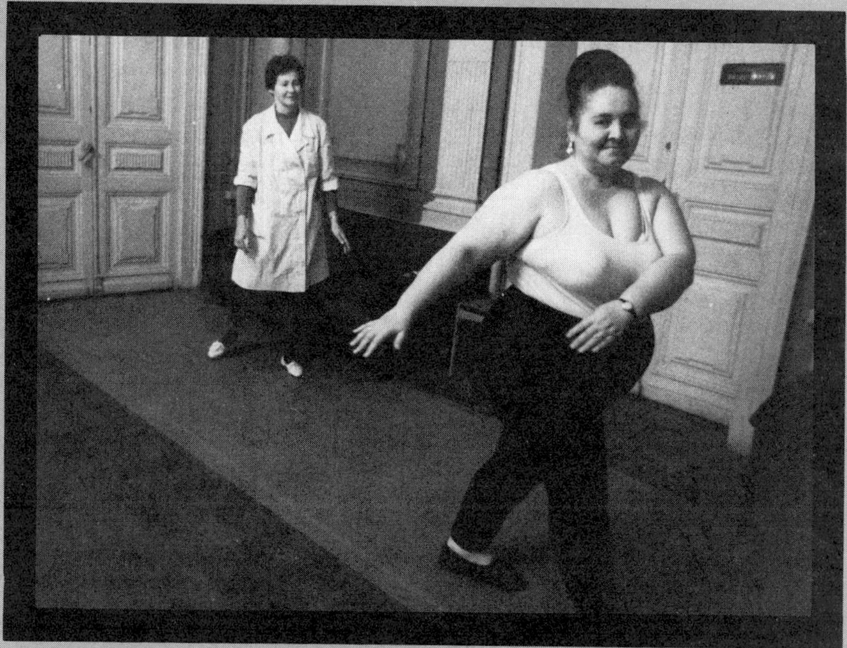

WHO photo by M. Jacot

nutrition factors in weight control

WEIGHT CONTROL OR THE ATTEMPT TO ACHIEVE NORMAL or desirable weight for height seems to be an American and Western World preoccupation. Television and popular magazines promote the thin, glamorous look for women and the lean, muscular look for men. Physicians and epidemiological surveys have pointed out the numerous chronic diseases for which obesity is an added health risk. At the same time, thin or underweight infants and young children in the developing countries are at greater risk of infection and life-threatening illnesses than are their counterparts with adequate reserve of subcutaneous fat. So weight control, whether for overweight or underweight, is important for psychosocial and health reasons.

Control of body weight requires maintenance of a level somewhere between excessive leanness and fatness. This maintenance level is the normal standard or desirable body weight. A person can survive with a 200 percent increase in body weight, but only a 25 percent loss by a lean body. In the United States the majority of the adult population varies between less than 5 percent below standard and less than 20 percent above standard weight (see Table 9–1).

We will discuss excessive weight or obesity which is the more common problem in our society, first, and then the problem of underweight. One is not more important than the other, because both can have serious consequences for the individual in all areas of life. And both, as we will see, are complex conditions without clear-cut causes or simple solutions.

ENERGY METABOLISM

Control of body weight is based on the amount of energy consumed and how the sources of energy are metabolized within the cells of the body. The major sources of energy in foods are fats, carbohydrates, protein, and alcohol. The energy value of a food can be measured by burning the food in a bomb calorimeter and adjusting for the percentage of efficiency within the human body. The Atwater method can be used to calculate the energy available from a food based on 9 calories per gram from fat, 7 calories per gram from alcohol, and 4 calories per gram from protein and carbohydrate. These figures are useful in a mixed diet; however, they become less accurate in specialized diets.

Carbohydrate, fat, protein and alcohol provide energy for the cells through the processes of metabolism. There are different initial pathways for each. Glycolysis for carbohydrates and β-oxidation for fat are common examples. The major pathways are interrelated in a process called intermediary metabolism. An understanding of energy metabolism is necessary to understand weight control. An abbreviated sketch of metabolism, Figure 9–1, is given as a basis for the discussion of weight control. The pathway for alcohol is presented in Chapter 10.

The digestive tract reduces complex carbohydrates to simple sugars. Because the liver converts fructose and galactose to glucose, the metabolism of carbohydrates is primarily the metabolism of glucose. A major pathway for producing energy in the cell is shown in Figure 9–1. The first steps (called glycolysis) from activation of glucose with phosphate to pyruvate is called an anaerobic pathway because of the absence of oxygen and occurs in the cell cytoplasm. The aerobic pathway, which requires oxygen, functions in the mitochondria and is known as the tricarboxylic acid (TCA) cycle or the Krebs cycle. The metabolism of lipids and protein is related to that of carbohydrate in providing energy. Vitamins and minerals serve as cofactors to activate the various steps.

When cellular energy requirements have been met, fatty acids are formed and stored in fat cells. (A small amount of carbohydrate is converted to glycogen and stored in muscle and liver cells.) The fat cell can thus be a major reservoir for energy; however, the ability of a cell to metabolize fat is dependent on the amount of oxaloacetate available. Glucose and certain amino acids are sources of oxaloacetate, so fat metabolism depends on carbohydrate and protein. During starvation, muscle mass may be catabolized to provide the necessary carbohydrate or amino acid precursors. Glucose and certain amino acids are necessary for the metabolism of fat by producing oxaloacetate to combine with acetyl coenzyme A (CoA), because the metabolism of acetyl CoA depends upon the amount of oxaloacetate.

Fat is stored as triglycerides. When needed to provide energy, the triglycerides are separated into fatty acids and glycerol. Glycerol is metabolized in the glycolysis pathway. Fatty acids are broken down and converted to acetyl CoA units in a process termed β-oxidation. The acetyl coenzyme A generated in this oxidation enters the Krebs cycle.

Figure 9–1 shows where certain amino acids enter the energy cycle. For amino acids to be used for energy, the nitrogen-containing group is removed, usually by transamination. Some amino acids can enter the pathway through acetoacetate to acetyl CoA, while the other amino acids contribute to the glucose pathways. With a deficit of oxaloacetate, acetyl CoA builds up and is synthesized as fat or converted to ketone bodies or cholesterol. An intricate network of hormones, enzymes, and metabolic feedback systems determines which route predominates. Ultimately, the solution to weight control will be found in understanding the multiple factors involved in the control of energy metabolism and the appetite feedback mechanism.

TABLE 9–1. Percent Distribution of Persons 20 Years of Age and Over by Body Weight,[a] According to Selected Characteristics: United States, 1977

characteristic	total[b]	10 percent or more below desirable weight	5–9.9 percent below desirable weight	plus or minus 4.9 percent of desirable weight	5–9.9 percent above desirable weight	10–19.9 percent above desirable weight	20–29.9 percent above desirable weight	30 percent or more above desirable weight
All persons 20 years of age and over	100.0	9.1	9.1	23.5	12.5	20.2	11.1	14.5
SEX								
Male	100.0	5.2	6.8	21.6	16.3	24.4	14.0	11.7
Female	100.0	12.2	10.9	24.9	9.5	16.9	8.9	16.7
RACE OR ETHNICITY								
White	100.0	9.4	9.4	24.3	12.8	20.2	11.0	13.1
Black	100.0	6.0	6.2	20.1	9.7	20.1	13.0	25.0
Hispanic	100.0	5.8	8.6	19.0	11.6	23.2	13.0	18.8
AGE								
20–34 years	100.0	13.0	12.8	27.6	12.4	16.6	7.6	10.0
35–44 years	100.0	6.8	8.5	23.2	13.2	21.4	11.8	15.0
45–54 years	100.0	5.1	6.4	20.8	13.3	23.5	13.4	17.5
55–64 years	100.0	5.3	6.4	19.6	12.3	22.1	14.8	19.6
65 years and over	100.0	10.2	6.4	20.5	11.4	22.2	12.8	16.4

TABLE 9-1. (Continued)

characteristic	total[b]	10 percent or more below desirable weight	5–9.9 percent below desirable weight	plus or minus 4.9 percent of desirable weight	5–9.9 percent above desirable weight	10–19.9 percent above desirable weight	20–29.9 percent above desirable weight	30 percent or more above desirable weight
INCOME								
Less than $5,000	100.0	11.5	8.8	20.5	9.8	18.9	11.4	19.2
$5,000–$9,999	100.0	9.2	9.0	22.9	11.5	19.7	11.1	16.5
$10,000–$14,999	100.0	9.0	8.3	23.1	12.8	21.2	11.0	14.5
$15,000–$24,999	100.0	8.0	9.7	24.4	13.5	20.3	11.3	12.6
$25,000 or more	100.0	8.9	10.3	26.0	14.0	20.5	10.7	9.5
EDUCATION OF INDIVIDUAL								
Less than 12 years	100.0	7.8	6.5	18.5	11.0	21.1	14.0	21.0
12 years	100.0	9.3	9.2	24.4	12.2	20.6	10.7	13.5
More than 12 years	100.0	10.3	11.5	27.6	14.4	18.7	8.7	8.8

[a] Desirable weight modified from 1960 Metropolitan Life Insurance Company data.

[b] Excludes unknown height or weight.

SOURCE: Advancedata from Vital and Health Statistics, National Center for Health Statistics, DHHS, PHS No. 64, 1980.

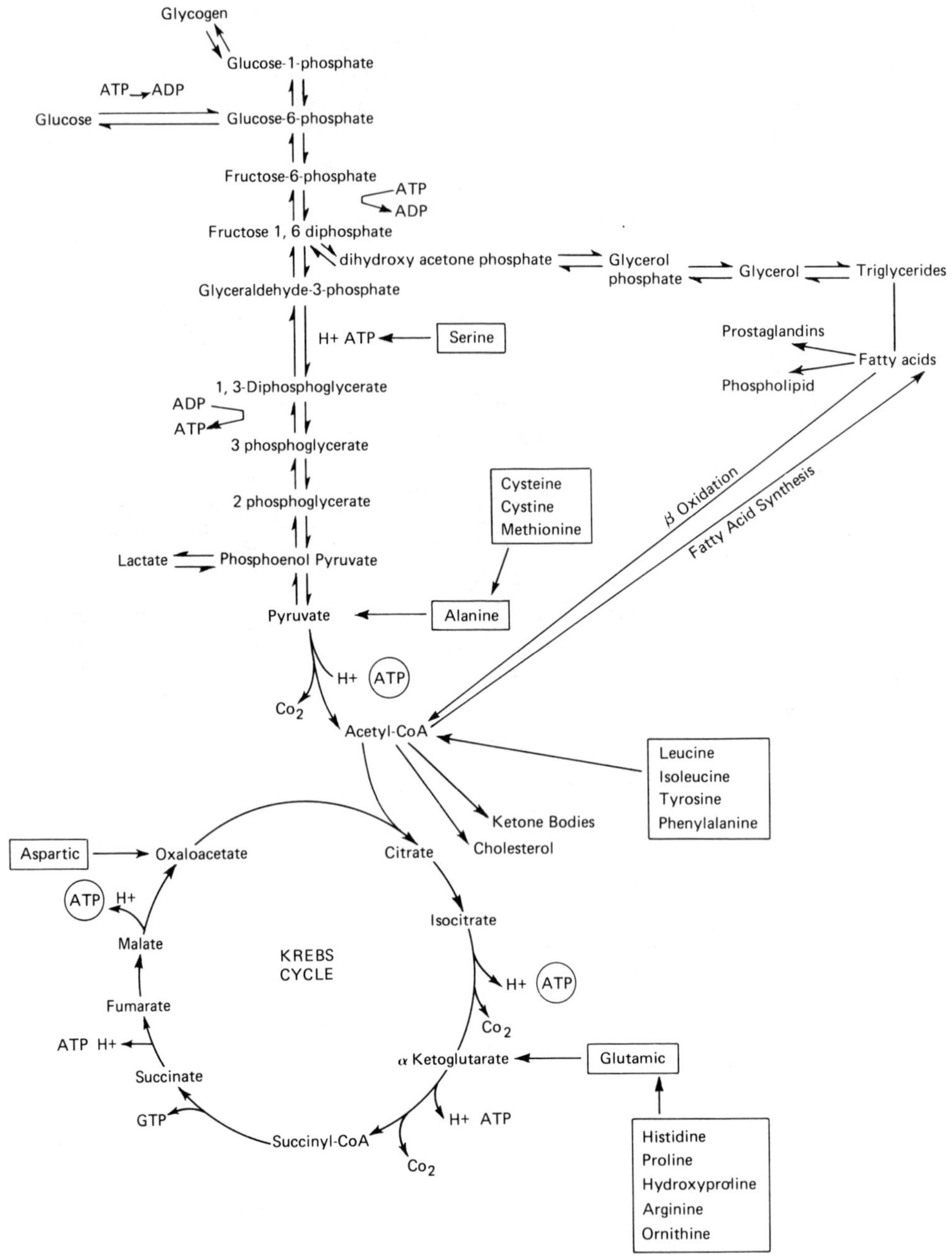

FIG. 9–1. Schematic diagram of the major final common pathway of energy metabolism for glucose, triglycerides, and amino acids.

OBESITY

Obesity, the condition of excessive body fatness, is associated with social stigma and adverse effects to health (1). We know that obesity results from an imbalance between caloric intake and output, but its causes and methods of treatment are still unproved hypotheses (2). Simple solutions to the problem are just not available. Obesity is a complex disorder related to social class, eating habits, exercise patterns, other behavioral patterns, physiological functions, and probably hereditary factors. The nutritional solution to the problem is more than simply eating less since few obese people are able to attain permanent weight loss by any method. In most studies less than 15 percent of the obese have maintained the weight loss for five years, and many weigh more than their pre-diet weight.

standards

The standards for obesity are somewhat arbitrary. Overfatness generally means above 20 percent body composition as fat in young men and above 30 percent in young women. Under research conditions a number of methods are available to determine body fatness; for general use, the most practical methods are height, weight, and skinfold measurements (3).

HEIGHT AND WEIGHT. One widely used chart for evaluation of weight and height is shown in the Appendix. Frame size is estimated in this chart. Because average weights for men and women increase with age in the United States, which is not considered desirable, the standards are based on weights in the young adult years. Current data for the height and weight of adults from NCHS are shown in Tables 9–2 and 9–3. Because weight is relative to height, the body mass index (wt/ht^2) has been suggested as a replacement for the common height-weight charts inasmuch as it produces an independent measure of relative weight.

SKINFOLD MEASUREMENTS. Because no measure of relative weight can reliably estimate obesity, it is generally considered more accurate to estimate fatness by skinfold measurements using a caliper. Triceps and subscapular muscle areas are the two most frequently measured. Because fat is located under the skin, care must be taken to measure only skinfold and not muscle tissue. Skinfold measurements of more than 30 mm for a double thickness skin indicate excessive body fatness for the adult. (Techniques for measuring and standards are shown in Chapter 7.)

fat cells

Fat is stored primarily as triglycerides in *adipocytes* (adipose or fat cells), as shown in Figure 9–2. Much of the current research on obesity has focused on factors related to fat cell size and number. Adipose tissue increases in two ways: by

TABLE 9-2. Height in Inches of Adults Aged 18–74 Years, by Sex, Race, and Age, 1971–1974

sex, race, age	sample size	estimated population (in thousands)	mean	standard deviation	standard error of the mean	percentile						
						5th	10th	25th	50th	75th	90th	95th
MEN												
White	4,343	54,109	69.1	2.8	0.08	64.6	65.6	67.2	69.1	70.9	72.7	73.6
18–24 years	625	9,849	69.8	2.8	0.20	65.3	66.3	67.9	69.8	71.4	73.4	74.5
25–34 years	672	11,191	69.7	2.8	0.13	65.3	66.3	67.7	69.7	71.7	73.4	74.3
35–44 years	570	9,857	69.2	2.6	0.13	64.8	65.9	67.5	69.3	71.1	72.6	73.4
45–54 years	628	10,117	68.9	2.6	0.14	64.7	65.6	67.2	68.9	70.7	72.5	73.3
55–64 years	504	8,125	68.3	2.6	0.17	64.2	65.1	66.7	68.2	70.1	71.7	72.5
65 years and over	1,344	4,970	67.3	2.6	0.09	63.2	64.2	65.6	67.3	69.1	70.6	71.7
Black	847	5,730	68.6	2.8	0.16	64.1	64.8	66.8	68.6	70.6	72.4	73.3
18–24 years	132	1,287	69.5	2.8	0.45	64.6	65.3	67.4	69.8	71.7	72.9	73.6
25–34 years	119	1,377	68.6	2.9	0.38	64.1	64.4	66.6	68.6	70.6	72.6	73.7
35–44 years	87	820	69.1	3.1	0.44	62.4	65.6	67.2	69.2	71.3	72.8	74.3
45–54 years	130	1,087	68.2	2.4	0.26	64.5	65.4	66.6	67.9	69.5	71.3	72.3
55–64 years	85	672	68.2	2.3	0.32	64.1	64.4	66.6	68.1	70.1	70.9	71.8
65 years and over	294	486	67.3	2.4	0.18	63.1	64.2	65.6	67.5	69.1	70.2	70.9
WOMEN												
White	6,758	59,482	63.7	2.5	0.05	59.5	60.6	62.0	63.7	65.3	66.8	67.8
18–24 years	1,165	10,298	64.3	2.5	0.09	60.3	61.3	62.7	64.3	65.9	67.4	68.4
25–34 years	1,539	12,338	64.1	2.5	0.08	60.2	61.2	62.4	64.1	65.8	67.3	68.3
35–44 years	1.301	10,250	64.1	2.5	0.09	60.1	60.9	62.4	64.1	65.7	67.3	68.4
45–54 years	705	11,091	63.6	2.4	0.11	59.9	60.6	62.0	63.7	65.2	66.7	67.3
55–64 years	552	8,905	62.8	2.4	0.11	58.6	59.7	61.2	62.8	64.5	65.6	66.6
65 years and over	1,496	6,601	62.3	2.4	0.09	58.2	59.2	60.7	62.3	63.9	65.3	66.2
Black	1,557	7,268	63.7	2.5	0.09	59.6	60.6	62.1	63.7	65.3	66.8	67.8
18–24 years	329	1,618	64.0	2.4	0.20	60.2	60.9	62.4	64.0	65.4	66.9	68.1
25–34 years	335	1,540	63.9	2.3	0.20	60.2	61.2	62.3	63.7	65.3	67.1	67.8
35–44 years	334	1,354	64.2	2.5	0.19	59.8	60.7	62.8	64.3	65.6	67.7	68.8
45–54 years	126	1,131	63.8	2.2	0.30	60.2	60.7	62.3	63.6	65.6	66.8	67.6
55–64 years	115	971	62.8	2.6	0.24	58.4	59.5	61.3	62.8	64.7	66.2	66.9
65 years and over	318	654	62.6	2.4	0.18	58.7	59.6	61.2	62.5	64.1	65.5	66.2

NOTE: Height was measured without shoes.

SOURCE: *Weight and Height of Adults 18–74 Years of Age: United States, 1971–74.* National Health Survey, Series 11, No. 211, DHEW Publication No. (PHS) 79-1659 (Hyattsville, Md.: U.S. Department of Health, Education and Welfare, 1979).

TABLE 9-3. Weight in Pounds of Adults Aged 18–74 Years, by Sex, Race, and Age, 1971–1974

sex, race, age	sample size	estimated population (in thousands)	mean	standard deviation	standard error of the mean	percentile						
						5th	10th	25th	50th	75th	90th	95th
MEN												
White	4,343	54,109	173	30	0.75	129	138	153	171	190	211	224
18–24 years	625	9,849	165	28	1.89	125	133	146	162	182	205	222
25–34 years	672	11,191	177	32	1.40	134	142	155	173	194	217	232
35–44 years	570	9,857	178	29	1.66	133	145	160	177	195	211	224
45–54 years	628	10,117	176	29	1.23	129	141	158	176	193	214	225
55–64 years	504	8,125	171	29	1.49	125	136	153	171	187	208	220
65 years and over	1,344	4,970	164	27	0.99	123	131	148	164	180	198	210
Black	847	5,730	171	40	2.54	125	134	145	163	189	217	239
18–24 years	132	1,287	166	37	4.04	123	131	142	159	176	202	227
25–34 years	119	1,377	175	51	8.17	124	134	148	162	193	219	235
35–44 years	87	820	182	37	4.59	130	137	151	180	201	236	255
45–54 years	130	1,087	168	32	3.75	135	136	145	162	185	220	230
55–64 years	85	672	172	41	6.34	119	138	145	163	186	237	249
65 years and over	294	486	161	30	2.31	121	127	137	156	179	205	218
WOMEN												
White	6,758	59,482	142	31	0.59	104	110	121	136	157	182	199
18–24 years	1,165	10,298	132	26	0.82	100	106	115	128	142	162	177
25–34 years	1,539	12,338	138	31	1.02	104	109	118	131	150	179	201
35–44 years	1,301	10,250	146	34	1.29	109	114	124	137	159	191	213
45–54 years	705	11,091	147	30	1.32	109	113	126	143	162	188	204
55–64 years	552	8,905	147	30	1.35	103	111	127	143	164	187	201
65 years and over	1,496	6,601	145	28	1.08	105	113	126	142	162	180	192
Black	1,557	7,268	156	41	1.53	104	111	129	148	176	207	228
18–24 years	329	1,618	138	34	2.47	100	107	114	130	150	184	203
25–34 years	335	1,540	149	37	3.20	100	108	127	141	170	190	226
35–44 years	334	1,354	165	39	2.68	112	121	136	158	185	216	238
45–54 years	126	1,131	169	42	4.53	115	128	139	162	186	215	244
55–64 years	115	971	168	48	6.37	104	118	139	156	191	215	297
65 years and over	318	654	155	36	3.28	94	109	133	153	177	202	219

NOTE: Total weights of all clothing ranged from 0.20 to 0.62 lb, which is not deducted from weight shown in table.

SOURCE: *Weight and Height of Adults 18–74 Years of Age: United States, 1971–74.* National Health Survey, Series 11, No. 211, DHEW Publication No. (PHS) 79-1659 (Hyattsville, Md.: U.S. Department of Health, Education and Welfare, 1979).

enlarging existing fat cells (hypertrophy) and by increasing the total number of fat cells (hyperplasia), which can also be enlarged. In humans, moderate adult-onset obesity is likely to be hypertrophic (4), and excessive obesity is probably hyperplastic and hypertrophic.

Because the technique developed measures only mature fat cells, the older research on influence of fat cell size and number has not considered the differentiated but unfilled preadipocytes in tissues. With methods to measure these, our information on the age of fat cell formation is changing. The ability of adults to increase fat cell number may exist or may result from failure to measure preadipocytes. There is a relationship between fat cell number and size that is related to overeating and possibly genetics. Many studies support the traditional concept of stability in the number of adipocytes in adults, while other reports demonstrate an increase in number of fat cells in adult animals (5). Pregnancy and old age may be periods of increase for the number of fat cells.

Early nutritional alterations have long-term effects on the number of fat cells in animals. Human studies under controlled dietary conditions are not available, but we do know that fat cell development proceeds at a continuous rapid rate in obese children until they are 14 or 16 years of age. Children and adolescents who have exceeded normal adult values for cellularity often retain their fat. Children whose fat cell numbers are within the normal range tend to reduce to normal weights more easily (6).

From studies of weight loss in obese children, there are two possible inter-

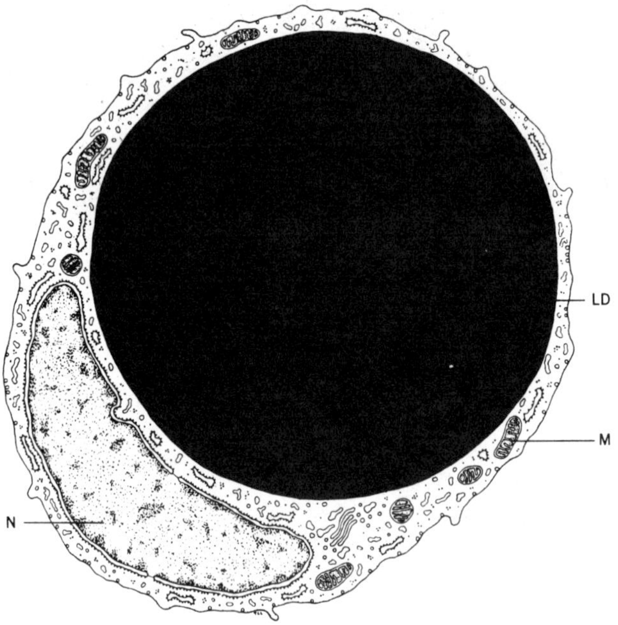

FIG. 9–2. White Adipose cell. N = nucleus; M = mitochondrion; LD = lipid droplet. *Source:* T. L. Lentz, *Cell Fine Structure* (Philadelphia: Saunders, 1971).

pretations of the data that need further study. It may be possible to modify the effect of genetic determinants by lowering the caloric balance, or it may be that people with the strongest genetic trait cannot reduce successfully. The first would indicate treatment of childhood obesity and could prevent adult hyperplastic obesity; the other shows little hope for this. Adult obesity with the largest fat cell numbers has a very poor treatment record.

Studies have shown that severely obese women were 2.4 times more likely to have been fat children than normal weight women (7). This suggests a greater risk of the fat child developing severe obesity. Hirsch's adipose cell hypothesis is often used to explain why some people stop gaining while others do not (8). In a family with tendencies toward obesity, early overfeeding of the baby increases the number of fat cells. The weight of a person who is genetically destined to be obese can be modified by early feeding in moderation. The means by which nutrition can have effects later on obesity is not completely understood. There may be critical periods in life when fat cells are sensitive to nutritional, hormonal, metabolic, or other factors that influence cell division and development.

The extent of adipose tissue cellularity is generally related to age of onset of obesity; however, this is not a precise relationship, and is often overestimated (9). Studies have shown increases of fat cell number at all ages in children and adult women. The techniques used for measuring the fat cells may account for different results. But there is a definite relationship between fat cell number and severity of obesity at any age (10). The fat cell number may continue to rise with continuing obesity, and at any age overfeeding may result in an elevated fat cell number. Although increased fat cell numbers are more common in early-onset obesity, some individuals with late-onset obesity show hypercellularity. A few people with early-onset obesity have little hypercellularity, but accurate retrospective histories of weight are difficult to obtain (4).

Van Itallie et al. indicate that nonobese animals keep a preferred body mass over the long term and that a hypothalamic coordinating center monitors adipose stores (11). Regulation may be for the total energy reserve or fat content of the body rather than for fat cells. Thus, attainment of a maximum fat cell size could cause development of new fat cells so more energy could be stored. Some work with animals and infants supports this, but much research remains to be done.

In an average adult woman, the size of individual fat cells increase up to a level of approximately 30 kg of total body fat. After this, the number of fat cells increase to accommodate more fat. So all fat people have hypertropic obesity, including those with hyperplastic obesity. Therefore, the long-term solution to adult obesity seems to be some means of reducing cell number. Careful life span documentation on early life feeding practices on obesity awaits longitudinal data collection and analysis. At present, early modification of diet, exercise, and heredity are principal areas of study.

factors in obesity

METABOLIC CHANGES. Stricker has suggested a dual model of obesity caused by overeating secondary to fat metabolism alterations, or by hyperphagia (14). Hormones related to lipid mobilization, lipolysis, have been studied in relation to obesity (13). The serum of obese children contain more factors related to lipid synthesis than breakdown (14). Insulin levels, for example, are two to five times higher in the obese than in leaner subjects. Levels are high in obesity because of the increased insulin resistance of the enlarged fat cells that interferes with the biological effectiveness of insulin, requiring more insulin to be secreted. The response in other tissues may be very different. A high sugar intake in insulin-resistant individuals seems to stimulate an overresponse. Hypocaloric diets with reduced soluble carbohydrate intake result in a lower insulin response. Hyperinsulinism is associated with the onset of obesity rather than being a long-term consequence of overweight (15). Studies with obese children show a hyperinsulinism related to the degree of obesity, but not to the duration. But the origin of hyperinsulinism and the mechanism of insulin resistance remain obscure. Other hormones, such as epinephrine, norepinephrine, growth hormones, and glucagon have been studied (16). Information in this area changes rapidly, and the means of controlling appetite or fat cell synthesis may come from research on basic hormonal interactions.

Others have suggested that the naturally occurring opiate β-endorphin plays a part in the development of obesity through overeating (17).

THERMOGENESIS. Cellular thermogenesis and other metabolic aspects of obesity are now under intensive research. It has been suggested that obesity may be caused by a thermogenetic defect. Animal studies with genetically obese mice have shown that overweight animals retain a greater percentage of ingested energy than do lean controls and demonstrate altered thermogenetic responses (18). Likewise, at least one human study has shown an impaired thermogenetic response in the obese. Rate of energy use may prove to be an important distinguishing characteristic of the obese population (19, 20). One research group has detected low levels of the enzyme adenosine triphosphatase (ATPase) in red blood cells of obese individuals (21). Since ATPase may account for 10 to 50 percent of the body's heat energy production, it is possible that some overweight persons may burn fewer calories as heat and store more calories as fat.

HEREDITY. Genetic influences may determine fat cell number, regulate the efficiency of metabolic processes, and establish the sensitivity of different parts of the central nervous system to nutrient deprivation and repletion. In humans, obesity as a result of a defect in a single gene is rare; most human obesity is polygenic and presents a difficult problem for study. In studies using twins, genetic factors seem to be of primary importance: from 74 to 88 percent of weight variance seems to be accounted for by heredity (9). On the other hand, Garn proposes that human obesity is primarily of environmental origin. The correlation coefficient between the skinfold thickness of marital partners is almost as high as that between parents and children who share common genes and environment. Adoption studies do not resolve the difference, since the studies show opposite results, with one supporting inheritance and another supporting environmental factors (9).

SET POINT. Another theory is that the body may have a *set point* of physiological regulation, and the obese may have a higher set point than lean individuals. Rather than just maintaining a constant body weight, there is a defense of the set point for body weight when it is artificially raised or lowered (9). Regulation results from changes in caloric intake and in energy expenditure. Weight loss triggers increased food intake and reduced energy expenditure, while weight gain results in the opposite response. The Minnesota semistarvation studies and the overfeeding experiments in Vermont, both conducted using healthy young men, seem to support this proposition of dual control of body weight. If obese individuals are defending an obese set point of body weight, this would explain why they remain obese no matter how hard they try to lose weight.

SOCIOECONOMIC FACTORS. Epidemiological studies show that children at the poverty level and below tend to be leaner, and those at median income and above tend to be fatter in both black and white males and females in America, Britain, and France (22). In adult females, the relationship changes: During youth, poor girls are leaner than the more affluent girls, while women of middle income and above are leaner than poor women in adult life. This argues against the fat child, fat adult hypothesis for obesity.

It is true that fat parents tend to have fat children and lean parents tend to have lean children. If both parents are fat, the children become fatter until age 17. They are three times as likely to be fat as children of two lean parents. These parent-child data are consistent with the genetic hypothesis. In addition, there could be an effect from learned eating patterns, inasmuch as obese husbands tend to be married to fatter wives.

PHYSICAL ACTIVITY. Many researchers have emphasized the importance of physical activity in weight control as a means of increasing the caloric requirement or the energy needed (23). Among obese children and adults, low energy expenditures are common (Table 9–4 shows calories and activity levels). Figure 9–3 shows fuel stores in the obese adult. Long-term and moderate increases in physical activity do not greatly increase the appetite, so physical activity is a useful means of weight reduction. Exercise increases the potential of adipose tissue cells to release free fatty acids in response to epinephrine stimulation (24). Although exercise has only a small effect on cell number, it may cause a significant decrease in cell size.

The metabolic response of adipose tissue to exercise appears to be related to the oxidative adaptation occurring in skeletal muscles. Increase in the ability of adipose tissue to synthesize triglycerides and mobilize free fatty acids after

TABLE 9-4. Calories and Activity Level

food	calories	Sedentary	Light	Moderate	Vigorous	Strenuous[b]
		level of activity (in minutes)[a]				
2 8-inch celery stalks	15	10	7	4	3	2
2 medium graham crackers	55	35	25	16	12	8
2 tbsp. fruit-nut snack	70	47	32	20	14	10
2 tbsp. peanuts	105	72	49	33	22	17
1 cup plain low-fat yogurt	145	96	70	44	30	25
1 cup split-pea soup	195	132	90	57	40	35
1 cup fruit-flavored yogurt	225	153	105	68	46	39
1/2 cup crunchy cereal with coconut	280	198	130	82	57	47
Hamburger (3-oz. patty on bun)	365	248	169	109	75	62
12-oz. chocolate milkshake	430	289	198	128	89	72

[a] Minutes of activity needed to "burn up" food calories are approximations.

[b] The calorie value of strenuous activity was calculated using a rate of 350 calories per hour. Some strenuous activities may require more than 350 calories per hour and would take less time to burn up energy or calories.

SOURCE: Adapted from Food, Home and Garden Bulletin No. 228, Science and Education Administration, U.S. Department of Agriculture.

vigorous physical exercise may be a secondary adaptation to increased ability of the skeletal muscles to oxidize fatty acid and ketone bodies during exercise. Adipose tissue plays a central role in the adaptation to physical training and the stress of exercise. Numerous reports have shown cyclic AMP to be involved in a variety of metabolic control mechanisms. The stimulation of free fatty acid release by adipose tissue is related to cellular mechanisms involving cyclic AMP and a lipase (25).

PSYCHOLOGICAL FACTORS. Much research has gone into psychological factors related to obesity (26), but the reports are conflicting. Some studies indicate that obese people have psychological disorders that lead to obesity; other studies do not show the same results.

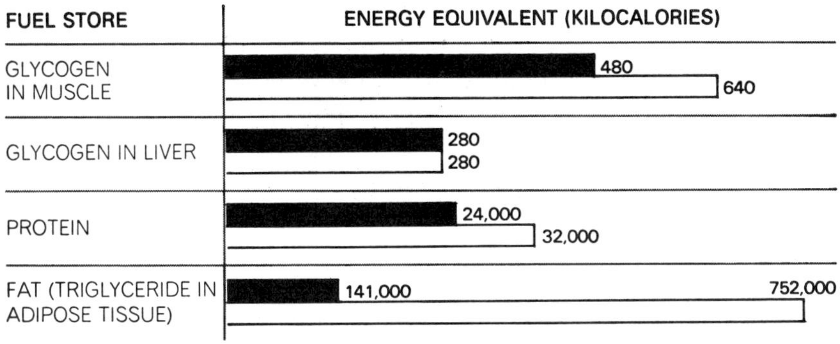

FIG. 9–3. Fuel stores in normal adult (black bars) and obese adult (white bars) are compared. Each pair of bars is on a different scale. The main store is fat, and in obese people this store is five or six times larger than in normal people. *Source:* V. Young and N. Scrimshaw, "The Physiology of Starvation." Copyright © 1971 by Scientific American, Inc. All rights reserved.

Obesity may be the result of faulty learning about the internal signals of the body (9). By relating food to all distress signals, an infant or child can be taught faulty interpretation of signals. The theories of classical conditioning can be related to satiety. The conditioned stimulus for satiety can be the body, the food, the time, the place, and the social context combined. The obese are more responsive to external stimuli for food consumption, according to psychologists. But externality is not peculiar to obese people, for many normal-weight individuals respond to external cues (9).

In our society, attitudes toward obesity are negative. There is much job discrimination and rejection of the obese individual, although food is important in social situations, and people are constantly encouraged to eat. The obese person is thus placed in great conflict. The stage at which obesity develops in the life cycle of an individual seems to have much to do with that person's self-concept. In addition, the attitudes of the people around the obese individual affect the self-concept. For those who have been obese in childhood, obesity may be accepted, or it may be a means of self-rejection. Families contribute much to a person's attitude about obesity; psychological case reports often provide information on mothers who overfeed and then criticize their children for being overweight. In addition, for some adults, obesity may provide an important psychological crutch. Increased body size may give a person a sense of security, and for some individuals, it has been suggested that it may provide a means of protecting themselves from sexual advances.

Psychological factors may also lead to the development of obesity. Food may be used as a tool for satisfying oneself over and above hunger needs. People may overeat when they are tired or angry, and problems are frequently dealt with through the consumption of food. These behaviors may be learned very early in life. Infants and children who are given food for every physiological and psychological need, whether it is food related or not, may learn to utilize food in this manner. The term *environmental obesity* has been used to describe the relative ease with which highly palatable food is available in the United States, and people's use of this abundant food supply for reasons unrelated to nourishment (27). Psychological techniques such as behavioral modification have been used effectively for the treatment of obesity (28, 29). Behavioral modification is based on the principle that one behavior is substituted for another; and that overeating is simply an incorrectly learned set of behavioral patterns.

health hazards of obesity

Life insurance studies demonstrate an inverse relationship between length of life and degree of overweight. The number of degenerative diseases increases with obesity, and normal body functions may be changed. Symptoms of many established diseases may be lessened by reducing adipose tissue. Arthritis, for example, is more physically limiting in the obese. Toxemia of pregnancy, chronic neuritis, and surgical risk are increased by obesity. Diabetes also appears to be more prevalent in populations with a substantial incidence of obesity (30). Of particular concern is the close association between obesity and hypertension. Obese hypertensive patients have a greater risk of coronary heart disease than nonobese hypertensives, and mortality rates for obese hypertensive individuals are high (31).

Several studies have reported a positive correlation between obesity and gallstones (32). Gallstones of obese patients are composed predominately of cholesterol. Cholesterol precipitation and gallstone formation are favored when bile contains more cholesterol than can be held in stabile solution by available bile acids and phospholipids. Obesity is also associated with an increased production of cholesterol. Saturation of gall bladder bile is increased in obesity as the result of enhanced secretion of cholesterol. With restriction of energy intake, saturation can increase because of decreased output of bile acids and phospholipids and the mobilization of cholesterol from adipose stores. Some subjects are transiently at risk of gallstone formation during active weight reduction, but that risk decreases when a lower weight is established and maintained.

life cycle obesity

CHILDHOOD. The incidence of childhood obesity varies from 3 to 20 percent, depending upon the population studied and the method used to determine obesity (33, 34). When caliper measurement of skinfold thicknesses as opposed to weight for height is used as the guideline, the incidence drops to the lower levels. Not all overweight children are overweight due to body fat. A very small percentage of childhood obesity is caused by disease state—for example, the Prader-Willi or the Pickwickian syndromes (35).

Longitudinal growth data on children who developed obesity during childhood support the hypothesis that overnutrition accelerates growth; the greater the positive energy balance, the taller in relative terms the child becomes (36). The children studied had a modest increase in lean weight, in addition to a large increase in fat. Since obese children grow rapidly, they obviously must take in enough protein and other essential nutrients to provide for their accelerated statural growth and their generous lean weight.

In a study of 963 children whose weight data were available from the first year of life on, it was shown that the factors which determined weight gain in infancy were no longer operative at ages between 7 and 10.5 years (37). Similar results have been found in another study indicating that fat infants were heavier and taller than the standards, but these children at school age were no longer heavier in relation to height than the standards. Therefore, the fat baby may not be doomed to be a fat child or a fat adult.

In a retrospective study, relative obesity was determined by the use of the obesity index, weight divided by height, for 73,523 members of a weight reduction club (7). Each person was asked, "Were you considered a fat child?" to indicate the presence of childhood obesity. Errors exist in this method, but the size of the sample would be more likely to obscure any relationship found. There was a definite relationship between adult and childhood obesity, with 2.4 times more severely obese women having been fat children than normal women. Similar findings have been found in a prospective study using 50 obese girls (5). At least 80 percent were also obese as adults, whereas only 18 percent of the 50 normal-weight juveniles were obese adults. Juvenile obese girls were 4.4 times as likely to become obese adults as normal-weight girls. Physical activity must also be evaluated, as studies have shown that the obese children are less physically active than normal weight children and consume the same number of calories.

In a society where there is a bias against the obese individual, obese children often suffer psychological problems (26). Studies indicate, for example, that the obese are less likely to be chosen for games. Negative feelings about body image can be carried into adult life. And eating habits learned in childhood are difficult to change in adult life.

ADOLESCENCE. Estimates of the incidence of obesity in adolescents range from 10 to 35 percent of the population. Studies have shown that obese teenagers actually eat less and consume fewer calories than normal weight teenagers, but are less active physically (38). The fat teenager is therefore more vulnerable to malnutrition when he or she limits food intake in an attempt to reduce. Girls, especially, often try bizarre fads, and "instant weight loss" regimens that can compromise their nutritional status.

In early to middle adolescence, when growth is still intense, sharp restriction of calories may result in large losses of lean body mass. For this reason, and because of the metabolic complications inherent in nutrient restriction and the physiological and/or psychological stress generated by food withdrawal, severe caloric restriction for long periods is not recommended for adolescents. Only restriction of clear excesses through portion control is advisable (22).

The adolescent being treated for obesity needs reinforcement from the family in order to develop a positive attitude toward food restriction (39). Treatment requires a program that can deal with the complexities of adolescence and obesity. A rigid approach to weight control based on parental enforcement of diet and exercise should be avoided (26). Especially in early adolescence, parental coercion may so intensify the normally strained parent-teenager relationship that the product of a well-intentioned therapeutic endeavor is a sullen, angry, rebellious youngster who is gaining rather than losing weight. Teenagers and their parents need to understand that all adolescents gain weight while growing. Increased adipose tissue is the problem, and it must be separated from normal weight gain. For the moderately obese, a realistic goal is the prevention of further gains in body fat. Well motivated teenagers are able to withstand the biological and psychological stress of food deprivation for the long periods required for weight loss.

Methods of evaluating body composition are complex, so the analysis of obesity in the adolescent is difficult. Some are heavy because of large muscle mass and/or heavy skeleton, the truly obese, however, have an excess of adipose tissue. In the prepubescent period, obesity is generally defined for both males and females as a weight/height ratio greater than the 95th percentile on the NCHS growth chart. During puberty, the individual height and weight percentile should not differ by more than 15 percentile points from the chronological age. The adolescent whose weight gain is in excess of the 15 percentile points above the height percentile should be evaluated for potential obesity. Other experts use 20 percent above ideal weight for height, which may be the 50th percentile of weight for age (40).

Exercise is another consideration. The obese adolescent gets less exercise than the nonobese even when performing the same physical activities. Movies of physical activity in the studies mentioned above showed that the obese move slowly and tend to be more withdrawn (41, 42, 43). Many choose more sedentary activities, such as reading and watching television, both of which tend to encourage or offer opportunities for more eating. Some are self-conscious and reluctant to participate in activities requiring undressing because they fear ridicule by peers (44).

Traditionally, emphasis has been placed on the quantitative aspects of energy intake rather than on energy expenditure. Many nutritionists have underestimated the benefits of exercise. In addition to its direct caloric contribution to energy expenditure, exercise may increase both the specific dynamic action of food and the postexercise metabolic rate (45). For this reason, encouraging physical activity and exercise is usually more profitable than dietary regimens alone. Recent reviews indicate that new and innovative treatments are needed for the adolescent because significant weight loss is rare with current methods (46, 47). These authors point out that the most promising therapies are combinations of dietary counseling, exercise programs, total environmental management, and behavior modification techniques.

Prevention of obesity would seem to hold greater potential for success than treatment of obesity in adolescence. In addition, weight reduction during the rapid growth period should be undertaken with extreme caution and only under close medical supervision.

ADULTHOOD. The percentage of those who are overweight increases in the adult age ranges. Among the adult population in the United States, more than 30 percent are obese. Among the very old, obesity is less common. Mortality rates in the earlier decades may account for this decline, or there may be a relationship between smaller food intake and long life, or weight loss and advancing age. Obesity may represent a potential health problem for a large segment of adults, since those who maintain body weight at a level suitable for their height at age 25 tend to live longer.

Reduced physical activity seems to be a major factor in the development of adult obesity. A sedentary life style contributes to an undesirable yearly weight gain. In industrialized countries, physical activity has decreased rather than food intake increasing, but the result has been the same: a definite increase in adult obesity.

PREGNANCY. Maternal obesity is regarded as a risk factor in pregnancy. Antepartum complications related to hypertension and diabetes mellitus are increased in the obese mother. Infants of obese women are larger than average, which may lead to complications in delivery. Induced labor and Cesarean sections are more common in obese women (48). Fewer low birth weight infants are born to obese mothers, although some obese women have inadequate pregnancy weight gains. The obese mother is less likely to deliver preterm and more likely to deliver postterm than the nonobese, so there is less risk of premature labor.

weight reduction

The method of weight reduction selected should be based on the severity of the obesity and related health complications. Of prime importance in treating obesity is selecting a method of weight control that provides the lowest level of physical and psychological risk to the person at the least expense possible. The method should result in weight reduction that can be maintained for many years. Unfortunately, the success rate for maintenance after weight loss is low. Only about one-fourth of those treated reduce successfully, and there is a high rate of recurrence (9). Only when low-risk methods are ineffective and the degree of obesity is great should the higher-risk treatments such as fasting, drugs, or surgery be selected. These methods are properly reserved for those whose lives are endangered by their obesity.

Successful and permanent weight reduction is accomplished slowly, and even under the best of circumstances requires discipline, determination, and motivation. A guide for selecting a weight reduction diet is shown in Table 9–5.

TABLE 9–5. How To Select a Weight Reduction Diet

factors to consider	reject diet if
Calculate the nutrient content	
Compare nutrient content with the RDA	Less than two-thirds RDA
Figure the approximate cost of the diet for the period it must be consumed	Too expensive
Compare the cost of the diet with ability of the person to purchase the diet	
Determine the availability of the food included in the diet	
a. Seasonal foods	
b. Preparation time and effort required	
c. Sources for purchase	
Compare the work habits, time, and ability of the person with the availability of the diet	Too difficult
Evaluate the diet in relation to the current food patterns of the person	Food not conveniently available
Evaluate the diet in relation to the health status of the individual	Includes too few current food likes
a. Allergies	
b. Other diet therapies	

The foundation diet should be based on a variety of foods. In the amount recommended for adults, about 1200 kilocalories are provided. A dietary plan based on the USDA Food Guide is shown in Table 9–6. Most adults respond to a structured or planned diet in the early phase of weight reduction. After success and weight loss, the diet can be liberalized. Exchange lists developed for diabetics can be used as guidelines for making food choices with similar calorie contents (see Appendix table).

Dieting causes stress for many people who maintain a body weight lower than their set point. The constant physiological hunger may be a source of frustration and a drain on the ability to cope emotionally. People who maintain a lower body weight by restrained eating are probably in a state of stress or arousal. This could affect behavior, emotions, or physical well-being (9). Such a person may be tense and irritable for no apparent reason.

Care must be taken in weight reduction plans for children (36), because drastic reduction in caloric intake will result in decreased growth. With children who are only moderately obese the emphasis should be on maintaining a stable weight rather than on reduction; then height gain can bring the weight into balance. In addition, physical activity must be increased. Postponing reduction to

TABLE 9-6. USDA Daily Good Guide Used for Weight Control

words for calorie counters

Do you have a weight problem? Have you ever tried to diet, and then V-ROOM! gained back most of the weight you lost? Worrying about weight is a popular diversion for Americans, and frankly, many people *should* be concerned about their weight.

The problem is *what* and *how much* to eat. Certain foods have more calories than other foods, so you should eat smaller or fewer portions of high-calorie foods. The calories in a pie aren't any more fattening than the calories in an apple—there are just more of them in the pie.

You should choose your calories for the "nutritional company" they keep—that is, pick foods which in addition to calories provide some of the vitamins, minerals, and protein you need. The Guide can help you to do this. Use it when selecting foods—keeping a cautious eye on the fifth group—Fats-Sweets-Alcohol—whose main contribution is calories.

If you are trying to control your weight, follow these guidelines:

1. Cut down on high-fat foods such as margarine, butter, highly marbled or fatty meats, and fried foods. Salad dressings, cream sauces, gravies, and many whipped dessert toppings are also high in fat.
2. Cut down on sugary foods such as candies; soft drinks and other sugar-sweetened beverages such as ades and punches; jelly, jam, sirups, honey; fruit canned in heavy sirup; pies, cakes, and pastries.
3. Cut down on or eliminate alcoholic drinks.
4. Cut down on portion sizes. Portions of some foods, such as meats, are hard to estimate. For example, a 3-ounce serving of cooked lean meat without bone is equivalent to a 3- by 5/8-inch hamburger pattie. What is your usual portion size?
5. Use whole milk or whole-milk products (most cheeses and ice cream) sparingly. Lowfat and skim-milk products, such as ice milk and skim-milk cheeses, provide fewer calories than their whole-milk counterparts.
6. Select cooking methods to help cut calories. Cook foods with little or no added fat and avoid deep-fat fried foods, which are high in calories because of the fat absorbed during cooking. For meat and poultry, trim off visible fat; either broil or roast on a rack. If braised or stewed, drain meat to remove fat. For fish, broil or bake. For vegetables, steam, bake, or boil; for an occasional change, stir-fry in a small amount of vegetable oil.
7. Be sure to count the nibbles and drinks enjoyed during social events and throughout the day as part of your day's calorie allotment.

calorie countdown[1]

Calorie Countdown illustrates how foods vary in calories. Use it to help you select foods. If you need another serving from the Milk-Cheese group, for example, but want to take it easy on calories, choose ice milk rather than a milkshake. Other examples show how added fats, sugars, sauces, and other ingredients increase calories. Three calorie levels are shown for each type of food.

TABLE 9-6. (Continued)

VEGETABLE/FRUIT GROUP		
Lower	In-Between	Higher
1 cup raw vegetable salad without dressing (40)[1]	3/4 cup raw vegetable salad with 1 tablespoon French dressing (95)	1/2 cup potato salad (125)
1/2 cup cooked cabbage (15)	1/2 cup coleslaw (60)	2 rolls stuffed cabbage (260)
1 medium baked potato (95)	2/3 cup mashed potatoes prepared with milk and butter (125)	1/2 cup hashed brown potatoes (170)
1 medium raw apple (80)	1 sweetened baked apple (160)	1/8 of 9-inch apple pie (300)
1/2 cup fresh citrus sections (40)	1/2 cup jellied citrus salad (120)	1/2 cup lemon pudding (145)
1/2 cup cooked green beans (15)	1/2 cup stir-fried green beans (35)	1/2 cup green bean-mushroom casserole (70)
1/2 cup diced fresh pineapple (40)	1/2 cup canned pineapple chunks in natural juice (70)	1/2 cup canned pineapple chunks in heavy sirup (95)

BREAD/CEREAL GROUP		
Lower	In-Between	Higher
1 cup plain corn flakes (95)[1]	1 cup sugar-coated corn flakes (155)	1/2 cup crunchy cereal (280 to 290)
1/2 cup steamed or boiled rice (85)	1/2 cup fried rice without meat (185)	1/2 cup rice pudding (235)
1 slice of bread (55 to 70)	1 corn muffin (125)	1 Danish pastry (275)
1/2 cup cooked noodles (100)	6 cheese ravioli with sauce (175)	1 cup lasagna (345)

MILK/CHEESE GROUP		
Lower	In-Between	Higher
1/2 cup (single dip) ice milk (95)	1/2 cup (single dip) ice cream (135)	1 cup vanilla milkshake (255)
1 oz. Cheddar cheese (115)	1 cup cheese souffle (260)	1 cup macaroni and cheese (430)
8 fl. oz. carton plain lowfat yogurt (145)	8 fl. oz. carton vanilla flavored yogurt (195)	8 fl. oz. carton yogurt with fruit or 2 dips frozen yogurt (225 to 240)

MEAT/POULTRY/FISH AND BEANS GROUP		
Lower	In-Between	Higher
2 oz. broiled chicken (95)	1/2 fried chicken breast (2-3/4 oz.) or 2 drumsticks (2-1/2 oz.) (160 to 180)	8 oz. individual chicken pot pie (505)

TABLE 9-6. (Continued)

3 oz. lean hamburger (without bun) (185)	3 oz. regular hamburger (without bun) (235)	3-1/2 oz. cheeseburger (without bun) (320)
3 oz. lean roast beef (205)	3 oz. Swiss steak (315)	2/3 cup beef stroganoff over noodles (525)
2-1/2 oz. broiled cod with butter or margarine (120)	2-1/2 oz. fried, breaded ocean perch (160)	2-1/2 oz. baked stuffed fish (1/2 cup bread stuffing) (325)
1/2 cup boiled navy beans (95)	1 cup navy bean soup (170)	1 cup baked navy beans (310)
3 oz. boiled shrimp (100)	3 oz. fried breaded shrimp (190)	1/2 cup shrimp Newburg (285)
	FATS/SWEETS/ALCOHOL GROUP	
Lower	In-Between	Higher
1 teaspoon sugar (15)	2 tablespoons pancake sirup (120)	12 fl. oz. cola (145)
12 fl oz. light beer or 3-1/2 fl. oz. dry wine (85 to 95)	12 fl. oz. regular beer or 3-1/2 fl. oz. sweet wine (140 to 150)	Tom Collins—1 fl. oz. gin & 6 fl. oz. Tom Collins mix (195)
3 oz. popsicle (70)	1/2 cup (single dip) sherbet (135)	1.2 oz. milk chocolate candy bar (175)

[1] Calorie values are shown within parens.

SOURCE: *Food, Home and Garden Bulletin*, No. 228, Science and Education Administration, U.S. Department of Agriculture.

the adult years may be less successful because of the number of fat cells or established habits in eating.

BEHAVIOR MODIFICATION. Behavior modification is based on the premise that social factors exert a major influence on eating, and that these factors can be changed to control excessive food intake (28, 49). Effective programs include keeping accurate records of food eaten and the other events surrounding food intake. Modifications are then made in current behaviors that contribute to overeating. Having low-calorie snacks available, planning meals ahead of time, and establishing one designated eating place are standard techniques. Many programs are based on a reward system, either monetary or praise. Control of the stimulus for eating can be effective for prolonged weight loss and more permanent control.

Overeating is the target behavior controlled by the reinforcer, which is either positive (reward) or negative (aversive stimuli). Effective reinforcers are different for each individual and must be carefully selected for maximum effect. The goal of extinction is attained by eliminating the need for reinforcement.

Stuart has developed a guide for self-management of behavior modification (29) in which the individual does not depend on another person for management. Unfortunately, few studies have been done on this self-management approach. Stunkard has reported excellent results in the use of behavior modification for treatment of obesity (9). In a review of outpatient treatments of obesity, Wing and Jeffery concluded that, on the basis of available data, behavioral therapy produces the best maintenance of weight losses (50). Currey et al., however, reported disappointing results with behavioral treatment of chronically obese women experiencing medical complications (51). Weight loss from behavior modification was similar to other methods of weight control. It may be that medically referred older, obese persons are less responsive to behavioral techniques than volunteers.

DRUGS. Most of the weight-control drugs used in humans produce marked effects on brain neurotransmitters like monoamines. Drugs that suppress food intake seem to alter the activity of amines in the brain.

Different drugs affect different neurochemicals. Catecholamines play a dominant role in the action of amphetamines, while the action of fenfluramine seems to be mediated by serotonin-related systems. Amphetamine may inhibit hunger, and fenfluramine may stimulate satiety. Fenfluramine reduces the amount of a meal eaten, amphetamine delays the meal. Amphetamine decreases all components of the diet; fenfluramine spares protein. In animals, the stress produced by overeating is reduced by fenfluramine but not amphetamine (9).

The many chemical agents affecting appetite vary widely in chemical structure, mechanism of activity, associated side effects, and potential for abuse. Fenfluramine, dextroamphetamine, diethylpropion hydrochloride, and mazindol have been studied most extensively and are usually prescribed along with a low-calorie diet. The value of such drugs is as a short-term adjunct to help maintain the prescribed diet. Hormones used for weight reduction include human chorionic gonadotrophic (HCG) and thyroid preparations. The highly controversial HCG regimen consists of daily hormone injections and a rigid 500 kilocalorie diet (9).

SURGERY. Individuals 100 percent or more over desirable body weight are called *morbidly obese.* This degree of obesity enhances the risk of premature death from heart disease, stroke, and diabetes mellitus (52). Such persons are the only appropriate candidates for surgical procedures.

Intestinal bypass surgery reduces the length of the small intestine. Weight loss is accomplished by reduced food intake and altered eating patterns. The benefits to the morbidly obese include significant weight loss, improved glucose tolerance, normalization of the Pickwickian syndrome, lowering of serum lipids, and the pleasure of social acceptability. Weight may stabilize above the projected ideal weight. Heavier patients (over 300 lbs) lose weight more rapidly and reach a weight plateau at a later time. The majority reach a plateau between 12 and

24 months. Some weight, about 20 to 30 percent, may be regained after five years. The complications of intestinal bypass surgery are related to major abdominal surgery and to metabolic disorders. The death rate is 0.5 to 7 percent. Other problems are electrolyte abnormalities, infections, kidney stones, arthritis, diarrhea, dizziness, weakness, and other subjective complaints. The persistent diarrhea can lead to malnutrition. Over 60 percent of patients show significant weight loss without major complications. Generally, these successful weight losses are obtained by lighter, younger, more vigorous people who have a positive outlook.

Stomach surgeries include gastric bypass and gastroplasty (stomach stapling). These procedures reduce the size of the stomach, and thereafter care must be taken to consume small volumes of food and to avoid drinking liquids while eating. Since only small amounts of food can be consumed, the nutritional quality of the diet must be high, and vitamin and mineral supplementation may be necessary. The major complication is perforations that can result in peritonitis and death.

Jaw wiring is another extreme procedure, but weight is usually regained after unwiring. A combination of gastric surgery and wiring is more effective.

OTHER METHODS OF WEIGHT REDUCTION. Total fasting, semi-starvation, the protein-sparing modified fast, and similar regimens remain more suited to inpatient treatment, which allows continuous medical supervision and ongoing laboratory evaluation. Weight reduction utilizing such esoteric approaches as acupuncture, psychotherapy, and hypnosis await further investigation and experimentation in controlled settings before their value can be assessed (53, 54, 55).

On the other end of the weight control equation, several low-calorie bulking agents are undergoing testing and may prove useful in the preparation of palatable and acceptable low-calorie desserts and snacks. But the desirability of these nutritionally unnecessary items must be weighed against their higher ingredient and preparation cost. One such product, sucrose polyester, has been shown to have a low-calorie use and to possess characteristics as a synthetic fat substitute. Agents such as isolated cellulose and other dietary fibers have been used as bulking agents for carbohydrate replacement with varying amounts of success. Polyols such as mannitol, sorbitol, and xylitol are frequently used as sucrose replacements in chewing gums and dietary foods, although their caloric use varies from 50 to 100 percent of that of sucrose.

Underweight (Undernutrition)

Thinness or leanness as measured by weight for height ratios and other anthropometric measures has genetic origins similar to obesity (56). Environmental factors play a role, since whole families tend to have similar food and eating habits. Family eating patterns may predispose to leanness by offering a minimum of calories or by terminating eating with satiety. Active or athletically inclined parents tend to have children who are also physically active, and a life style that includes adequate energy expenditure to prevent storage of excess calories.

Little has been written about the underweight or undernourished individual except for infancy, where weight gains and losses are the most closely monitored nutritional parameter. Even small weight losses can be significant in the lean infant, who has a greater proportion of body surface area to weight. This is particularly important in maintaining approximate body temperatures, because some subcutaneous fat is essential to the regulation of normal temperature. Chronic failure to gain adequately in infants has been described as "failure to thrive" and serves as an excellent model to show the complexities of weight control (57, 58). The majority of these infants are described as having less than adequate intakes of nutrients. This may be due to ignorance, lack of available resources, neglect, or abuse on the part of the caretaker. Some of these infants can be fed adequate nutrients and still not grow, indicating the significant relationship of psychological and emotional factors to the achievement of adequate nutritional status. The fact that many of these infants did not "bond" or enter into a close maternal-child relationship played a role in their failure to thrive (59). One would assume that this condition would exist only in the dependent stage of infancy. However, studies have shown the same syndrome occurring in orphanages, residential centers, and family groups where adequate emotional support was lacking or negative (60). Although early infancy is a critical time for the effects of emotional security on nutritional status, they can occur at other ages (61).

Thin children and adolescents are especially conscious of their body composition and suffer as much ridicule from being "skinny" as do their fat peers. Boys suffer more psychologically than girls because society expects boys to be heavy and strong-not skinny and weak. Weakness is wrongfully associated with body size because the lean or thin individual may have good musculature and strength.

factors in underweight

Underweight is frequently associated with chronic diseases at all ages. Disease may impose such increased metabolic demands on the body that it is impossible for an individual to consume enough calories to maintain adequate weight without intensive nutrition counseling. In these cases, calorically dense foods should be used so that greater amounts of nutrients can be consumed in less volume. This is especially true for children, who have less capacity and tolerance for increased volumes. Meal frequency must also be increased.

Lack of or poor appetite may be a contributory cause of undernutrition. As stated earlier, appetite is a complex mechanism. Various techniques may be tried to improve or increase appetite: regularity of food offerings, improving the esthetic quality of food offered, reducing sweet snacking, and changing the eating environment.

In the adolescent male the "spurt" in height growth is more intense than that in weight, and many young men are physiologically "thin." At the same time, they may have excessive energy expenditures without adequate rest. Increasing caloric intake may not be possible because at this time they are usually "eating constantly" and are unwilling to give up activities for rest. Weight gains to keep up with gains in height are not possible, and the male stays thin. The genetically thin—both male and females—will have the same difficulties gaining additional weight. Gaining is more complicated than just a simple balance of calorie intake being greater than caloric output; many thin persons will consume considerably more calories and still not gain weight.

Even though more time is usually devoted to techniques of weight reduction, the problems of gaining weight are just as important and often as difficult to solve for the underweight person. Methods for gaining weight must be as carefully chosen as those for weight reduction. As with weight reduction, therapy should be undertaken only after a complete physical examination and under medical supervision. Assessing nutritional status, including a good dietary history, is an important first step. This may help to pinpoint the causes of decreased intake and may be useful in making recommendations for increasing food intakes.

For some, the solution is as simple as providing a source of food. Others may need different combinations of foods. Increases in feeding should be gradual so that the individual has an opportunity to adjust over a period of time (62). Excessive amounts of food may lead to stuffing, vomiting, and gastrointestinal disturbances that serve to further decrease weight. Vitamin supplementation is not recommended unless the amount of food the individual is able to consume is less than enough to provide adequate vitamins. Increased caloric intake is an obvious adjunct to weight gain. Generous amounts of fats should be used as tolerated to increase calories while at the same time not making the total amount of food required excessive.

Changes in weight do not occur quickly in any except infants; therefore, underweight individuals should be prepared for slow gains at best after changes are made in eating behavior.

anorexia nervosa

Anorexia nervosa is excessive thinness that results from a morbid fear of gaining weight. By definition a neurosis with severe psychologic disturbance is a part of this disease; therefore, it must be treated with expert psychotherapy (63). Teenagers with this disease are emaciated and have extreme difficulty eating. Self-induced vomiting is often associated with eating, as well as hiding food to avoid eating. Sufferers may have grossly distorted body images and see themselves as grossly overweight and further restrict food. They view their continued weight loss as a measure of success (26, 64).

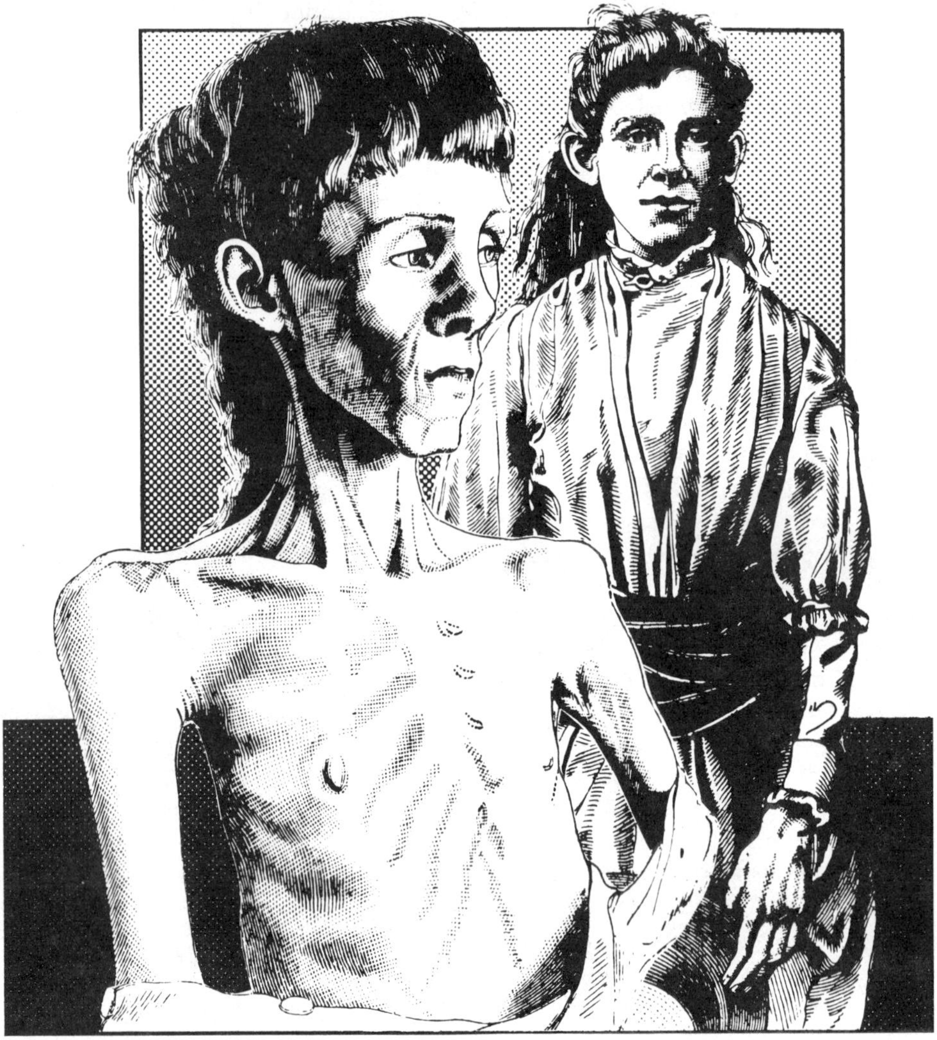

FIG. 9–4. Woodcuts accompanying Sir William Gull's article "Anorexia Nervosa" in Volume 1 of *Lancet,* 1888: illustration of the dramatic changes possible in patient with anorexia (left) after appropriate treatment (right) for what Gull called a "morbid mental state." Woodcuts courtesy National Library of Medicine.

The condition usually occurs in white, middle-class girls aged 12 to 18 at the rate of one in 200 American girls, and is fatal in 10 to 15 percent of the cases. Only 4 to 6 percent of the incidence is among boys. Sir William Gull named the illness in 1874 (see Figure 9–4). Organic vulnerability and environmental stress reflect the multifaceted aspects of anorexia nervosa. The general characteristics are obsessive pursuit of thinness, very small food intake or huge food intake followed by vomiting, hyperactivity, cessation of menstruation, and a distorted body image.

Bruch (26) defines anorexia nervosa as a psychological disorder accompanied by excessive weight loss that leads to emaciation and sometimes death. In the weight history of a person who develops anorexia nervosa there may be evidence of previous obesity, or fear of obesity. Dietary modification must be combined with psychological treatment of the individual and the family.

Future Considerations

Neither obesity nor excessive underweight are unitary disorders. Identifying and classifying the various forms of obesity or underweight will lead to a better understanding and more precise treatment of the disease. Although genetic predispositions and traumatic intervention are important, environmental factors related to food intake may well prove to be the most important in body weight manipulation.

Many questions remain to be solved before clinical problems in obesity and thinness can be approached intelligently. For those persons who are already obese, research must determine methods to influence the number and size of adipose cells or to develop satiety. The focus must be on finding a physiologically feasible metabolic method for control of the mechanism of adipose cellular division and fatty acid synthesis. Tissue cultures may be a means of studying key metabolic processes in glucose and fatty acid metabolism and thermogenesis and could lead to better weight control measures for both extremes. The development of caloric and nutrient dense formulas that are palatable, inexpensive, and without side effects would be a benefit to the underweight. Studies must be designed to attempt to answer the question of why some people are lean and some are fat even with similar caloric intakes and activity regimens.

Summary

Weight control is a preoccupation in the Western world. It is dependent upon a balance between energy consumed and expended. Protein, carbohydrates, and fats, along with alcohol, are the energy sources. Obesity is excessive body fatness. Some standards for obesity include height, weight, body mass index, and skinfold measurement. Lipids are stored in the fat cell, and fat cell development is a continuing topic for research.

Factors in the development of obesity include metabolic changes, thermogenesis, heredity, socioeconomic conditions, physical activity, and psychological factors. Obesity presents several health hazards. The effects and treatment of obesity vary during the life cycle.

A number of methods are used for weight reduction. The method selected should be effective in producing weight loss with the lowest level of physical and psychological risk and the least expense possible. Some techniques used are the low-calorie diet, exercise, behavior modification, and surgery, or combinations of these. Underweight is a serious problem. Anorexia nervosa is excessive thinness resulting from a morbid fear of obesity, and is a serious psychological disorder.

references

1. *Obesity and Health.* PHS Publication No. 1485, National Center for Chronic Disease Control, Public Health Service. Washington, D.C.: U.S. Department of Health, Education and Welfare, 1968.
2. SELTZER, C. C., and J. MAYER, "A Simple Criterion of Obesity." *Postgraduate Medicine* 38(1965): A101.
3. MONTOYE, H. J., F. H. EPSTEIN, and M. O. KJELSBERG, "The Measurement of Body Fatness: A Study of a Total Community." *American Journal of Clinical Nutrition* 16 (1965): 417.
4. SJOSTROM, LARS. "Fat Cells and Body Weight," in Stunkard, A. *Obesity*. Philadelphia: Saunders, 1980.
5. BRAY, F., and B. ZACHERY. "Eating Patterns of Massively Obese Individuals." *Journal of the American Dietetic Association* 72(1977): 24.
6. GARN, S. M. "The Origins of Obesity." *Archives of American Journal of Diseases of Children* 130(1976): 465.
7. RIMM, I., and A. RIMM. "Association between Juvenile Obesity and Severe Adult Obesity in 73,532 Women." *American Journal of Public Health* 66(1976): 479.
8. HIRSCH, J. "The Adipose Cell Hypothesis." *New England Journal of Medicine* 295 (1976): 389.
9. STUNKARD, A. J. *Obesity.* Philadelphia: Saunders, 1980.
10. KIRTLAND, J., and M. I. GURR. "Adipose Tissue Cellularity: A Review. 2. The Relationship between Cellularity and Obesity." *International Journal of Obesity* 3(1979): 15.
11. VAN ITALLIE, T. B., N. S. SMITH, and D. QUARTERMAIN."Short-term and Long-term Components in the Regulation of Food Intake: Evidence for a Modulatory Role of Carbohydrate Status." *American Journal of Clinical Nutrition* 30(1977): 742.
12. STRICKER, E. M. "Hyperphagia." *New England Journal of Medicine* 298(1978): 1010.
13. KASTIN, A. J., et al. "Lipid-Mobilizing Hormones of the Hypothalamus and Pituitary." *Pharm. Biochem. Behavior* 3, suppl. 1(1975): 121.
14. ASKEW, E. W., et al. "Adipose Tissue, Cellularity and Lipolysis." *Journal of Clinical Investigation* 56(1975): 521.
15. DESCHAMPS, I., B. J. GIRON, and H. LESTRADET. "Blood, Glucose, Insulin and Free Fatty Acid Levels during Oral Glucose Tolerance Tests in 158 Obese Children." *Diabetes* 18(1977): 89.
16. NEWSHOLME, E. A. "A Possible Metabolic Basis for the Control of Body Weight." *New England Journal of Medicine* 302(1980): 400.

17. MARGULES, D. L., et al. "β-endorphin Is Associated with Overeating in Genetically Obese Mice (ob/ob) and Rats (fa/fa)." *Science* 303(1978): 988.

18. CHLOVERAKIS, C. "Induction of Obesity in Obese-Hyperglycaemic Mice on Normal Food Intake." *Experentia* 26(1970): 1262.

19. JUNG, R. T., et al. "Reduced Thermogenesis in Obesity." *Nature* 279(1979): 322.

20. SIMS, E. A. H., et al. "Endocrine and Metabolic Effects of Experimental Obesity in Man." *Recent Progress in Hormone Research* 29(1973): 457.

21. DELUISE, M., G. L. BLACKBURN, and J. S. FLIER. "Reduced Activity of the Red-Cell Sodium-Potassium Pump in Human Obesity." *New England Journal of Medicine* 303 (1980): 1017.

22. MAYER, J. *Overweight: Causes, Cost, and Control.* Englewood Cliffs, N.J.: Prentice-Hall, 1968.

23. MANN, G. V. *The Management of Obesity-Medical and Social.* Produced and Published by CRC Forum on Obesity, Cleveland, Ohio, 1977.

24. OSCAR, L. B., et al. "Exercise on Food Restrictions: Effect on Adipose Tissue Cellularity." *American Journal of Physiology* 227(1974): 901.

25. ROBINSON, G. A., R. W. BLUTCHER, and E. W. SUTHERLAND. "Catecholamine." In *Biochemical Actions of Hormones,* ed. C. Glitwack. New York: Academic Press, 1972.

26. BRUCH, H. *Eating Disorders: Obesity, Anorexia Nervosa, and the Person Within.* New York: Basic Books, 1973.

27. VAN ITALLIE, T. B. "Obesity: The American Disease." *Food Technology* 33(1979): 43.

28. STUART R. B. "Behavior Control of Overeating." *Behavior Research and Therapy* 5 (1967): 357.

29. STUART, R. B., and B. DAVIS. *Slim Chance in a Fat World.* Champaign, Ill.: Research Press, 1972.

30. *Statistical Bulletin* (Metropolitan Life Insurance Company) 41(1960): 5.

31. KEYS, A. "Overweight and the Risk of Heart Attack and Sudden Death." In *Obesity in Perspective,* ed., G. A. Bray. DHEW Publication No. (NIH) 75-708.

32. BENNION, L. J., and S. M. GRUNDY. "Effect of Obesity and Caloric Intake on Biliary Lipid Metabolism in Man." *Journal of Clinical Investigation* 56(1975): 996.

33. FORBES, G. B. "Prevalence of Obesity in Childhood." In *Obesity in Perspective,* ed. G. A. Bray. DHEW Publication No. (NIH) 75-708.

34. COLLIPP, P. J. "Obesity in Childhood." In *Obesity,* ed. A. J. Stunkard. Philadelphia: Saunders, 1980.

35. STOOL, S. E., et al. "The Chubby Puffer Syndrome." *Clinical Pediatrics* 16(1977): 43.

36. FORBES, G. B. "Nutrition and Growth." *Journal of Pediatrics* 91(1977): 40.

37. MELLBIN, T., and C. J. ZUILLE. "Weight Gain in Infancy and Physical Development between Seven and Ten and a Half Years of Age." *British Journal of Preventive and Social Medicine* 30(1976): 233.

38. STEFANIK, P. A., P. HEALD, and J. MAYER. "Caloric Intake in Relation to Energy Output of Obese and Non-Obese Adolescent Boys." *American Journal of Clinical Nutrition* 7(1959): 55.

39. HANNAR, S. L., M. N. CAMPBELL, and V. A. CAMPBELL. "An Interdisciplinary Study of Adolescent Obesity." *Journal of Pediatrics* 80(1972): 373.

40. HAMILL, P. V. V., T. A. DRIZD, C. L. JOHNSON, R. B. REED, and ALEX F. ROCHE. "NCHS Growth Charts, 1976." *Monthly Vital Statistics Report, Health Examination Survey Data.* NDHW Publication No. (HRA) 76–1120, 25(June 1976).

41. BULLEN, B. A., R. B. REED, and J. MAYER. "Physical Activity of Obese and Non-Obese Adolescent Girls Appraised by a Motion Picture Sampling." *American Journal of Clinical Nutrition* 14(1964): 211.

42. MAYER, J. "Obesity during Childhood." In *Childhood Obesity,* ed. M. Winick. New York: Wiley, 1975.

43. SPARGO, J. A., F. P. HEALD, and P. S. PECKOS. "Adolescent Obesity." *Nutrition Today* 1(1966): 2.

44. KAUFMAN, M. A., R. POZNANSKI, and K. GUGGENHEIM. "Eating Habits and Opinions of Teenagers on Nutrition and Obesity." *Journal of the American Dietetic Association* 66 (1975): 264.

45. ALLEN, D. W., and B. M. QUIGLEY. "The Role of Physical Activity in the Control of Obesity." *Medical Journal of Australia* 2(13) (1977): 434.

46. COATES, T. J., and C. E. THORENSEN. "Treating Obesity in Children and Adolescents: A Review." *American Journal of Public Health* 68(1978): 143.

47. HEALD, F. P. "Treatment of Obesity in Adolescence." *Postgraduate Medicine* 51 (1972): 109.

48. GROSS, T., R. J. SOKOL, and K. C. KING. "Obesity in Pregnancy: Risk and Outcome." *Obstetrics and Gynecology* 56(1980): 446.

49. BROWNELL, K. D., and A. J. STUNKARD. "Behavioral Treatment of Obesity in Children." *American Journal of Diseases of Children* 132(1978): 403.

50. WING, R. R., and R. W. JEFFERY. "Outpatient Treatments of Obesity: A Comparison of Methodology and Clinical Results." *International Journal of Obesity* 3(1979): 261.

51. CURREY, H., et al. "Behavioral Treatment of Obesity." *Journal of the American Medical Association* 237(1976): 2829.

52. "Symposium on Surgical Treatment of Morbid Obesity." *American Journal of Clinical Nutrition* 33(1980): Supplement.

53. SOONG, Y. S. "Treatment of Exogenous Obesity Employing Auricular Acupuncture." *American Journal of Clinical Medicine* 3(1975): 285.

54. WICK, W., R. SIGMAN, and M. V. KLINE. "Hypnotherapy and Therapeutic Education in the Treatment of Obesity: Differential Treatment Factors." *Psychoanalytical Quarterly* 45(1971): 234.

55. AJA, J. H. "Brief Group Treatment of Obesity through Ancillary Self-hypnosis." *American Journal of Clinical Hypnosis* 9(1977): 231.

56. ABRAHAM, S., C. L. JOHNSON, and M. F. NAJJOR. *Height and Weight of Adults 18–74 Years of Age in the United States.* Advance data, U.S. DHEW, No. 3, Rockville, Md., November 19, 1976.

57. SMITH, C. A., and W. BERENBERG. "The Concept of Failure to Thrive." *Pediatrics* 46 (1970): 46.

58. Whitten, C. F. "T. L. C. and the Hungry Child." *Nutrition Today* 7(1972): 10.

59. Pollitt, E. "Behavior of Infant in Causation of Nutritional Marasmus." *American Journal of Clinical Nutrition* 26(1973): 264.

60. Widdowson, E. M. "Mental Contentment and Physical Growth." *Lancet* 1(1951): 1316.

61. Graham, G. G. "Environmental Factors Affecting the Growth of Children." *American Journal of Clinical Nutrition* 25(1972): 1184.

62. Goplan, C., et al. "Effect of Caloric Supplementation on Growth and Undernourished Children." *American Journal of Clinical Nutrition* 26(1973): 563.

63. Lucas, A. R., J. W. Duncan, and V. Peins. "The Treatment of Anorexia Nervosa." *American Journal of Psychiatry* 133(1976): 1034.

64. Lipton, M. A., and F. J. Kane. "Psychiatry." In *Nutritional Support of Medical Practice*, eds. H. A. Schneider, C. E. Anderson, and D. B. Coursin. Hagerstown, Md.: Harper and Row, 1977.

CHAPTER 10

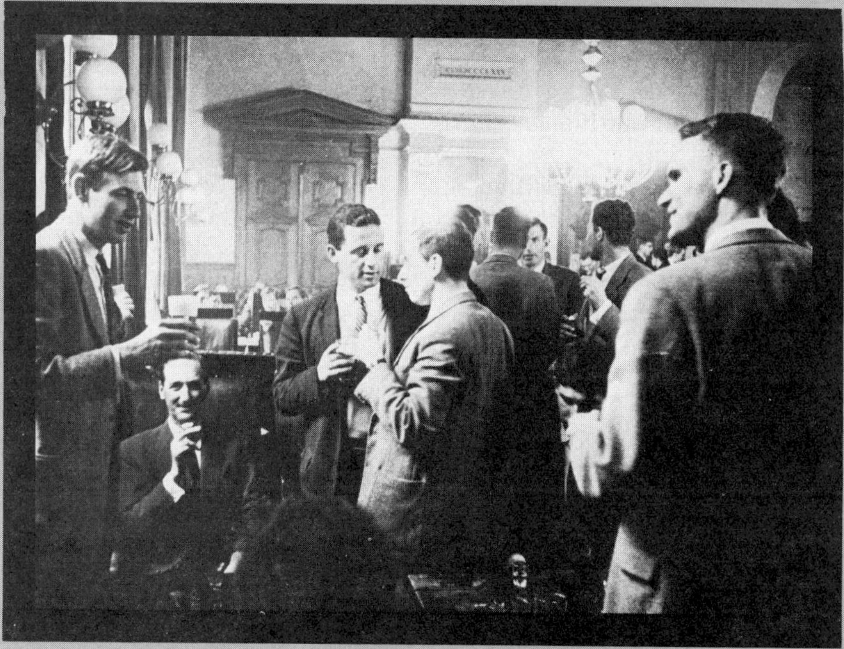

WHO photo by Jean Mohr

alcohol and other drugs

Americans have increased their use of drugs not only for medical reasons, but for recreational and social purposes. Alcoholic beverages, coffee, tea, cola drinks, tranquilizers, aspirin, and antacids are drugs, and all can have an effect on the body and on our nutritional status, depending on how we use them. Alcohol, for example, can provide energy, and used in moderation can be a relaxant. Used to excess, it can have destructive effects on the body and, when it is used as a substitute for food, add malnutrition to a host of other physical problems.

Many drugs interact with one another or with food to produce a new metabolic or physiological effect on the body—often an unintended effect. We are just beginning to learn about this synergism, and about the range of synergistic effects that can result when different foods and drugs are ingested in quantity and in combination.

In this chapter we will look at the effect on nutritional status of some of the more common drugs Americans use: alcohol, caffeine, and some common medicines. We will also look at what can happen when alcohol is combined with other drugs.

Alcohol

Alcohol's impact on a person's nutritional status depends upon the amount consumed. The effect of a given quantity of alcohol also varies among individuals. Small amounts have beneficial effects for relaxation, and possibly for heart disease or disorders of the circulatory system. Consumption of large amounts of alcohol is usually described as alcohol abuse. An alcohol problem or alcoholism describes frequent, consistent, and intensive overuse of alcohol. The National Council on Alcoholism has defined alcoholism as a pathological dependency on ethanol.

A large proportion of the adult population of the United States consumes alcoholic beverages (see Table 10–1). The level of consumption varies from a few ounces yearly to 8 or more ounces daily. In the United States, the average daily energy consumption from alcohol equals 210 kcal for persons of drinking age. In 1975, the average age at first drink was 12.9 years, with 40 percent having tasted alcohol by age 10. The lowest level of consumption is found in the South and the highest in the West. Drinking of alcohol is greater in metropolitan than

TABLE 10–1. Alcohol and Drug Use in the United States in 1979

type of drug	youths (%) 12–17		young adults (%) 18–25		adults (%) 26 and older	
	EVER USED	CURRENT[a] USER	EVER USED	CURRENT[a] USER	EVER USED	CURRENT[a] USER
Analgesics	3.2	0.6	11.8	1.0	2.7	*b*
Stimulants	3.4	1.2	18.2	3.5	5.8	0.5
Sedatives	3.2	1.1	17.0	2.8	3.5	*b*
Tranquilizers	4.1	0.6	15.8	2.1	3.1	*b*
Alcohol	70.3	37.2	95.3	75.9	91.5	61.3

[a]Persons who used drugs at least once within the month prior to this study. National sample of 2,165 youths, 2,044 young adults, and 3,015 older adults.

[b]Less than 0.5 percent.

SOURCE: U.S. Bureau of the Census, *Statistical Abstract of the United States: 1980.* Washington, D.C., 1980.

in rural areas. In the adult population, 7 percent are problem drinkers; among 14- to 17-year-olds, 19 percent are problem drinkers.

Table 10–2 presents information on alcohol consumption of persons 20 years of age and over during 1977. It is interesting to note that alcohol consumption increased as income went up and as education of the individual increased. Those aged 20–34 consumed more alcohol than did other age groupings. Differences in consumption with regard to race and sex are also given.

Alcohol is a drug that depresses the central nervous system. The alcohol in beverages for human consumption is ethanol or ethyl alcohol. Its general effects are shown in Table 10–3. Like other drugs, alcohol has toxic effects on body tissues. Unlike other drugs, it can be consumed in amounts that provide significant energy. Each gram provides about 7 kilocalories. We will look at this drug in relation to its effect on absorption, metabolism, metabolic alterations, and health factors.

absorption and distribution

Although most ethanol is absorbed through the small intestine, autopsy studies have demonstrated that ethanol can diffuse through the stomach wall (1). Ethanol is absorbed by simple diffusion, possibly by active transport (2). Factors affecting the absorption of alcohol include the concentration in the gastrointestinal tract, the nature and surface of the absorption area, the blood flow through the mucosa capillaries, the rate of stomach emptying, and the type and amount of food in the gastrointestinal tract (3). If ethanol is consumed rapidly a much higher blood

TABLE 10-2. Persons 20 Years of Age and Over: Frequency of Alcohol Consumption and Percent of Those Who Drink Alcohol Who Consumed Five or More Drinks at One Sitting in Past Year, United States, 1977

characteristic	TOTAL[a]	alcohol consumption: NEVER	OCCASIONALLY	1 OR 2 TIMES A WEEK	3 OR MORE TIMES A WEEK	5 OR MORE DRINKS AT ONE SITTING
All persons 20 years of age and over	100.0%	28.6%	41.9%	15.5%	14.0%	29.4%
Sex						
Male	100.0	21.5	35.9	20.2	22.5	43.1
Female	100.0	34.2	46.7	11.8	7.3	18.5
Race or Ethnicity						
White	100.0	26.2	42.7	15.9	15.2	30.3
Black	100.0	34.1	40.2	15.2	10.5	26.4
Hispanic	100.0	32.1	43.2	15.3	9.4	32.2
Age						
20–34 years	100.0	18.9	47.3	19.5	14.3	43.1
35–44 years	100.0	24.5	43.5	17.3	14.7	33.7
45–54 years	100.0	27.3	40.7	14.8	17.2	26.7
55–64 years	100.0	36.0	37.7	12.6	13.6	18.4
65 years and over	100.0	48.6	33.3	8.2	9.9	7.2
Income						
Less than $5,000	100.0	46.2	35.0	10.3	8.5	20.4
$5,000–$9,999	100.0	34.3	40.9	13.6	11.2	26.2
$10,000–$14,999	100.0	26.4	44.6	16.1	12.9	32.2
$15,000–$24,999	100.0	21.1	45.5	17.1	16.3	33.4
$25,000 or more	100.0	14.9	42.5	20.7	21.9	36.8
Education of Individual						
Less than 12 years	100.0	42.1	35.2	12.0	10.7	22.1
12 years	100.0	25.7	45.5	15.6	13.2	31.1
More than 12 years	100.0	17.0	45.0	19.2	18.8	35.4

[a] Excludes alcohol consumption.

SOURCE: *Advancedata from Vital and Health Statistics.* National Center for Health Statistics, DHHS, PHS No. 64, 1980.

TABLE 10-3. Effects of Blood Alcohol Concentration on Behavior

blood concentration (percent)	effect	probable intake to produce this level in 2 hours[a] (whisky)
0.03	Mild depression; relaxation.	1.5–2 oz
0.05	Depresses uppermost level of brain; reduces inhibitions, restraint, and judgment (takes personal and social liberties).	2–3 oz
0.10	Depresses lower motor area of brain; staggers slightly; difficulty dressing; slurred speech; reduced digital dexterity; decreased auditory and visual discrimination; speed of motor response drops.	4–5 oz
0.15	Legal intoxication in many states.	6–8 oz
0.20	Entire motor area of brain disturbed; mid-brain affected (controls emotional behavior); horizontal position; needs help walking.	10 oz
0.30	Lower brain affected; stupor.	16 oz
0.40–0.50	Coma; anesthesia.	
0.60–0.70	Control of breathing and heartbeat affected; death.	

[a] Exact level is dependent on rate of consumption, absorption, metabolism, and lean body mass.
NOTE: One ounce of whisky per hour can be metabolized by the average adult man.
SOURCE: L. A. Greenberg, "Alcohol in the Body," *Scientific American*, 65:86, 1961.

concentration results than when it is sipped slowly. In addition, the total concentration of the alcohol in the beverage influences the blood concentration; the higher the alcoholic content, the greater the blood concentration. Older evidence suggests that different alcoholic beverages have varying rates of absorption, with beer absorbed more slowly than whiskey or brandy. Such studies have not been conducted using recent techniques and may be related to alcohol concentration (3).

The absorption of alcohol is influenced by food composition as well as the size of the meal (4). Carbonation like that in sparkling wines or sodas enhances the absorption of alcohol. The general observation that milk consumption reduces intoxication has had some scientific support in a study on a limited number of subjects (5). Sedman (4) studied and documented the effects of food on slowing gastric emptying rates and decreasing alcohol absorption. Decreased absorption lowered blood alcohol concentration. Higher fat meals delay gastric emptying. The higher the volume of food consumed, the slower the transit times regardless of the kind of food consumed.

Alcohol affects the digestive system, and can cause malabsorption. Ethanol can cause acute gastritis and impair gastric emptying. The effects of alcohol on ulcers and chronic gastritis is controversial. In the intestine enthanol may produce lesions, alterations in mucosal enzymes, and malabsorption of nutrients. The folate depletion that often accompanies chronic alcohol consumption impairs intestinal absorption. Alcohol increases intestinal waves, which can result in diarrhea.

The distribution of alcohol in the body is proportional to the water content of the various tissues. At equilibrium, most organs contain 70 to 80 percent of plasma concentration. Bone and fat are low in water content and have little alcohol. An obese person would have a higher blood alcohol concentration than a normal weight individual with the same intake of alcohol per kg of body weight.

metabolism

The liver is the major organ for the metabolism of alcohol; the kidney and skeletal muscles also metabolize small amounts. The initial oxidat ion of ethanol to acetaldehyde may be catalyzed by different enzyme systems. The speed of oxidation is dependent on the amount of enzymes present, which is limited. The major enzyme systems are alcohol dehydrogenase and microsomal ethanol-oxidizing (MEO). As much as 80 percent of the ethanol is metabolized by hepatic dehydrogenase. Much smaller percentages may be metabolized by MEO, which is a mixed function oxidase. Catalase is a minor system. A very small percentage of alcohol is excreted in urine and sweat and through expired breath.

Further oxidation converts acetaldehyde to acetic acid. Acetic acid is activated by adenosine triphosphate (ATP) to acetyl-coenzyme A, which is metabolized through the Krebs cycle to carbon dioxide and water (see Figure 10–1). The oxidation of ethanol is an effective source of energy, 7 kcal/g; however, the metabolic effects of alcohol may inhibit fat synthesis unless other sources of energy—fat, protein, or CHO—are provided (6). The MEO system uses metabolic energy rather than producing energy as occurs in the alcohol dehydrogenase system (7).

In the alcohol dehydrogenase dependent pathway the enzyme combines with nicotinamide adenine dinucleotide (NAD). Ethanol is oxidized and NAD+ accepts the liberated hydrogen ($NADH+H^+$). The formed acetaldehyde is released, and the reduced coenzyme NADH is detached from alcohol dehydrogenase. Alcohol dehydrogenase then reenters the cycle. The rate of alcohol metabolism depends upon the rate of NADH reoxidation by the respiratory chain. The resultant increase in the NADH/NAD ratio has marked metabolic effect and leads to several metabolic abnormalities, including altered lipid metabolism (8).

Alcoholic hypoglycemia is often a result of heavy drinking with no food intake. Children or those with alcoholic liver disease are especially vulnerable.

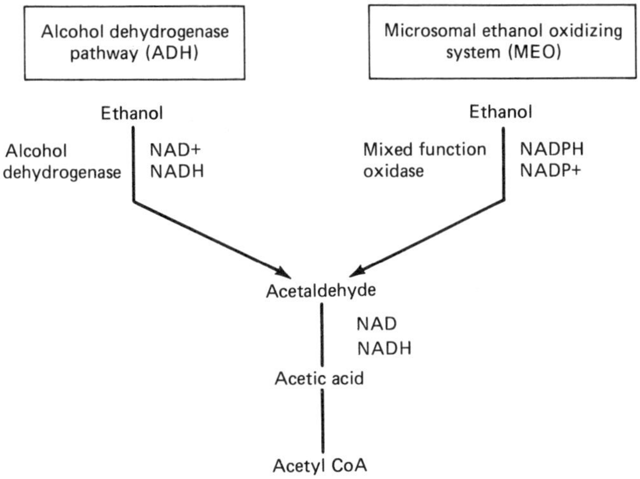

FIG. 10–1. Metabolism of alcohol. Alcohol dehydrogenase (ADH) is the major pathway, and microsomal ethanol oxidizing (MEO) depends on alcohol intake.

Ethanol, via the altered NADH/NAD ratio, inhibits gluconeogenesis by suppressing pyruvate carboxylase (9). In addition, there is depletion of liver glycogen, which is a source of glucose. Alcoholic hypoglycemia is similar in symptoms to diabetic hypoglycemia, including weakness, tremulousness, mental confusion, bizarre behavior, incoherent speech, sweating, and tachycardia, which can be followed by coma.

After a person drinks alcoholic beverages, the blood uric acid concentration increases, which disposes an individual to an increase in gouty attacks. Blood uric acid results from an increase in liver uric acid production (10). The increased NADH/NAD intercellular ratio leads to an increase lactate/pyruvate ratio, which results in hyperlactacidemia. The hyperlactacidemia reduces the kidneys' capacity to excrete uric acid and causes the development of hyperuricemia. This type of uricemia leads to the classic attacks of gout precipitated by alcohol binges.

Administration of ethanol to normal men who have fasted for 56 hours results in a slight fall in glucose levels, suppression of circulating insulin to values indistinguishable from zero, and a dramatic stimulation of glucagon secretion. The stimulation of glucagon secretion compares to that usually seen with a sharp drop in glucose after insulin administration. The extremely low insulin levels probably accentuate the glucagon response (11). Ingestion of ethanol increases oxygen consumption in normal and alcoholic subjects, which indicates that ethanol increases the metabolic rate. This may be the result of stimulation of the MEO system, which involves oxidation without phosphorylation.

The rate of alcohol metabolism varies with consumption patterns, lean body mass, nutritional status, and race. The general rate is about 10 ml of alcohol an hour for a 70 kg man, but the rate of oxidation is reduced by low protein intake

(3). The rate may decrease by 30 to 50 percent when dietary protein is reduced from 120 to 20 g in the same subject. There are differences among ethnic groups in response to alcohol. Wolf first reported a greater sensitivity of Orientals and American Indians to alcohol when compared to people of European ancestry (12). No significant differences have been found between Chinese and Europeans in rate of alcohol metabolism, but there have been appreciable differences in acetaldehyde levels, with higher ones in Orientals. The difference in the rate of metabolism is unclear; if the variation is not due to enzymes or activity, anatomical variation may be important (13).

metabolic alterations

The intake of alcohol has a number of effects on the body. For some people, ethanol represents from one-third to one-half of the energy ingested. Alcoholic beverages do not contain important vitamins, minerals, and protein (see Table 10–4). Many abusers of alcohol ingest little or no food during drinking bouts, resulting in depleted body stores of some nutrients.

The nutritional difficulties associated with alcohol intake include these: interference with absorption of nutrients, including thiamin, folate, B_{12}, amino acids, and calcium; impaired absorption of water, electrolytes, and glucose; interference with the absorption and transport of fat; altered carbohydrate metabolism; decreased synthesis of albumin in the liver; reduced conversion of thiamin, riboflavin, and pyridoxine to the active form where they serve as cofactors; and catabolic loss of zinc, calcium, and magnesium (3). Alcohol dehydrogenase in tissues other than the liver may function on other alcohols such as retinol. Retinol plays a vital role in vitamin A related functions, such as spermatogenesis and the visual process. A high intake of ethanol may result in a competition between ethanol and vitamin A for the alcohol dehydrogenase and contribute to vitamin A deficiency symptoms (14).

Alcohol is closely associated with hematological abnormalities, cardiomyopathy, peripheral neuropathy, acute and chronic muscle disorders, central nervous system degeneration, chronic pulmonary disease, certain malignancies, intestinal malabsorption, hypoglycemia, ketosis, hyperuricemia, gout, alterations in drug metabolism, increased susceptibility to infection, and malnutrition (15). Alcohol has a direct toxic action on the erythroblast with the development of megoblastic anemia. The same anemia develops with folate deficiency. Macrocytosis disappeared in patients who stopped consuming alcohol but persisted with folate therapy for over six months with continued consumption of alcohol.

Folate absorption is decreased in malnourished alcoholics and improves with feeding even with continued alcoholic intake. Experimental, clinical, and epidemiological evidence indicates that even when adequate diets are consumed, ethanol exerts an adverse effect on the liver. Alcoholics have seven times more cirrhosis than nondrinkers. In the United States, the death rate from cirrhosis fell during Prohibition and rose again after repeal. Ten to 20 percent of heavy

TABLE 10–4. Nutrient Content of Selected Alcoholic Beverages

beverage	alcohol (oz)†	amount (oz)	water (%)	food energy (Calories)	protein (g)	CHO (g)	CA (mg)	phosphorus (mg)	iron (mg)	sodium (mg)	potassium (mg)	thiamin (mg)	riboflavin (mg)	niacin (mg)
Beer (4.5% alcohol by vol.; 3.6% by wt.)	0.54	12.0	92.0	151	1.1	13.7	18	108	Trace	25	90	0.01	0.11	2.2
Gin, rum, vodka, whisky, 80 proof (33.4% alcohol by wt.)	0.60	1.5*	66.6	97	—	Trace	—	—	—	Trace	1	—	—	—
86 proof (36% by wt.)	0.60	1.5*	64.0	105	—	Trace	—	—	—	Trace	1	—	—	—
90 proof (37.9% by wt.)	0.64	1.5*	62.1	110	—	Trace	—	—	—	Trace	1	—	—	—
94 proof (39.7% by wt.)	0.70	1.5*	60.3	116	—	Trace	—	—	—	Trace	1	—	—	—
100 proof (42.5% by wt.)	0.75	1.5*	57.5	124	—	Trace	—	—	—	Trace	1	—	—	—
Wine														
dessert (18.8% by vol.; 15.3% by wt.)	0.67	3.5	76.7	141	0.1	7.9	8	—	—	4	77	0.01	0.02	0.2
Table (12.2% alcohol by vol.; 9.9% by wt.)	0.42	3.5	85.6	87	0.1	4.3	9	10	0.4	5	94	Trace	0.01	0.1

*Jigger.

†Calculated from percent by volume.

SOURCE: C. Adams, *Nutritive Value of American Foods*, Agriculture Handbook No. 456 (Washington, D.C.: U.S. Department of Agriculture, 1975).

drinkers develop cirrhosis, which is related to the duration and amounts of alcohol intake (15). Although severe protein malnutrition is related to the development of human cirrhosis, protein fortification for alcoholics is not an effective remedy if alcohol abuse continues (16). Although low-protein diets are commonly associated with cirrhosis, diets relatively rich in protein do not preclude the development of alcoholic cirrhosis. Daily intakes of alcohol as low as 40 g in men and 20 g in women have resulted in a statistically significant increase in the incidence of cirrhosis (8). In a well-nourished population, even with adequate diet, the amount of alcohol considered to be innocuous may harm the liver. The incidence of advanced liver disease seems higher among men than women with a similar-history of alcohol abuse (17). Under controlled conditions in a metabolic unit, administration of large amounts of ethanol causes a fatty liver and a striking increase in liver triglycerides (18). These results can be found when alcohol is administered with adequate supplements of vitamins and minerals or with a high-protein diet. The response to ethanol varies as a function of hereditary associated diseases, dose, and duration of alcohol intake (19).

The role of alcohol toxicity and of malnutrition in the pathological development of cirrhosis are not fully understood. Patek presents a strong case for the importance of adequate nutrition in the prevention of cirrhosis of the liver but further study is needed to clarify these relationships (1).

The integrity of the mucosa lining of the stomach and small intestine can be compromised by chronic intermittent exposure to ethyl alcohol. Digestive and absorptive functions in the small intestine may be impaired with the development of malabsorption and malnutrition. The permeability of the mucosal lining to foreign macromolecules is increased, with the consequence of exposing the body to undesirable toxins, antigens, and pathogenic organisms (20).

Alcohol ingestion itself does not appear to be carcinogenic (21), but excessive alcohol ingestion coupled with a nutritional deficiency or some other insult may be carcinogenic. Alcohol and the accompanying nutritional deficiencies associated with heavy consumption have been shown to be immunosuppressive, and there is a strong relationship between immunocompetency and neoplasis. Ethanol is a depressant for the central nervous system, so prolonged abuse of alcohol can lead to serious neurological disorders (22).

Heavy drinkers are twice as likely to develop hypertension. When all other factors are eliminated statistically, the association between above average alcohol intake and elevated blood pressure remains.

Serum concentration of triglycerides and high-density lipoprotein (HDL) cholesterol are positively associated with alcohol ingestion. The increase in plasma triglycerides is greater in people who must be genetically susceptible. The increase in HDL may have a protective effect in heart disease, although this is unclear because of the difference in types of HDL. There is neither a strong nor a consistent association between alcohol intake and atherosclerotic disease.

Alcohol consumption can lead to caloric excesses, because alcohol provides 7 calories for every gram of alcohol. But a high level of energy consumption from alcohol reduces the percent of nutrient intake which can affect body metabolism (14). No close relationship has been found between body fatness and alcohol intake, although this may differ with socioeconomic class (3).

Alcohol is not an efficient source of calories. Although alcohol liberates about 7 calories per gram upon combustion, it does not provide food value equal to carbohydrates. Use of ethanol to replace carbohydrate at 50 percent of the total calories in a balanced diet resulted in a decline in body weight. Ethanol produces less weight gain than calorically equivalent food when given as supplemental calories. Ethanol may increase the energy requirement, based on rat and human studies showing increased oxygen consumption with ethanol feeding (23).

fetal alcohol syndrome

The pattern of malformation in infants born to women with severe chronic alcohol intake has been identified as *fetal alcohol syndrome* (24). Children born of mothers with excessive alcohol intake show characteristic facial features (see Figure 10–2). Note the low nasal bridge with a short or upturned nose, a long, convex upper lip, wide mouth, prominent ears, and the eyes. Chronic maternal alcohol abuse has been one of the most recognizable causes of mental deficiency. The current prevalence of chronic alcohol abuse is between 0.40 and 1.25 cases per 1000 pregnancies. In addition to mental retardation, there is a decreased growth in height and weight, increased frequency in malformation, and psychomotor disturbances. Perinatal mortality is at the level of 17 percent, and 44 percent of the surving children of alcoholic mothers are mentally deficient.

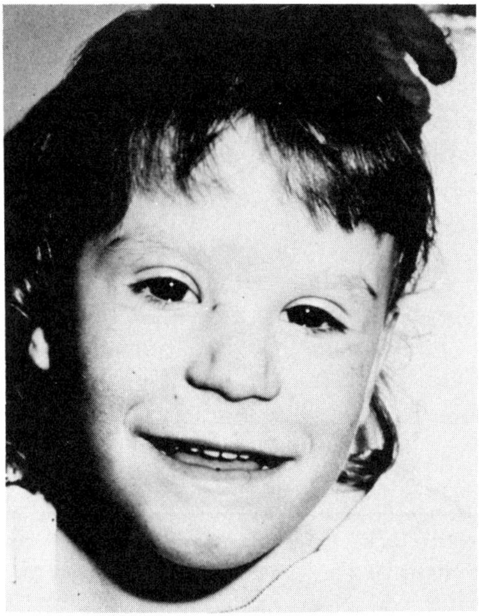

FIG. 10–2. Four-year-old child born of a chronically alcoholic woman who has moderate mental and growth deficiency. Facial features include short palpebral fissures, smooth philtrom and upper lip, and relatively small maxilla. Courtesy of David W. Smith.

Affected children often fail to survive. Hyperactivity and irritability may be found during the neonatal period. Fine motor dysfunction and developmental delay may be permanent. Mental deficiency of varying severity is the most serious clinical consequence and is related to the degree of growth deficiency in the brain. Abnormalities of the eye are common, as well as abnormalities of the joints and skeleton. The growth deficiency appears to be permanent.

Recent information indicates that the infant of even moderate drinkers shows some or all of the features of the fetal alcohol syndrome (25). During pregnancy, as little as 1 ounce of pure alcohol a day or the equivalent of two to three cocktails produce some characteristics of the syndrome. Symptoms can also be found in the infants of mothers who become drunk occasionally on 5 ounces of alcohol early in pregnancy. The symptoms seen include retarded growth, reduced size for gestational age, smaller head circumference, and multiple dysmorphic features—the broad nose spread, heart murmur, and ear abnormalities. A study of 1,529 mothers suggests that maternal drinking, even in moderate amounts during and after conception, is dangerous to the developing fetus. Maternal alcohol use before pregnancy and in late pregnancy is significantly related to decreased infant birth weight (26). Daily consumption of 1 ounce of absolute alcohol before pregnancy is associated with a decrease in birth weight of 91 grams; 1 ounce consumed daily in late pregnancy is associated with a decreased birth weight of 160 grams.

In a study of the relationship of drinking during pregnancy to spontaneous abortion, 25 percent of pregnant women drinking twice a week or more are likely to abort, compared to 14 percent of women who drink less often (27). The minimum harmful dose was 1 ounce of absolute alcohol. As shown in Table 10–3, this is usually less than two drinks. Other potentially confounding variables such as maternal age, prior spontaneous abortions, smoking, and nausea were controlled in the analysis. Drinking during pregnancy and spontaneous abortions did not vary with the factors. Moderate drinking during pregnancy is a risk factor for spontaneous abortion and may be a cause of acute or chronic fetal poisoning.

teenage drinking

In the 14 to 17 age group there are 3.3 million problem drinkers in the United States. With this age group, the problems tend to be acute rather than chronic. Early drinking behavior predicts adult habits. Adolescent problem drinkers are more likely to have similar problems 25 years later. Social attitudes, availability, and peer pressure encourage early drinking. The lowering of the legal drinking age makes alcoholic beverages available to younger adolescents, and the average age of the first drink is now 13.

There is increased consumption of alcoholic beverages by adolescents. The public health concern extends to the lack of documentation of the physiological effects of alcohol on the metabolism of the teenage body. Rapid growth and development may alter the utilization and effects of alcohol in cells. Alcohol abuse makes adolescents very susceptible to nutrient deficiencies because of the increased nutritional requirement of growth and development. Alcoholic beverages can displace food in the diet or decrease appetite for food.

Caffeine

Caffeine is a commonly consumed and widely available drug. Most of the caffeine comes from coffee, tea, cola drinks and cocoa. The general public and regulatory agencies have shown much interest in caffeine, but little research has been conducted to understand its physiological effects (28). Despite the worldwide consumption there have been few epidemiologic studies of the health effects.

Caffeine is absorbed rapidly and completely from the gastrointestinal tract and is distributed in proportion to the water content of the tissue. Caffeine is broken down rapidly in tissues with half of the amount absorbed degraded in 2.5 to 3 hours. The newborn cannot metabolize caffeine. The ability gradually improves, and by 6 years of age caffeine is metabolized rapidly.

Caffeine has a marked effect on some systems and tissues. It is a stimulant which increases cardiac central nervous system output and basal metabolic rate, induces diuresis (increased production of urine), and a variety of psychopharmacological effects. In the cardiovascular system, caffeine stimulates the force of contraction of the heart and increases cardiac output. The effect that dilates the blood vessels increases blood flow to muscles and the heart, but circulation of blood in the brain is decreased. Caffeine stimulates mental and motor activity. Fatigue and drowsiness are decreased. Stimulation may be followed by fatigue.

The adverse effects of caffeine use are insomnia, nervousness, stomach aches, and nausea. There is a wide variation in individual level of tolerance for caffeine. Excessive consumption may be associated with arrhythmia in a few people. Removal of caffeine and related alkyloids from the diet resulted in resolution of fibrocystic breast disease in more than half the women studied. The diuretic action of caffeine may produce an electrolyte deficit of minerals like calcium. This could affect bone formation. The risk of chromosome alterations from caffeine use is negligible in adults, except for pregnant women. Caffeine passes the placenta into the fetus, which may not be able to metabolize caffeine. Although we do not know its effects on humans specifically, there is no research indicating mutagenic, carcinogenic, or chromosome damaging effects.

Other Drugs

At the present time there is much interest in the interaction between drugs and nutrients. In some instances, marginal malnutrition along with the drug therapy may result in obvious nutrient depletion and deficiency symptoms. On the other hand, adequate nutritional status allows for a better therapeutic response to some drugs because of the individual's increased tolerance. This is particularly significant for individuals on long-term therapies, those who are chronic drug abusers, and those on multiple drug regimens (29). Individual differences exist in utilization of drugs as well as nutrients; therefore, some individuals require larger doses to get the desired response. The discussion of the relation of drugs to nutritional status can be divided into two sections: 1) the effects of drugs on nutritional status; and 2) alteration of drug response by nutrients. We will not attempt to delineate all the specific interactions known, but rather we will provide a general discussion of groups of drugs and refer the reader to other works for greater detail (30).

effect on nutritional status

One of the most obvious effects of drugs on nutritional status arises from decreased intake of food as a result of drug therapy. Evidence of the effects of drugs on appetite is inconclusive, although amphetamines have been used with varying results and side effects in the treatment of obesity. The entire concept of appetite is difficult to study because direct cause and effect relationships cannot be shown. The physiological, social, and economic factors that can alter food intake complicate studies of the effects of drugs on appetite.

We do know that drugs which have an unpleasant taste decrease desire for food. Some drugs may alter taste sensations to the point that all food "tastes the same" or that differences in intensity of flavors cannot be determined, so eating becomes boring and the individual may just stop. Nausea and vomiting, frequent side effects of drugs, can alter food intake significantly. Many of the chemotherapeutic agents used in the treatment of malignancies are said to cause changes in taste acuity. In some instances, the specific relationship may be related to zinc deficiencies caused by the therapeutic regimen (31). Bulking agents such as methylcellulose will absorb moisture and swell, giving the sensation of "being full," which may decrease further food consumption. Certain drugs, such as digitalis glycosides, biguanide, phenformin and penicillamine, can lead to weight loss in thin people, especially the elderly, by impairing appetite or taste. Oral diuretics may contribute to zinc depletion and loss of appetite, because some taste and smell dysfunctions occur with zinc deficiency. Taste and smell disorders stem from multiple causes. Some respond to zinc therapy, but many do not change with zinc supplements.

At therapeutic dosages, the antibiotic neomycin and the anti-inflammatory drug colchicine can damage intestinal mucosa, reducing fat, fat-soluble vitamin, and sugar absorption. Nutrient synthesis may be diminished with the use of antibiotics. For example, tetracycline inhibits bacterial synthesis of B complex vitamins in the gastrointestinal tract, and certain analogs (modified chemical structures) have been produced that block the action of B vitamins in their co-enzyme and energy release mechanism. Another antibiotic, chloramphenicol, has been shown to interfere with protein synthesis (33).

Other drugs, such as steroids, antihistamines, insulin, and psychotropic agents, tend to improve the appetite and thereby increase food intake to the point of excessive weight gain (32). These drugs are not used to improve appetite, but it is a side effect.

Changes in absorption of nutrients have been caused by drug therapy (34). Absorption of nutrients is largely dependent on enzyme activity, gastrointestinal secretions, and pH of fluids. Drugs that alter any of these systems may cause malabsorption of the nutrients. The drugs may be grouped as follows: 1) Those that affect intestinal mobility, namely cathartics and laxatives; mineral oil, for example, decreases the absorption of all fat-soluble vitamins, and some cathartics cause diarrhea (34, 35, 36). 2) Those that alter the histology of the small intestine; cytotoxic agents and antibiotics can act as irritants causing cellular damage. 3) Those that bind certain nutrients, altering their solubility or absorptive mechanisms; cholestyramine, for example, is a bile acid sequestrant that produces steatorrhea, and antacids bind minerals, causing them not to be absorbed. 4) Those that damage the pancreas, resulting in decreased synthesis and/or release of enzymes and subsequent malabsorption of carbohydrates, fats, and proteins.

In addition to malabsorption, drugs may increase excretion of nutrients by complexing nutrients and detaching them from binding sites, by replacing the nutrient on the binding site, or by producing a combination of these effects. Nutrients are excreted free or with the drug which alters nutrient efficiency as well as drug effectiveness. Certainly diuretics can increase the excretion of significant electrolytes (mainly sodium and potassium) to the point of deficiency.

Many drugs affect the metabolism of fats. They 1) cause steatorrhea, 2) increase fecal excretion of bile acids and salts, 3) inhibit cholesterol absorption, 4) affect lipoprotein lipase, 5) cause fatty livers, 6) affect free fatty acid release from adipose tissue, 7) lower plasma lipid concentration, and 8) increase plasma concentrations (37). Carbohydrate metabolism is altered by many different drugs. They can be classified as those which lower fasting blood glucose and those which raise fasting blood glucose (38). Metabolism of various vitamins and minerals is also altered with drug therapy. The more common drugs are the oral contraceptive agents, antacids, and anticonvulsant drugs (34, 39). Routine use of mineral oil in the treatment of constipation leads to deficiencies of the fat-soluble vitamins unless supplementation is instituted. Antacids are high in sodium, which may be contraindicated in some disease processes and drug therapy. Some common laxatives are high in magnesium, causing high blood levels if continued over long periods.

nutritional alteration of drug response

The alteration of drug response by nutrients may be summarized as follows: 1) foods change the rate of excretion of drugs by changing the pH of the urine; 2) pharmacologically active ingredients in foods may change the response of drugs taken simultaneously with food; 3) food may decrease or increase drug absorption; and 4) nutrients may alter drug metabolism. For the most part, these alterations are caused by nutrient-induced changes in the drug metabolizing enzymes. These changes may be stimulatory or inhibitory toward the activity of the drug enzymes. These enzyme systems are further affected by starvation, protein nutrition, and deficiencies or excesses of minerals, vitamins, and fats.

Some foods and nutrients have a specific cause and effect relationship on drug efficiency. For example, milk products eaten at the same time tetracyclines are given will bind with the drug causing mineral losses as well as ineffectiveness of the drug (40). An anticoagulant drug (griseofulvin) is much more effective with a high-fat meal (41). Because of these and other interactions, it is not always beneficial to mix certain drugs with liquids even to mask an unpleasant flavor. Alteration of pH, as with a fruit juice, can inhibit stability of the drug and alter its absorption. Strict adherence to the directions on drug labels is necessary to achieve the best results from the drug while minimizing negative nutrient influences. Most labels give directions for the best time for drug administration with regard to meals, foods, and beverages.

Controlled studies are needed in many of the areas discussed in this chapter to provide more complete information on the risks of drug-induced malnutrition. In addition, studies need to be undertaken to evaluate the effects on nutritional status of long-term drug therapy, as with malignancies, the use of oral contraceptive agents, or long-term usage of drugs by the elderly. The elderly are most likely to be on multiple drug regimens. Controlled studies with humans are difficult to devise and those with animals are not always transferable.

alcohol combined with other drugs

Alcohol use combined with other drugs accounts for 20 percent of the total number of accidental and suicidal deaths each year that are drug-related (42). More morbidity than is recognized may be related to the ingestion of drugs and alcohol, especially in a drug-oriented society such as ours. Many commonly prescribed drugs have altered or adverse therapeutic effects when taken with alcohol, including sedatives, hypnotics, narcotics, antidepressants, tranquilizers, antihistamines, analgesics, anticoagulants, and anti-infective agents (43). Minor tranquilizers and other central nervous system (CNS) depressants in combination with alcohol may produce adverse medical consequences. CNS depressants can impair tasks requiring alertness, like driving.

The microsomal system for oxidation of alcohol is similar to the microsomal drug detoxifying system (23). Competition between these systems may explain the reduction in drug metabolism with the intake of alcohol. Alcoholics have delayed clearance of some drugs when drugs and drinking are combined, especially the depressant drugs. For some chronic alcoholics, there is increased metabolism of barbituates, anesthetics, and others. The pattern and history of alcohol consumption needs to be carefully documented in individuals who need drug treatment. The dietitian can play an important role in alerting other members of the health care team about potential alcohol and drug problems.

SUMMARY

Alcohol and drugs are widely used and may have a marked effect on nutrition. The frequency and amount consumed are factors related to the intensity of the effect.

Alcohol is a drug that provides significant amounts of energy. Alcohol is absorbed through the stomach and intestines and distributes in the body water. The content of the food in the digestive tract affects the rate of absorption. Most alcohol is metabolized in the liver. Alcohol consumption can lead to a number of nutritional difficulties. Fatty liver is associated with alcohol abuse. Other problems are malnutrition, water-soluble vitamin and mineral deficiencies, obesity, and hypertension.

Fetal alcohol syndrome is found in the children of alcoholic mothers. Even moderate alcohol consumption may harm the fetus.

Caffeine is a widely used drug obtained from coffee, tea, cola beverages, and cocoa. In moderate amounts it causes alertness and relieves fatique. In some people there are the side effects of nervousness, insomnia, stomach aches, and nausea.

Drugs can affect nutritional status directly, or nutrients can alter the response to drugs. Drugs can change taste, routes for metabolism of nutrients, or alter absorption.

Alcohol combined with other drugs can emphasize the effects of both. Patterns of alcohol consumption need to be considered with drug treatment.

references

1. Patek, A. J. "Alcohol Malnutrition and Alcohol Cirrhosis." *American Journal of Clinical Nutrition* 32 (1979): 1304.
2. Pleuckhahn, D. D., and B. Ballard. "Diffusion of Stomach Alcohol and Heart Blood Alcohol Concentration at Autopsy." *Journal of Forensic Science* 12 (1967): 463.
3. Roe, D. A. *Alcohol and the Diet.* Westport, Conn.: AVI Publishing, 1979.
4. Sedman, A. J., P. K. Wilkinson, E. Sakmar, D. Weidler, and J. G. Wagner. "Food Effects on Absorption and Metabolism of Alcohol." *Quarterly Journal of Studies on Alcohol* 37 (1976): 1197.
5. Miller, D. S., J. L. Sterling, and J. Yudkin. "The Effects of Ingestion of Milk on Concentrations of Blood Alcohol." *Nature* 212 (1966): 1051.
6. Lieber, C. S., and N. Spritz. "Effects of Prolonged Ethanol Intake in Man: Role of Dietary Adipose in Endogenously Synthesized Fatty Acids in Apthogenesis of Alcoholic Fatty Liver." *Journal of Clinical Investigation* 45 (1966): 1400.
7. Boeker, E. A. "Metabolism of Ethanol." *Journal of the American Dietetic Association* 76 (1980): 550.
8. Lieber, C. S., R. Teschke, Y. Hasumura, and L. M. DeCarli. "Differences in Hepatic and Metabolic Changes after Acute and Chronic Alcohol Consumption." *Federation Proceedings* 34 (1975): 2060.
9. Golding, D. N. "Alcohol Induced Hypoglycemia in Childhood." *British Medical Journal* 1 (1970): 278.
10. Grunst, J., D. Dietz, and M. Wicklmays. "Effects of Ethanol on Uric Acid Production of Human Liver." *Nutrition and Metabolism* 21 (1977): 138.
11. Palmer, J. P., and J. W. Ensinck. "Stimulation of Glucagon Secretion by Ethanol Induced Hypoglycemia in Man." *Diabetes* 24 (1975): 295.
12. Wolf, P. H. "Ethnic Differences in Alcohol Sensitivity." *Science* 175 (1972): 449.
13. Hanna, J. M. "Metabolic Responses of Chinese, Japanese, and Europeans to Alcohol, Alcoholism." Clinical and Experimental Research 2 (1978): 89.
14. Thompson, J. N. "Some Aspects of the Metabolism in Biochemistry of Vitamin A." *Proceedings of the Nutrition Society* 24 (1965): 160.
15. Spritz, N. "Appraisal of Alcohol Consumption as a Causative Factor in Liver Disease and Atherosclerosis." *American Journal of Clinical Nutrition* 32 (1979): 2654.
16. Lieber, C. S. "Ethanol and the Liver: A Decreasing Threshold of Toxicity." *American Journal of Clinical Nutrition* 32 (1979): 1177.

17. MORGAN, M. Y., and S. SHERLOCK. "Sex Related Differences among 100 Patients with Alcoholic Liver Disease." *British Medical Journal* 1 (1977): 939.

18. LIEBER, C. S., and E. RUBIN. "Alcoholic Fatty Liver in Man on a High Protein and Low Fat Diet." *American Journal of Medicine* 44 (1968): 200.

19. LELBACH, W. K. "Cirrhosis in the Alcoholic and Its Relation to the Volume of Alcohol Abuse." *Annals of the New York Academy of Science* 252 (1975): 85.

20. WORTHINGTON, C. S., et al. "Effect of Daily Ethanol Ingestion on Intestinal Permeability to Macromolecules." *American Journal of Digestive Diseases* 23 (1978): 23.

21. VITALE, J. J., and L. S. GOTTLIEB. "Alcohol and Alcohol Related Deficiencies as Carcinogens." *Cancer Research* 35 (1975): 3336.

22. OLSEN, R. E. "Nutrition and Alcoholism." In *Modern Nutrition in Health and Disease,* 5 th ed., eds. R. S. Goodhart and M. E. Shils. Philadelphia: Lea & Febiger, 1973.

23. SHAW, S., and C. S. LIEBER. "Nutrition and Alcoholism." In *Modern Nutrition in Health and Disease,* 6th ed., eds. R. S. Goodhart and M. E. Shils. Philadelphia: Lea & Febiger, 1980.

24. HANSON, J. W., K. L. JONES, and D. W. SMITH. "Fetal Alcohol Syndrome—Experience with Forty-one patients." *Journal of the American Medical Association* 235 (1976): 1458.

25. HANSON, J. W., Ed. Jaan Kangilaski. "Even Moderate Drinking May Be Hazardous to Maturing Fetus." *Journal of the American Medical Association* 237 (1977): 2585.

26. LITTLE, R. E. "Moderate Alcohol Use during Pregnancy and Decreased Infant Birth Weight." *American Journal of Public Health* 67 (1977): 1154.

27. KLINE, K., P. SHROUT, Z. STEIN, M. SUSSER, and D. WARBURTON. "Drinking during Pregnancy and Spontaneous Abortion." *Lancet* 2 (1980): 176.

28. "Third International Caffeine Workshop." *Nutrition Review* 39 (1981): 183.

29. BAKER, L. R., et al. "Iatrogenic Osteomalacia and Myopathy due to Phosphate Depletion." *British Medical Journal* 1 (1974): 150.

30. HATHCOCK, J. N., and J. COON. *Nutrition and Drug Interrelations.* New York: Academic Press, 1978.

31. HENKIN, R. I., et al. "Idiopathic Hypogeusia and Dysgeusia, Hyposmia, and Dysomia." *Journal of the American Medical Association* 217 (1971): 434.

32. CLARK, M., et al. "The Effect of Chlorpromazine on Serum Cholesterol in Chronic Schizophrenic Patients." *Clinical Pharmacology and Therapy* 11 (1970): 883.

33. WILSON, C. W. M. "Vitamins and Drug Metabolism with Particular Reference to Vitamin C." *Proceedings of the Nutrition Society* 33 (1974): 231.

34. ROE, D. A. "Drug Induced Malabsorption. In *Drug-Induced Nutritional Deficiencies.* Westport, Conn.: AVI Publishing, 1976.

35. CUMMINGS, J. H., et al. "Laxative-Induced Diarrhea: A Continuing Clinical Problem." *British Medical Journal* 1 (1974): 537.

36. MORGAN, J. W. "The Harmful Effects of Mineral Oil (Liquid Petroleum) Purgatives." *Journal of the American Medical Association* 117 (1941): 1335.

37. TRUSWELL, A. S. "Drugs and Lipid Metabolism." *Proceedings of the Nutrition Society* 33 (1974): 215.

38. MARKS, V. "Effect of Drugs on Carbohydrate Metabolism. *Proceedings of the Nutrition Society* 33 (1974): 209.

39. REYNOLDS, E. H. "Iatrogenic Nutritional Effects of Anti-convulsants." *Proceedings of the Nutrition Society* 33 (1974): 225.

40. GREENBERGER, N. J. "Effects of Antibiotics and Other Agents on the Intestinal Transport of Iron." *American Journal of Clinical Nutrition* 26 (1973): 104.

41. CULLEN, S. I., and P. M. CATALANO. "Griseofulvin-Warfarin Antagonism." *Journal of the American Medical Association* 199 (1967): 582.

42. *Alcohol-Drug Interaction.* FDA Drug Bulletin 9: 2. Rockville, Md.: U. S. Department of Health, Education and Welfare, 1979.

43. KISSIN, B. "Interaction of Ethyl Alcohol and Other Drugs." In *The Biology of Alcoholism.* Vol 111, *Clinical Pathology,* eds. Bard H. Kissin and E. A. Begeites. New York: Plenum Press, 1974.

CHAPTER 11

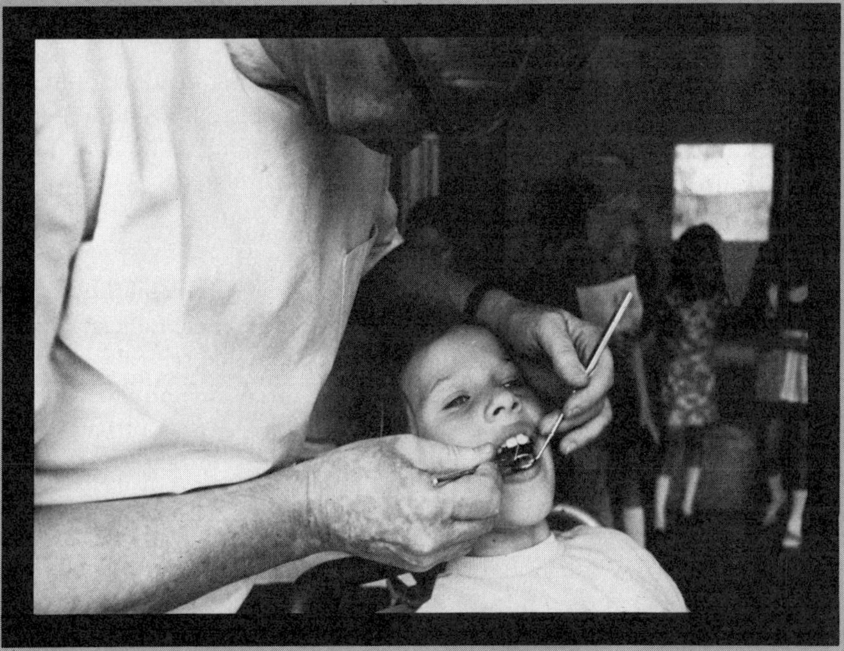

WHO photo by M. Jacot

nutrition and dental health

NUTRITION PLAYS A VITAL ROLE IN THE DEVELOPMENT OF teeth, gums, and the supporting jaw structure. The quality of nutrients available during the developmental period influences the strength of the teeth for the person's entire lifetime (1). In addition, several oral problems are related to nutrition, including dental caries, periodontal disease, and mucosal lesions.

GROWTH AND DEVELOPMENT

Tooth development begins prenatally and continues into childhood, as shown in Figures 11–1 and 11–2. Prenatal and neonatal nutritional deficiencies affect subsequent resistance to oral disease. Miller has designated critical periods that affect the prenatal, neonatal, and later posteruptive phases in childhood (2). Malnutrition at such periods can result in irreversible damage to oral tissues or structure. The role of neonatal malnutrition in dental caries is more precisely defined than its role in malocclusion or periodontal disease. Alterations in the structure, size, composition, alignment, eruption, and caries susceptibility of teeth have been linked to numerous nutritional problems. Pitting and striations on tooth surfaces, irregular ragged edges, and white opalescent spots are indications of systemic stress during tooth development (3). A defect built into the tooth cannot be repaired, but remains for the entire life of the tooth.

Once the tooth has formed and erupted, the enamel becomes one of the least sensitive parts of the body and is metabolically inactive. The cells which lay down the enamel atrophy so that no further metabolic change occurs in the tooth enamel. The odontoblasts which lay down the dentin do not atrophy. Secondary dentin can be laid down, but the dentin already formed is not modified. Only physiochemical or chemical changes that do not depend on enzymes of the tooth occur. There is no cellular repair once tooth eruption, formation, and calcification has occurred. The stages in the development of the tooth occur in fixed order and must be followed in sequence for normal structure to result. For the enamel and dentin, a protein matrix is laid down first and then calcified. A defect in protein matrix can lead to abnormal calcifications or abnormal structure of the tooth. Even if the matrix is normal, faulty calcification can result in a poorly formed tooth. Nutrition is very important in these developmental processes.

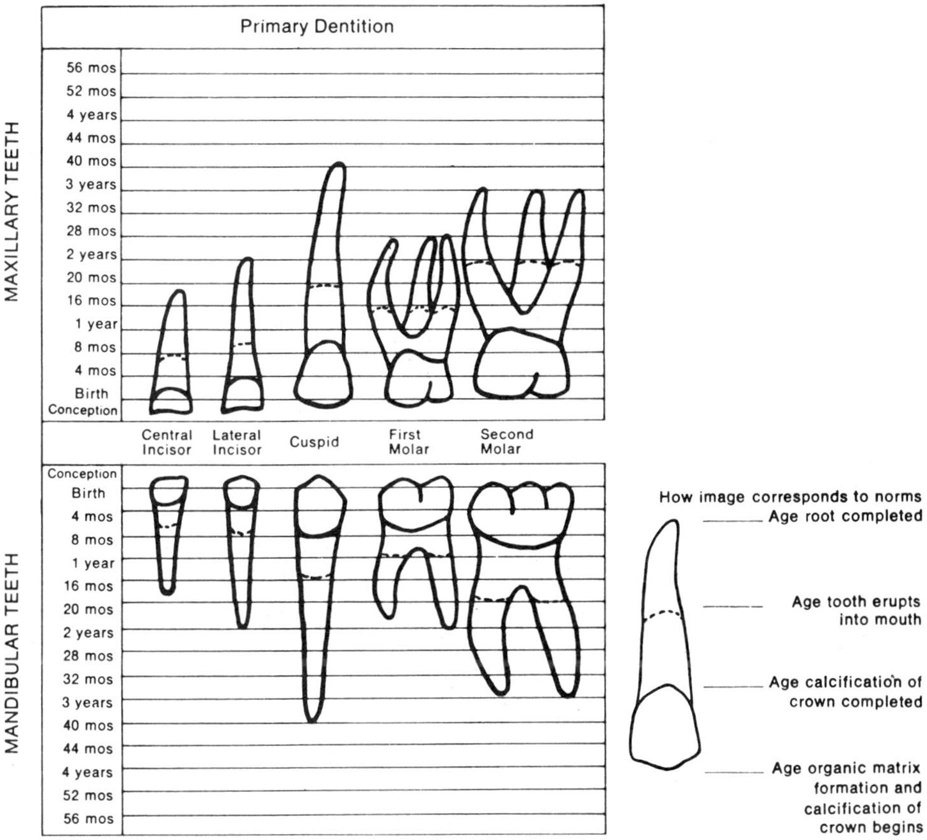

FIG. 11–1. Chronologic development of primary teeth. *Source:* D. F. Bowers, *Children Are Different: Developmental Physiology.* T. R. Johnson, W. M. Moore, and J. E. Jefferies, Eds. Columbus, Ohio: Ross Laboratories, 1978.

Much of our evidence has come from studies on animals under extreme conditions of deprivation of one essential nutrient to demonstrate the effects of nutritional imbalance, and application of this information to humans is limited.

The animal models may not be like human beings, and it is rare to have a deficiency or severe imbalance of only one nutrient in a human diet; however, these studies do point to the importance of nutrients in tooth formation (4). Vitamin A is involved in the formation of the matrix of the enamel; vitamin C in the collagen matrix of dentin; vitamin D is related to calcification; calcium, phosphorus, and the ratio of calcium and phosphorus influence the quality of calcification (5). Dietary magnesium is related to cell formation. Optimum fluoride makes a stronger enamel, while excess fluoride in the diet can interfere with enamel formation and result in mottled enamel. In the human being, the teeth are somewhat less sensitive to dietary deficiencies than other organs of the body. For example, a person with moderately severe rickets whose bones show considerable

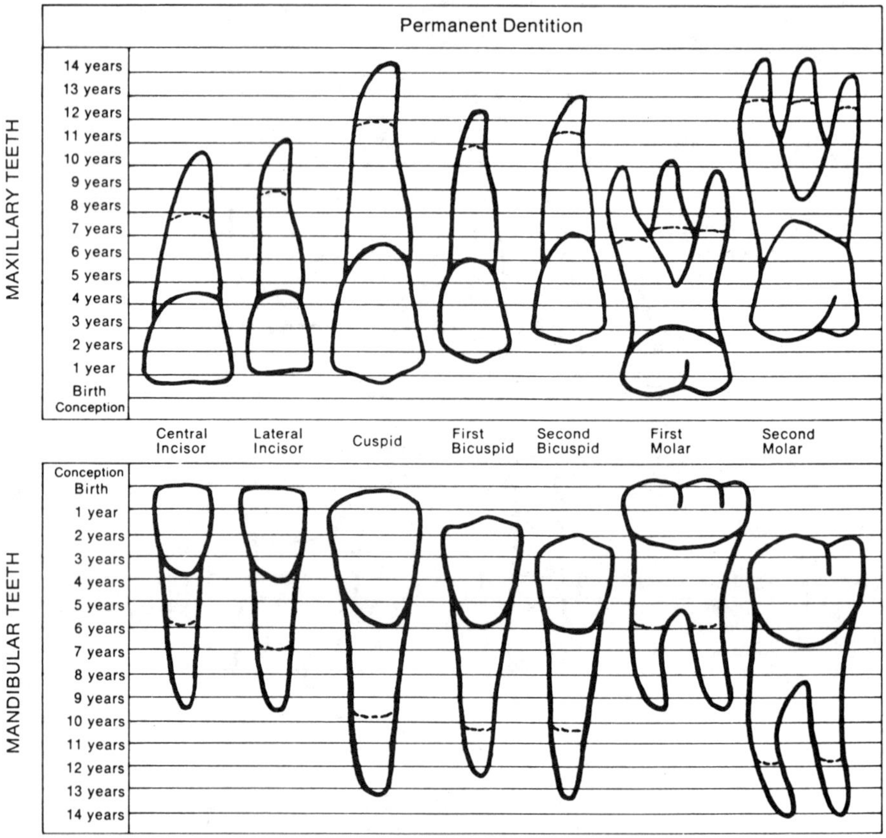

FIG. 11–2. Chronologic development of permanent teeth. *Source:* D. F. Bowers, *Children Are Different: Developmental Physiology.* T. R. Johnson, W. M. Moore, and J. E. Jefferies, Eds. Columbus, Ohio: Ross Laboratories, 1978.

injury, may appear to have normal teeth. Nutritional deficiency associated with other stress such as chronic disease, fever, or severe injury may damage the teeth. Greater mottling of enamel occurs with a diet deficient in calcium than one with adequate calcium intake in high fluoride areas (6). Deficiencies of protein or high intake of dietary fat may enhance the fluorosis. Mild nutritional deficiencies produce subtle changes in tooth structure that may make teeth more responsive to substances causing erosion and caries.

Small amounts of fluoride produce a stronger tooth surface that is less vulnerable to caries. Fluoride available prenatally or in the early months of postnatal life is important. In addition to the systemic effects fluoride can have in early life, the use of topically applied fluorides or fluorides in tooth paste or mouth rinses can reduce caries in formed teeth. The typical effect of fluoride continues to the latter stages of the life cycle; however, the effect is less as we age, since absorption of fluoride decreases. Incorporation of fluoride in teeth and bones is much less in adults than in young children.

Various investigations have been carried out in an attempt to identify trace mineral elements that might result in making the teeth more or less likely to develop caries. Some inconclusive evidence shows that increased intake of selenium or cadmium may result in greater susceptibility to caries, while increased levels of magnesium, molybdenum, vanadium, or boron may reduce susceptibility (7). Dietary studies assessing the effects of trace mineral elements other than fluoride have been complicated by not knowing quantitatively and qualitatively the amount of supplement or the total dietary intake of trace minerals in human populations.

tooth structure and growth

Teeth are hard, calcified structures consisting of a crown and root which are anchored to the jawbone. Teeth are composed of: enamel, which covers the crown; cementum, a bonelike substance covering the root; dentin, which forms the body of the tooth; dental pulse, which occupies the pulse chamber in the crown; and the root canal in the root (see Figure 11–3). The tooth is held in place by the peridontal membrane, composed of fibers attached to the root on one side and the wall of the socket on the other. The enamel is 99.5 percent inorganic matter; the dentin 77 percent, and the cementum 70 percent. This inorganic material is complex salts of calcium and phosphorus which are insoluble in water but soluble in dilute acids (3).

Genetic inheritance determines many dental characteristics, such as arrangements of teeth in the arch, eruption time, occlusal fissure patterns, cusp arrangement, and tooth size.

Growth of the bone structure supporting the teeth depends on heredity and other factors. The muscle contractions of sucking, mastication, swallowing, and speech draw the bone to its adult form. The kind of food eaten and the amount of chewing can affect the jaw. These developmental patterns can be altered by severe local or metabolic disturbances during tooth formation.

The tooth grows and develops in three stages—the proliferative cellular developmental phase, the preeruptive maturation phase, and the posteruptive maturation phase. The teeth are under the influence of the vascular system until eruption. During the developmental stage, the enamel-forming cells (ameloblasts) and the dentin-forming cells (odontoblasts) lay down an organic matrix and liberate minerals that harden the enamel and dentin. This process continues until about the age of 8. Thus, during the first eight years of life the enamel surface is vulnerable to internal stresses, including improper nutrition. The most sensitive periods are 10 months, 2.5 years, and 5 years, but the effects of nutritional stress continue through the life cycle.

During the preeruptive maturation stage, mineralization occurs by a chemical transformation to crystalline hydroxyapatite. It is during this period that systemic fluorides exert their major influence in further converting the hydroxyapatite to fluorapatite, which is much more resistant to future demineralization.

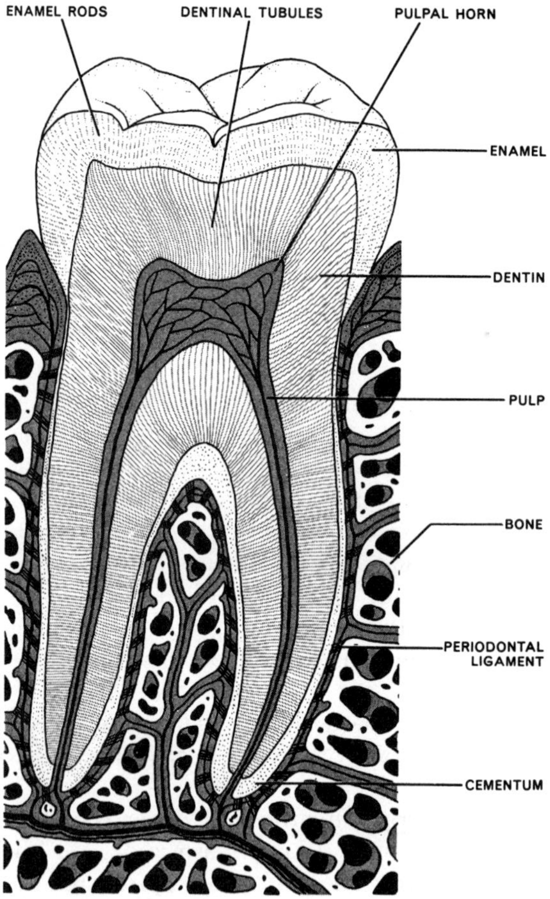

FIG. 11–3. The anatomy of the tooth and surrounding structures. Source: L. W. Morrey and R. J. Nelsen, *Dental Science Handbook* (Washington, D.C.: Superintendent of Documents, 1970).

In order to have this effect, systemic fluorides must be provided from birth until the eruption of the second molar at about 13 years. Immediately after the tooth breaks through the gum and erupts into the oral cavity, a chemical maturation reaction occurs between the immature outer enamel surface and the oral environment for about two or three years. At this stage, topical or oral fluorides can combine in small amounts with the tooth mineral to form fluorapatite until about the age of 16 or 17 years.

Development of the crown begins about the sixth week of pregnancy and continues through adolescence, when the third molars are forming, as shown in Figures 11–1 and 11–2. The stages of growth being on the thirty-fourth day of embryonic life. By the sixth week of intrauterine life, the tooth buds of the primary teeth begin development. These buds develop into layers that become the parts of a tooth. Between the fourth and sixth month, calcification begins. Following the laying down of dentin and enamel, the roots form. Tooth buds for the permanent teeth form from 5 months in utero to 10 months after birth. As a child grows, the crowns of the permanent teeth develop and the roots of the primary teeth are resorbed (4).

The dental life cycle encompasses growth, calcification and maturation, eruption of primary teeth, primary teeth root resorption, eruption of permanent teeth, and finally attrition. A regular sequence of eruptions is important to the development of normal occlusion. Malocclusion can result from genetic, functional, or muscular reasons. Mixed heredity and improper care of the primary teeth are common causes. Malocclusion can have long-term effects on nutrition. Children may have difficulty biting and chewing meat or other foods, and change their food intake. Parents are often unaware that a child cannot bite or chew because the child selectively alters food intake, consuming only those foods that do not require biting and chewing. Parents should have occlusion checked when children consistently prefer liquids and soft foods and exclude raw fruits and vegetables or foods requiring chewing, such as meats. In adult and later life, malocclusion results in a higher level of periodontal disease. Food collects in spaces surrounding the teeth and results in gum infections.

dental plaque

Dental plaque is a soft, white, tenacious material consisting of a dense aggregation of microorganisms imbedded in a matrix of protein and carbohydrate that is approximately 20 percent dry weight and about 80 percent water. Following ingestion of a fermentable carbohydrate, such as sugar, acid is formed rapidly within the plaque. Following exposure to sugar, plaque becomes an acid sponge in close approximation to the tooth. Dental plaque acts like a permeable membrane and obeys the laws of diffusion. Simple sugars are soluble and readily diffuse through the dental plaque that adheres to the enamel surface. The rate of sugar diffusion depends on its concentration and solubility. Solutions of table sugar often have a high concentration and diffuse readily. Fresh fruits have a sugar gradient that is too weak to penetrate the plaque. As the sugar passes through the plaque it is converted to organic acids, generally lactic and pyruvic, by the bacterial enzyme. These acids demineralize the enamel by producing soluble calcium phosphate, calcium lactate, and water. They create micropores that allow for the invasion of the proteolytic bacteria which break down the organic portions of the tooth. The enamel rods, which have now lost supporting structure, then collapse and form a cavity.

Each ingestion of carbohydrate is followed by a rapid fall in pH to values often as low as 4.0 The enamel calcium begins to dissolve when a value of 5.5 or lower is reached. The frequency of consuming sugar is much more important than the total amount consumed according to Nizel (3). Once dental plaque is formed, it can be removed only by brushing, flossing, or scaling and polishing. High-phosphate diets increase buffering power within the plaque by raising plaque phosphate levels to a height that lowers tooth solubility. This topical, local effect may be a result of detergent action by reducing adherence of the plaque bacteria. Research is still needed to determine the form and amount of phosphate needed for an anticaries effect in humans (3).

Dental Caries

Dental caries has been described as the most prevalent chronic disease in the United States. Caries is generally thought to be an infectious disease caused by cariogenic organisms (streptococci, lactobacilli, or gram-positive filamentoses rods) excreting lactic acid, which results in demineralized enamel. White has stated this differently by emphasizing the relationship of the tooth to bacterial and environmental factors; the role of caries-causing bacteria; and environmental effects on the bacteria and teeth (8). Of 3- and 4-year-old children, 40 to 55 percent have some tooth decay and 90 percent by age 12. Dental caries affects 98 percent of the people in the United States at some time in their lives (3). Although caries does not endanger life, it is troublesome, incapacitating, and expensive. Pain, infection, facial disfigurement, chewing and speech impairment, and malnutrition can result. The formation of caries depends upon three concurrent factors: (a) the state of the tooth itself; (b) the presence of fermentable carbohydrates; and (c) the presence of specific bacteria. Saliva is important in the prevention of dental caries for its buffering, rinsing, antibacterial, and remineralization properties.

Carbohydrates play an important role in caries. Dental caries is caused by a specific group of bacteria, the cariogenic streptococci, which act on specific carbohydrates. Sucrose has the highest cariogenicity (9). Starches, fructose, lactose, glucose, and sorbitol are lower. Sugar supplied in the diet is rapidly fermented to form an acid that dissolves the tooth structure. The form of the carbohydrate and the material with which it is mixed are important; once teeth erupt, the relationship of diet to caries depends upon the stickiness of the substance and the fermentable materials present in the food. Dietary supplements have no systemic effect on the tooth; the only systemic effect occurs within the gum. The amount of fluid associated with the carbohydrate-containing material affects caries development. Sugar dissolved in water is less cariogenic than dry sugar. Foods that adhere to the enamel surface produce more caries than those that do not. Certain substances, such as amino acids, provide buffering action and seem to reduce the formation of caries. Dietary fat protects the surface of the enamel by decreasing oral carbohydrate retention and inhibiting glycolysis by the acid-forming microorganisms (10).

prevention

Fluorides are the cornerstone of any caries prevention program. Animal studies suggest fluoride may be an essential element (11). One of the most effective means of providing fluoride in urban and suburban areas is fluoridation of the central water supply in the approximate amount of one part per million (ppm) because fluoride is made available without regard to education or socioeconomic background. The cost is low on a per capita basis, usually between $0.10 and $0.50. A fluoridated water supply can prevent the formation of two out of three caries in the teeth of children. Caries prevention should result in fewer extractions throughout an individual's lifetime. In communities with fluoridated water, almost six times as many teenagers are caries-free as their counterparts in fluoride-deficient areas. In places where fluoridation is not feasible, tablets and lozenges are the most practical solution. Mottled enamel is not seen unless 2 ppm or more is ingested daily during the first eight or nine years of life.

The percentage of Americans aged 30 and over who wear one or two complete dentures has dropped from 35 percent in 1960 to about 25 percent in 1975. This is attributed in part to fluoridation. About 60 percent of Americans have fluoridated public water systems. The economic benefits of fluoride are evident if there is a reduction in the billions of dollars spent for dental bills and the taxes to support dental care programs. Fluoridation can reduce the professional time needed for dental care of children by half.

There is some question about the benefits of prenatal fluorides. Most of the mineralization and maturation of teeth occurs after birth, so the administration of dietary fluoride to pregnant women cannot be justified on the basis of dental caries prevention.

A number of factors influence the ability of foods to produce caries. The amount of enamel destroyed by fermenting foods is not directly proportional to the sugar content or the amount of acid produced; the relationship also depends on the acid-buffering capacity of the foodstuff and the presence of enamel protectors in the foods. Buffering capacity is important in such foods as graham crackers and gingersnaps, which have a lower demineralization capacity than other foods with comparable content. In some foods, no new acids may be formed, but the food itself may contain a larger portion of the acids that result in demineralization.

More enamel is destroyed in the presence of sorbitol than in the presence of sugar, for sorbitol speeds up enamel solubility. Tests on 180 snack foods and beverages showed widely different amounts of enamel dissolved on incubation in saliva. The highest enamel dissolution is produced by acid candy, beverages, and fruits without the formation of any fermentation acids. Items with high concentrations of sugar did not destroy as much enamel as those with lower concentrations of sugar in combination with starch, as in bread and cookies. Those with high concentrations of sugar were eliminated more rapidly from the mouth after eating. Nonsugar constituents of food, such as sorbitol or flavoring agents, can increase or reduce enamel destruction, depending upon buffering capacity (12). Other studies using primates have found sorbitol to have a low cariogenic potential. Sorbitol is an alcohol that is about 80 percent as sweet as sugar and is not readily fermented by oral microorganisms. Sorbitol-containing gum is minimally cariogenic.

Nizel was one of the first dentists to recommend nutritional counseling for caries prevention (13). The foundation of the counseling is a normal diet with modifications to reduce the frequency of food intake so that there are only three regular meals per day. The use of carbohydrates is decreased so that no more than 50 percent of the total calories is provided by carbohydrates. Sticky sweets like candies, cakes, pastries, and dried fruits are eliminated, and liberal use of firm detergent foods like raw fruits and raw vegetables is recommended. This aids the maximum oral clearance of food debris and provides for minimal accumulation of dental plaque. Nutrition counseling for caries prevention is consistent with good nutrition education. The immediate response of reduced caries over a six-month period may be better motivation than other sources of feedback for nutrition education. Madsen has developed a snack guide for caries prevention using the Basic Four (14) (see Table 11–1).

nursing bottle syndrome

Very young children who are put to bed with a nursing bottle of milk or other sweet liquid as a pacifier easily develop caries (15). Bottle-fed infants are also more likely to develop caries in the front teeth than breast-fed children. Late weaning from the bottle and the addition of sugar to the milk of bottle-fed infants is associated with caries. Any sweetened beverage will give similar results. The sugar-rich beverage pools around the upper teeth; the lower ones are somewhat protected by the tongue. When the child sleeps there is no appreciable salivary flow to clear the mouth of food and to neutralize acids. The best procedure is to avoid using a bottle as a pacifier, even for infants. If emotional dependence on the bottle from use as a pacifier exists, authorities suggest the use of plain or fluoridated water in the nighttime bottle until the pattern can be broken. Plaque should be removed by brushing or wiping away with a pad. Without prevention, the result is painful, unattractive, and carious teeth very early in life.

Nursing bottle syndrome is characterized by rampant decay of all upper teeth, but not the lower front teeth. The average 3-year-old has one decayed and filled (DF) tooth, the 4-year-old has 2.5. A child of 3 or 4 still using a bottle has more than 10DF. Pain and discomfort from the decayed and broken teeth will produce an irritable and fussy child. Teeth become abscessed and facial inflammation can result. Loss of front teeth will allow the child to thrust the tongue into the space, and this undesirable habit can cause malalignment and malocclusion of the permanent teeth. Speech problems may also develop. Without incisors, the usual biting and chewing cannot occur, so some foods, such as meat and some fruits and vegetables, cannot be eaten. Biting and chewing are painful, so the tendency is to consume only liquids. Malnutrition can result.

TABLE 11-1. How To Snack Wisely For Dental Health—A Guide Based on the Four Food Groups

Eating between meals or "snacking" can be beneficial, especially for young children, teenagers, and certain older adults. Done wisely, it provides added calories and nutrients for various ages or lifestyles without risking health. However, for most persons, habitual snacking, nibbling, or drinking between meals competes with eating of good meals and foods.

The same four-food-group guide used to plan meals is useful for planning snacking habits. For better dental health, especially caries prevention, it is of greatest importance to avoid habits that frequently expose the oral cavity to fermentable carbohydrates. Thus, in this snacking guide, some items are recommended only at mealtime when hazardous carbohydrates are usually eaten away. Safer and noncarbohydrate items are allowed between meals. Others must be modified or eliminated altogether.

Most individuals achieve dental benefits by redistributing their mealtime and snack foods. If at the same time they replace excess sugar and fat with nutritious starch foods and dietary fiber, they can benefit total health. This is done by replacing excess calories from dairy, meat, and nonfood groups with vegetable-fruit and bread-cereal foods. Otherwise, the indiscriminate use of this or other snacking guides could actually be harmful. As with fatty foods, any increase in the daily intake of salty foods should be avoided.

	good snacks (no added sugars)	better with meals*
Bread & Cereal Group	Popcorn and other seeds (lightly salted)	Bread and cereals of all kinds; crackers; pretzels; caramel corn; all sweet baked goods
Fruit & Vegetable Group	All raw, fresh, frozen or waterpack fruit or vegetables or their juices prepared without addition of sugars**	All items prepared or used with the addition of sugars**; dried fruits, for example, raisins; catsup
Meat Group	Meat of all kinds including luncheon meats, leftovers and smoked meat; hard boiled eggs; Nuts of all kinds; Peanut butter**; Bean dips**	Meats prepared with sugars**; candy-coated nuts
Dairy Group	Milk—whole, low-fat, skim, or buttermilk; all cheeses including cottage; plain yogurt; dips and spreads**; flavored drinks**	Chocolate milk; malts; shakes; cocoa; ice cream, ice milk, sherbet, and other dairy desserts; sweetened yogurt
	suitable between meals	**unsuitable between meals***
Nonfood Group Foods & Other Items	Sugarless gums and candies; Sugarless soft drinks and other liquids without sugar; dill or sour pickles; olives; some breath sweeteners**; some antacid gums or tablets**; margarine and other fats; some salad dressings**	All sugared gums, candies, mints, soft drinks or other sweet liquids; sugars; syrups; honey; jellies; jams; sweet pickles and relishes; jello; chips; coffee creamers; cough drops; sugared drugs (syrups and tablets)**

*The slow or continual sipping, chewing, sucking, or nibbling of these items makes them especially hazardous to dental health. Even if consumed rapidly they should be followed with brushing, flossing or, at least, mouth-rinsing.

**Check labels for added sugars. If unsure, write the manufacturer. Look for (cane, maple, brown) sugar (sucrose); molasses; invert sugar; honey; dextrose (glucose); (modified) corn (sugar, syrup, sweetener, solids); lactose; levulose (fructose); carob.

SOURCE: Kenneth O. Madsen, "The Future Role of Sugar Substitute in Dental Caries, Prevention of Dental Caries." *National Symposium on Dental Nutrition*, ed. Stephen H. Wei (The University of Iowa, 1979).

The relationship between nutrition and periodontal disease in humans is unclear. Once started, periodontal disease progresses more rapidly in the poorly nourished. Malnutrition cannot cause common inflammatory periodontal disease; however, it may either predispose the host to the disease process or modify the progress of preexisting lesions (16, 17, 18). The present trend is to deny or overstate the importance of nutrition in periodontal disease because the design flaws in early studies made their conclusions controversial.

Many factors are related to human inflammatory periodontal disease, including local irritants such as calculi, faulty restorations, poor tooth alignment, and systemic factors. These include age, and the immunological, nutritional, psychosomatic, and endocrinological status of the individual. Malnutrition may modify the potential mechanisms for host defense of periodontal tissue. But we still do not have solid research data on the fundamental interactions of nutrition, host resistance, and infection.

The antibacterial effect, the modification of bacterial adsorption, and the importance of saliva in the formation of plaque suggest that saliva is important in modifying the subgingival plaque and preventing periodontal disease. The protective aspects of saliva have less influence for the periodontal tissues than for the tooth (16). When salivary flow is decreased dental caries increase, but not periodontal disease. And dietary factors such as protein intake can modify the composition of saliva and reduce the effect of salivary pathogens.

Little or no gingival fluid is present in healthy, noninflamed periodontal tissue. Gingival fluid contains numerous antimicrobial agents, but it also provides the nutrients for the growth of certain subgingival microbes. Early gingival flow probably has a net protective effect on the periodontium, and nutrition can alter the quantity and quality of the gingival fluid. Certain microbial flora in healthy gingival crevices prevent the growth of pathogens by releasing products toxic to other bacterial species and consuming the available nutrient supply. Inflammatory periodontal disease can result from an overgrowth of the normal microflora (9).

The epithelial barrier minimizes the penetration of antigenic, toxic, or noxious substances from the outer epithelial surface to the underlying connective tissue. This penetration is the fundamental event in the beginning of periodontal inflammation. Nutritional deficiencies can affect the complex epithelial barrier system. Animal studies have shown that vitamin C deficiency increases mucosal permeability (17). In nutritionally healthy periodontal tissue a small amount of plaque may not initiate inflammatory disease until the host is nutritionally stressed. In the absence of plaque, even with nutritional stress, there can be no disease.

Nutrition plays a role in the healing capacity of many tissues, including periodontal tissues. Peridontal disease results from an imbalance between destruction and repair of tissues. If the repair process is reduced, the disease progresses more rapidly (16). Healing is important for the therapy of periodontal disease. All nutrients involved in formation and maintenance of healthy tissues are important, including protein, and vitamins A and C. Use of raw fruit and vegetables for mechanical action will stimulate gum tissues.

Life Cycle Concerns

Both the Ten-State Nutrition Survey and the HANES survey indicated a high incidence of missing, decayed, and filled teeth in American children and adolescents. Dental caries was determined to be a serious nutrition-related problem. No differences in incidence were seen among various ethnic or socioeconomic groups. Females had higher numbers of dental caries than males, with white adolescents having slightly more dental problems than black. The average number of decayed, missing, and filled teeth at age 12 was 4, and it increased to 8.7 by age 17. Only 6 percent of all subjects had no decay or fillings by age 17. Twenty-five percent of the teenagers in the lowest income group needed dental treatment for decay. A relationship was noted between the consumption of refined carbohydrates between meals and the DMF ratio, but no relationship was demonstrated when the same carbohydrates were consumed with meals. Other apsects such as dental hygiene and dental care are important in prevention of dental caries as well as nutrition.

The gradual loss of teeth is the result of dental caries and periodontal disease, both of which are preventable. A large number of the elderly in the United States have poor dental status, with lost teeth and poorly fitting dentures. Many older people accept poor dental health and discomfort as an inevitable burden of age. Many fail to seek treatment because of physical immobility, inability to communicate, fear of cost, and fear of treatment. But poor dental status can add to the nutritional problems of older people.

The effects of food intake and malnutrition on resistance to oral disease are shown graphically in Figure 11–4. In addition to dental caries and periodontal disease, severe nutrient deficiencies may cause mucosal lesions. Analysis of dietary intake and food habits is important and necessary before cause and effect statements can be made and before appropriate and effective nutritional counseling can be done. Certainly, frequency of eating and drinking is as important to the treatment of oral disease as the type of food consumed.

Summary

Nutrition and dental health are related, for nutrition is important in the development and maintenance of the teeth and supporting tissues from the prenatal period to the later years. The quantity and quality of the diet, the frequency of eating, and the availability of fluoride influence the development of caries.

Dental plaque is a combination of soft material and microorganisms. The consistency and texture of the diet affects plaque formation. Plaque and other factors lead to the development of dental caries. Carbohydrates play an important role. Overuse of nursing bottles with sweetened milk or other sweetened beverages leads to caries in infants and young children.

Periodontal disase is emphasized by malnutrition. The disease results from an imbalance between the destruction and repair of tissues surrounding the tooth.

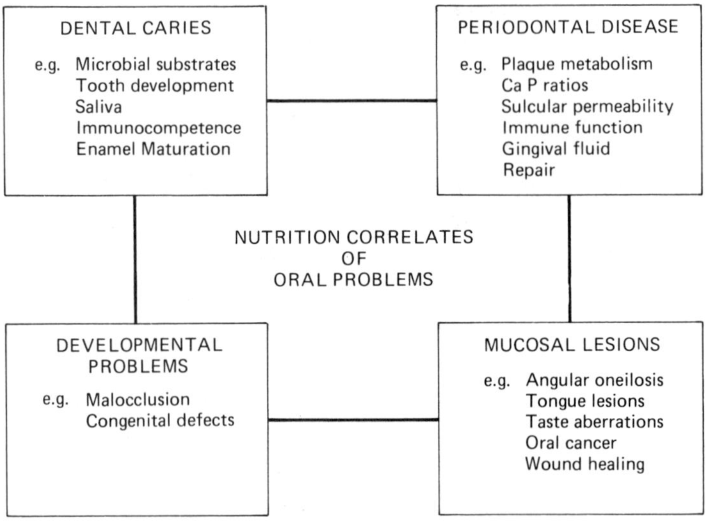

FIG. 11–4. Diagrammatic representation of the effect of nutrition on oral problems. *Source:* M. C. Alfano, "Effect of Diet and Malnutrition During Development on Resistance to Oral Disease." In *National Symposium on Dental Nutrition,* ed. Stephen H. Wei (Iowa City: University of Iowa, 1979), p. 29. Used with permission.

references

1. LEICETER, H. N. "Nutrition in the Tooth." *Journal of the American Dental Association* 52 (1956): 284.
2. MILLER, S. A. "Nutrition in the Neonatal Development of Protein Metabolism." *Federation Proceedings* 29 (1970): 1497.
3. NIZEL, A. E. "Preventing Dental Caries: The Nutritional Factors." *Pediatric Clinics of North America* 24 (1977): 141.
4. GOODHART, R. S., and M. E. SHILS. *Modern Nutrition in Health and Disease,* 6th ed. Philadelphia: Lea & Febiger, 1980.
5. IRWIN, M. I., and E. W. KIENHOLZ. "A Conspectus on Research on Calcium Requirement of Man." *Journal of Nutrition* 103 (1973): 1019.
6. MASSLER, M., and I. SCHOUR. "Relation of Endemic Dental Fluorosis to Malnutrition." *Journal of the American Dental Association* 44 (1952): 156.
7. CURZON, M. E. J., and F. L. LOSEE. "Dental Caries and Trace Element Composition of Whole Human Enamel: Eastern United States." *Journal of the American Dental Association* 94 (1977): 1146.
8. WHITE, G. E. *Dental Caries, A Multifactorial Disease,* Springfield, Ill.: Charles C Thomas, 1975.
9. MORHART, R. E., and R. J. FITZGERALD. "Nutrition Determinants of the Ecology of the Oral Flora." *Dental Clinics of North America* 20 (1976): 473.
10. DEPOOLE, D. P., and M. C. ALFANO. "Nutrition and Oral Health." *Nutrition Today* 12 (1977): 6.
11. NEWBURN, E. *Fluorides and Dental Caries.* Springfield, Ill.: Charles C Thomas, 1975.
12. BIBBY, B. G., and S. A. MUNDORFS. "Enamel Demineralization by Snack Foods." *Journal of Dental Research* 54 (1975): 461.
13. NIZEL, A. E. "Oral Problems." In *Nutritional Support of Medical Practice,* eds. Howard A. Schneider, C. E. Anderson, and D. B. Coursin. Hagerstown, Md.: Harper and Row, 1977.
14. MADSEN, K. O. "The Future Role of Sugar Substitute in Dental Caries, Prevention of Dental Caries." In *National Symposium on Dental Nutrition,* ed. Stephen H. Wei. University of Iowa, 1979.
15. FASS, E. S. "Is Bottle Feeding of Milk a Factor in Dental Caries?" *Journal of Dentistry for Children* 29 (1962): 245.
16. ALFANO, M. C. "Controversies, Perspectives and Clinical Implications of Nutrition in Periodontal Disease." *Dental Clinics of North America* 20 (1976): 519.

17. Alfano, M. C., S. A. Miller, and J. F. Drummond. "Effect of Ascorbic Acid Deficiency on the Permeability and Collagen Biosynthesis of Oral Mucosal Epithelium." *Annals of the New York Academy of Science* 258 (1975): 253.

18. Dawes, C. "Effects of Diet on Salivary Secretion and Composition." *Journal of Dental Research* 49 (1970): 1263.

CHAPTER 12

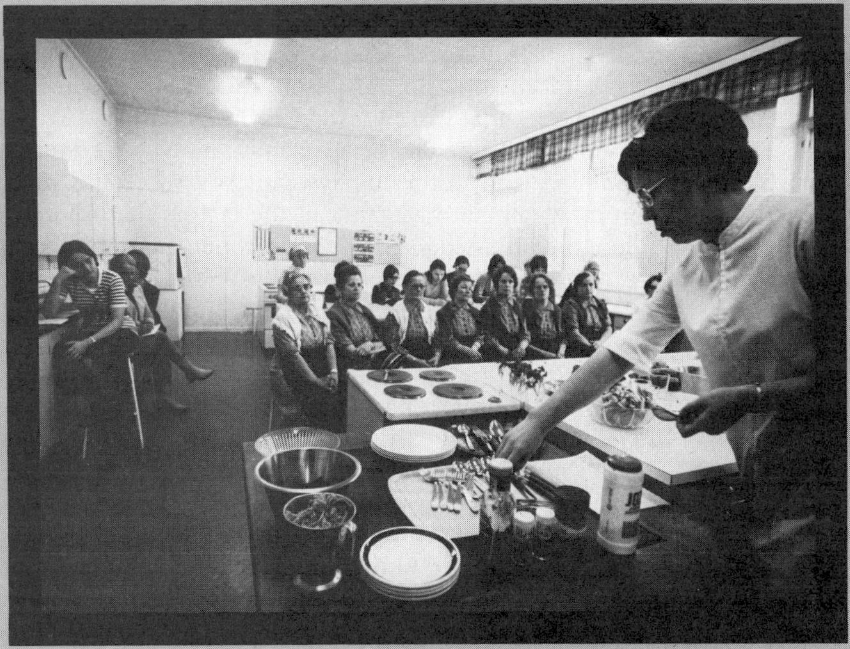

WHO photo by T. Farkas

nutrition education

THE KNOWLEDGE WE ACQUIRE ABOUT NUTRITION needs to be used for other people. This transfer of information to others, who subsequently change their behavior, is nutrition education. The uninformed are easy targets for fads or quackery. This final chapter presents information on the factors related to nutrition education and some of the techniques that can be used to spread it.

The food we eat is determined by the available supply, our culture, the time available, our knowledge, and our value system. Any successful program for nutrition education must take into account all the factors that influence eating behavior. In addition, the physiological functions of humans vary during the life cycle and from person to person. Food habits and life style are closely linked. Food choices result more from a lifetime of social, cultural, and marketing influences than from the knowledge one has. Money, accessibility of food, transportation, literacy, family structure, and tradition cannot be ignored. Food serves many purposes in a society in addition to providing nutrition.

Knowles has pointed out that each person has an obligation to preserve his or her health (1). Too many people do not worry about their health until they lose it. Exercising regularly, improving nutrition, going to the dentist, having screening examinations, practicing contraception, and ensuring harmonious family and work life are not considered until illness occurs. For a person to assume responsibility for his or her own health, information for the prevention of disease or disabilities must be provided. Nutrition education must be part of this system. It can contribute to reduced medical costs by decreasing the need for some high-cost, hospital-based technologies. Major advances in the health of the American people will be determined by what the individual is willing to do for healthy living for himself or herself and society (1). As Figure 12–1 shows, diet affects some but not all diseases (2). Nutrition education should focus on those diseases where diet is a major risk factor. But before considering education techniques, we need to review some of the many factors that influence nutritional status.

FACTORS IN FOOD CHOICES

educational level

In one study using a national sample, nutrition knowledge, food beliefs, and reported shopping behavior were positively associated and had a linear relationship (3). Level of educational achievement had the strongest association to nutri-

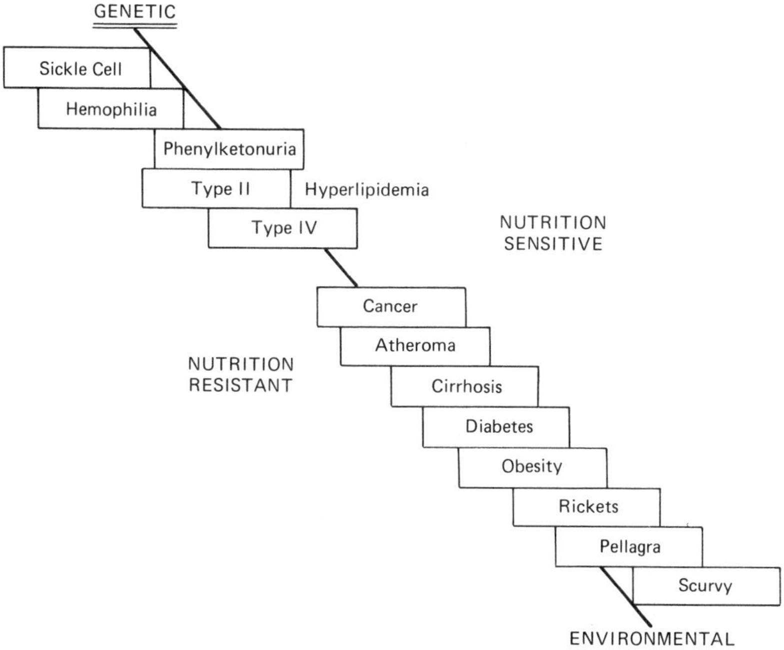

FIG. 12–1. Multiple bases of disease. Reciprocal genetic and environmental determinants of 13 diseases are shown on a linear scale. The extent to which nutritional intervention can modify the disease is indicated by the degree of displacement of each bar to the right of the line. *Source:* R. E. Olsen, "Are Professionals Jumping the Gun in the Fight against Chronic Disease?" *Journal of the American Dietetic Association* 74 (1979): 543.

tion knowledge. The findings indicated a particular need for education and facts about certain nutrients such as iron, thiamin, riboflavin, and vitamins A and D. Consumers with low knowledge tended to have low income and less prestigious occupations. Understanding nutrition requires some knowledge of human physiology and chemistry. Educational achievement through high school increases the opportunity for exposure to the sciences and nutrition information.

income

For some parts of the population in the United States and all over the world, lack of adequate income prevents the purchase of a nutritionally adequate diet. But money alone will not ensure an adequate diet. Middle- and high-income people can also be malnourished. Nutrition education programs can assist consumers to use food resources effectively. Although many low-income households make more efficient use of their food dollars than higher-income households, this too does not ensure good nutrition. Recently, greatly increased prices for food have affected the ordinary person's ability to buy an adequate diet. Education is even more necessary to aid people in selecting less expensive alternatives or in changing meal patterns.

cultural food patterns

Food is related to religion, customs, traditions, and celebrations, as well as survival. Social acceptance, status, and prestige are intertwined with food. Each group of people has important status foods and food taboos. Within a culture there may be status foods and taboos for certain groups, such as children or pregnant women. No culture has been known to consume all its potential sources of food. What is an acceptable food also varies from group to group; for example, horsemeat is popular in parts of France but not in the United States.

The geography of the United States varies from dense forests and lakes to arid desert lands, rugged mountains to rolling hills, fertile farmlands to rocky, untillable soils. But America's farmlands and cattle ranges, with modern, progressive agricultural methods and advanced food technology, produce a great bounty of food. With excellent transportation and marketing techniques, all types of foods are available in all sections of the country. New foods are constantly being brought to the American people by travel, education, and technology.

The early pattern of American food habits began with the American Indians and the early English, Dutch, and French settlers. Later German, Italian, Spanish, and Scandanavian influences were added. When the first European immigrants arrived, the colonies that survived adopted some of the food habits of the native American Indians. Each wave of movement of people into the United States has brought altered patterns of eating.

Although each major section of the country has its own strong regional overtones and individual variations, Americans basically follow a common dietary pattern: breakfast upon arising, a medium light lunch at noon, and dinner, the main meal, in the evening. The most common breakfast is fruit juice, eggs, meat, toast, and coffee. America devised the dry breakfast cereal, which is also eaten for breakfast with milk. Many Americans lead fast-paced lives, with little time for preparation or consumption of food. Fast food businesses serving hamburgers, fried chicken or fish, french fried potatoes, and soft drinks have developed to meet this need. The evening meal might be almost anything, but a general pattern is usually meat, with beef the most preferred, potato or substitute, vegetable, salad, bread, margarine or butter, dessert, and milk for the children, milk or iced tea for the adults, and often coffee.

Cummings has presented the historical development of American food habits from the formation of the country until the late 1930s (4). Agricultural developments, cultural food preferences, the growth of transportation and refrigeration have all altered the food intakes of people. Burk has added more recent information on economic and social factors affecting food consumption in the United States (5). Other authors have collected information on additional aspects of Americans' food habits (6, 7).

food habits

Mead reports that food habits do not occupy a special place among the attitudes of humans (8). A food habit is not a passing fancy, but a feature of society (9). Food habits are integrated into a structure of social values. They may have little or nothing to do with the principles of nutrition.

Many foods are rejected for cultural or religious reasons. Occasionally entire groups of food may be rejected, but usually it is only selected items. Established food practices tend to persist after movement to another social group. Habits change more easily than food taboos, which function more like a code of conduct. Because beliefs about food are often integrated into social behavior, a very subtle form of indoctrination occurs. A group of nutrients does not become a food until a community accepts it and gives cultural and psychosensory value to the food. Figure 12–2 shows this complex human behavior in graphic form.

Most people have an aversion to some food or method of preparing certain foods. These aversions are quite diverse. The greater the number of aversions, the more difficult the process of nutrition education. Certain foods have prestige value. This can have negative or positive implications. Making a food popular can be enhanced by raising the status of the food through consumption by the upper class. Meat consumption, for example, usually increases as the socioeconomic level of a country rises. Many Americans spend time avoiding eating, feeling guilty about eating, or drinking low-calorie drinks. Adequate nutrition education must emphasize the physiology of human beings, their habits, loves, hopes, and the way food is distributed in the home, as well as the nutrient and chemical properties of food.

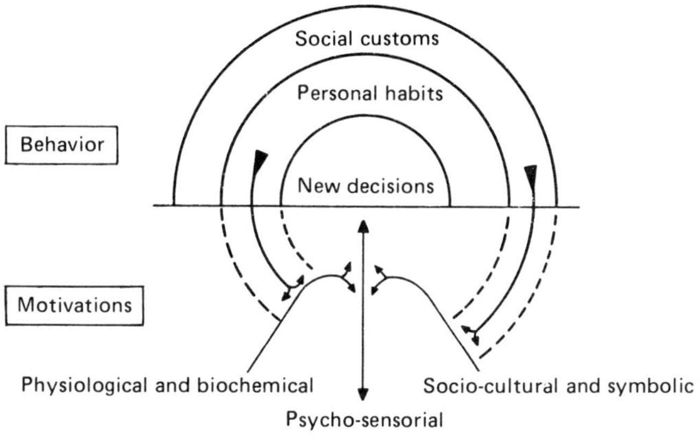

FIG. 12–2. Human feeding behavior. *Source:* J. Trémolièrs, "Nutrition and Public Health," *World Review of Nutrition and Dietetics* 18 (1973): 277–319.

faddism

The American Medical Association estimates between 50 and 80 percent of all human illnesses will cure themselves in time if merely left alone. This ability of the body to cure itself is the mainstay of the quack and faddist. As long as the faddist does not poison people, a large percentage will get well—usually less from the recommendations than from the fact they would have improved anyway (10).

Fads and fallacies may have harmful effects. Special products and health foods are usually more expensive than traditional foods. Usually foods of higher or comparable value can be obtained from ordinary markets. Fads can lead to inadequate or poorly balanced diets. Following a fad diet or food fallacy can lead to a false sense of security and prevent an individual from seeking medical assistance.

Many forms of faddism exist in the United States (11). Faddism is the number one problem of nutrition education among the well educated and higher socioeconomic groups. Table 12–1 summarizes the types of food faddists and the possible need such behavior serves.

instinct

People do not instinctively select an adequate diet without education or training. In primitive societies a dietary pattern is established by the survival of those who could adapt to the available food supply. To satisfy hunger, humans have eaten almost anything that could be chewed and digested. Trial and error developed a tradition for which foods caused illness or death, and which were acceptable. Biochemically, our dietary requirements were established millions of years ago. A balanced selection of food to achieve the requirement was found by primitive experimentation with edible and digestible things in the environment, and not by instinct.

The history of dietary deficiency diseases also demonstrates that people are not guided by instinct. No one instinctively knew that vitamin C was the cure for scurvy.

changing life styles

Since deficiency diseases are rare in the United States, nutrition education must focus on selecting an adequate diet from among the foods technology has made available. More than half of the foods we currently consume are processed. Advancing food technology will develop new foods which people must learn to use in obtaining an adequate diet.

TABLE 12-1. Types of Food Faddists and the Patterning of Needs Their Practices Serve, as Described by Beal

type of food faddist	need served by the fad
1. Miracle seeker	Patterning need to establish stability regarding health, energy, and so on. Accomplished by diets intended to forestall aging or restore organism to health. Ego defense need to reestablish positive self-concept and feeling of self-worth.
2. Antiestablishmentarian	Self-realization need to express self in a manner consistent with self-concept and value system.
3. Super health seeker	Ego defense need to forestall aging process. Accomplished by diet intended to give super health. Self-realization need to present front of strength and health.
4. Distruster of medical profession	Ego defense need to establish control over own destiny and not be dependent on unknown others.
5. Fashion-follower	Ego defense and patterning need to establish an identity to gain approval and acceptance from others.
6. Authority seeker	Self-realization need for recognition of self-competency, provided by apparent knowledge in area of food information.
7. Truth seeker	Patterning need to process existing claims concerning nutrition.
8. One concerned about uncertainties of living	Patterning need for anchors and stability concerning the world.

SOURCE: Based on V. A. Beal, "Food Faddism and Organic and Natural Foods," paper presented at National Dairy Council Food Writers' Conference, Newport, R.I., May, 1972. Reprinted from Robert Schafer and Elizabeth A. Yetley, "Social Psychology of Food Faddism," *Journal of The American Dietetic Association* 66 (February 1975): 131, by permission of The American Dietetic Association. Copyright © 1975 by The American Dietetic Association.

In 1977, 47 percent of all American mothers were working outside the home. Many more women work out of economic necessity. In 1977, about 5.5 million children under 18 lived in households headed by women with no husband present. Some results of these changes? Less time is spent in shopping and food preparation. Food purchasers include many men and children as well as women, those knowledgeable in buying food as well as the foolish. Larger numbers of meals are eaten away from home by children and adults. Family meals together are fewer. Individualized eating is popular. The eating-out industry is growing at four times the rate of the retail food industry. Thus, increasingly greater influences on children's behavior is exerted by forces outside the home.

Historical Aspects of Nutrition Education

Traditionally, nutrition education efforts have been directed almost entirely toward low-income groups and dietary modifications for disease conditions. Dietitians and nutritionists have spent more time on counseling for therapeutic effects than for prevention of disease conditions. But nutrition education must address the preventive aspects for all socioeconomic levels and age groups if it is to be effective in motivating behavioral changes.

Token efforts at nutrition education were previously made in schools by inclusion of nutrition units in health, science, biology, and home economics. Additional information sometimes accurate and reliable, and other times faddish and scientifically unsound, was given to athletes by coaches and physical education personnel. Some early nutrition education efforts were directed toward undernourished children, and several studies have shown improved food habits and resultant weight gain in underweight children after nutrition education (12).

Programs in over 20 countries have shown that nutrition education improves the food habits, the well-being, and the productivity of the population (13). McKenzie and Mumford noted in a review of nutrition education that the success of a program depended on the methods used, the personalities involved, and the circumstances in the area (14). They emphasized the need for social scientists and nutritionists to work in cooperation to develop methods for implementation and evaluation.

In the early years, nutrition education dealt only with cognitive knowledge; therefore, improvements in knowledge were easily shown. As we shift to behavioral emphases, evaluation of the effectiveness of programs becomes more difficult. The measurement of human behavior is complex, and errors and misinterpretations are easy to make. Since the advent of television and mass marketing techniques, the process of nutrition education and behavioral change is more complex. Few studies have approached this problem, although the effects have been considered.

Approaches to Nutrition Education

Physicians, dentists, nurses, and public health workers are usually seen as the most credible nutrition authorities, although some of these professionals may be the least knowledgeable and effective in providing nutritional guidance. For the person trained in nutrition, the development of communication skills to use with physicians and other professionals and the integration of education and communication techniques for counseling is critical to the success of nutrition education. This makes it necessary to have a background in the technical and scientific aspects of nutrition to be able to communicate with confidence and authority.

The challenge for nutrition education is to create a learning situation in which people will recognize their own nutritional problems. Effective nutrition education recognizes that the food supply is undergoing change. The nutritional status of some populations has been improved by increasing the available food, improving food production or distribution, or by food supplements. In a complex society, supplementation is difficult. Take the fortification of bread, for example. Some individuals will eat one slice of bread, others may eat six. Do you fortify for the one slice or the six slices? Either way, someone gets too much or too little.

Nutrition education must address the difficulty of defining nutrition because there is a *science* of nutrition and a *practice* of nutrition, and the same term is used for both (15). The science of nutrition draws on chemistry, physics, biology, and the social sciences. Its objective is to describe in detail, using basic scientific procedures, the relationship of food to health. The application of the knowledge obtained through the science of nutrition to human well-being at all stages of the life cycle is the practice of nutrition. The practice and science of nutrition are not mutually exclusive; many people participate in both to varying degrees. The American Dietetic Association defines *nutrition education* as "... the process by which beliefs, attitudes, environmental influences, and understanding about food lead to practices that are scientifically sound, practical, and consistent with individual needs and available resources" (16).

basic concepts and guides

Basic concepts for nutrition education were developed during the 1960s and distributed at a national conference in 1967. These concepts have been widely used in planning for nutrition education (see Table 12–2). Another National Conference on Nutrition Education, Directions for the 80's, was a jointly sponsored effort of the White House, the Department of Health, Education and Welfare, the Department of Agriculture, the Federal Trade Commission, and the Society for Nutrition Education. The population groups emphasized were these: pregnant women, children and adolescents, low-income and elderly populations, and persons with diet-restricted diseases (17). Government, demographic, scientific, and communications prespectives were presented. The ten issues of general concern raised in all four reports are as follows:

1. GOALS include nutrition messages on the prevention of diet-related disease as well as the promotion of health and treatment or support of medical therapies through food.
2. APPROACHES to nutrition education delivery include more targeting and focusing of messages to specific groups, outreach efforts, participant involvement, and greater use of the mass media.

TABLE 12–2. Basic Concepts for Nutrition Education

1. Nutrition is the food you eat and how the body uses it.
   - We eat food to live, to grow, to keep healthy and well, and to get energy for work and play.
2. Food is made up of different nutrients needed for growth and health.
   - All nutrients needed by the body are available through food.
   - Many kinds and combinations of food can lead to a well-balanced diet.
   - No food, by itself, has all the nutrients needed for full growth and health.
   - Each nutrient has specific uses in the body.
   - Most nutrients do their best work in the body when teamed with other nutrients.
3. All persons, throughout life, have need for the same nutrients, but in varying amounts.
   - The amounts of nutrients needed are influenced by age, sex, size, activity, and state of health.
   - Suggestions for the kinds and amounts of food needed are made by trained scientists.
4. The way food is handled influences the amount of nutrients in food, its safety, appearance, and taste.
   - Handling means everything that happens to food while it is being grown, processed, stored, and prepared for eating.

SOURCE: Developed by the Interagency Committee on Nutrition Education. Distributed at the National Nutrition Education Conference, Washington, D.C., February 20–22, 1967.

3. ADVOCACY by consumers as well as providers is seen as necessary to improve the status of nutrition education efforts.
4. COORDINATION among and within federal departments as well as state and local governmental levels and with voluntary and private groups is deemed necessary.
5. TRAINING of those who train the nutrition educators is seen as a necessary first step to take in improving nutrition education efforts.
6. FINANCING of nutrition education efforts, including counseling of patients, is seen as an essential prerequisite.
7. RESEARCH on nutrition education needs greater emphasis.
8. EVALUATION of nutrition education programs must be instituted on a more widespread basis.
9. FOLLOW-UP efforts to assure implementation of the recommendations is called for.

10. LINKAGES among nutrition education and food or income assistance, health, and education programs are needed at federal, state, and local levels.

Each task force drafted a position paper that was criticized, revised, and rewritten by the conference participants. The specific recommendations are shown in Table 12–12 at the end of this chapter and are worthy goals for nutrition education programs.

Curriculum guides have been developed for nutrition education in schools. A majority of the states and a number of large cities have guides that are available through the education department or agency in each state. USDA, through the National School Lunch Program, has provided impetus for curriculum development in nutrition as well as improvement in the quality of food service. An example of the concept for a comprehensive curriculum is shown in Table 12–3.

perspectives and techniques

Nutrition education must promote attitudinal and behavioral changes in addition to disseminating information. The nutrition educator must know how people learn and what influences their learning. The successful teacher must be sincere of purpose, have a sense of humor and a pleasant manner, and understand the background and goals of the learners (18).

Nutrition education should be conducted from a multidisciplinary perspective that includes human behavior, consumerism, food management, and food preparation. Basic knowledge of nutrition must be accompanied by the ability to select, buy, prepare, and/or serve nutritious foods in a setting that encourages consumption. This has implications for where nutrition education is provided and by whom.

The nutrition educator must know how to use a visually oriented medium such as television. Television is the primary source of information in the United States, yet little positive nutrition education is provided either in programming or advertising. Television ads are a major way to sell foods. Approximately one-fourth of TV advertising time is devoted to food and beverage items. The most time is devoted to nonnutritive beverages. The majority of the advertising is devoted to high-calorie food. Restaurant advertising is mainly of the limited-menu, fast-food type. Special concern must be given to advertising directed toward preschool children, who may not be able to discriminate between the program and the commercial or who may believe everything they see on TV. In addition, such early conditioning for acceptance of sweet beverages and high-calorie, low-nutrient-density snack foods may have lifetime effects.

The nutrition educator must use simple, clear language. Winston Churchill, a master of persuasion, used "blood, sweat, and tears," not "hemorrhage, perspiration, and lachrymation." Education requires clarity; educators should avoid fuzzy or misleading terms.

TABLE 12–3. Nutrition Concepts for a Comprehensive Curriculum for Schools, K to 12

A. NUTRIENTS ARE ESSENTIAL TO LIFE AND HEALTH.

1. Nutrients are chemical substances which are needed but either cannot be made or made in sufficient quantity by the body; nutrients are drawn from the environment.
2. The biological requirement for, and the obtaining of nutrient elements is a continuous process throughout the life cycle.
3. While the need for nutrients is lifelong, the relative amounts and proportions of nutrients needed are influenced by age, sex, body size, physical activity, specific conditions of growth, physical condition, state of health, and other individual variations.
4. Varying amounts, proportions and combinations of nutrients are found in plant and animal sources which serve as food from the environment.
5. Individuals can meet appropriate nutrient-intake needs by the judicious selection of foods derived from plants and animals.
6. Nutrients as body constituents are distributed throughout the body, concentrated or stored in varying amounts over time, and may be withdrawn from tissue for use.
7. Nutrient supplies for immediate use and reserves or stores need to be replenished on a regular basis in order to maintain normal body function and to prevent health impairment. Failure to consume adequate amounts of any essential nutrient with sufficient frequency will result in the physiological and/or mental dysfunction of the individual.
8. Nutrient excesses, greater than needed for immediate use and limited concentration or storage, are of no special nutritional benefit. In some cases, nutrient excesses actually may be harmful.
9. During critical periods of growth and development, pregnancy, lactation, and recovery from illness or trauma, the body is more sensitive to inadequate nutrition, with the increased probability of biological disadvantage as a result.
10. Identification and amounts of nutrients needed are determined by scientists whose findings provide the basis for recommended dietary allowances. These recommended dietary allowances are revised from time to time according to the latest research findings.

B. FOOD SERVES BIOLOGICAL, PSYCHOLOGICAL, SOCIAL, AND CULTURAL NEEDS.

1. Food can provide the nutrients to meet the biological needs of the healthy individual.
2. No one type of food found in nature contains appropriate amounts and combinations of nutrients to meet total nutritional needs. In general, a diet selected to include a variety of food choices is most likely to meet nutritional needs.
3. The way a food is handled influences the amount of nutrients in the food, its safety, appearance, flavor and cost. Handling means everything that happens to food while it is grown, processed, stored, and prepared for eating.
4. Non-nutritive fiber in food is valuable to the function and health of the gastrointestinal tract.
5. With skills, knowledge, and appropriate motivation and experience, individuals can select many different diets which meet biological, psychological, social and cultural needs, given adequate economic and ecological opportunities.

TABLE 12-3. Continued

6. While foods have given nutrient values, their nutritional benefit is best described in terms of how they contribute to meeting the total nutrient needs of the individual with specific food consumption patterns.
7. Foods included in a diet constitute a nutritionally valuable food pattern when they are selected within given periods of time to supply a balanced array of nutrients in appropriate quantities. While certain food patterns are conducive to good health, food patterns are just one of the many "inputs" to health and will not (in and of themselves) assure good health.
8. It may be desirable to adjust (reduce or increase) consumption of certain classes of foods with special nutritional properties at certain stages of life in order to promote long-term health and survival.
9. The energy value of one's diet and energy expenditure should be balanced to maintain normal body weight, or to modify over- or underweight toward a more normal weight, thus reducing risks of associated health disorders.
10. Foods play an important role in the physical and psychological health of a society or a nation just as it does for the individual, the family, or living unit.

SOURCE: Developed in the first phase of the Pennsylvania State University School Nutrition Education Curriculum Study, supported by the Heinz Endowment funded through the Nutrition Foundation, 1975. © The Pennsylvania State University 1980.

mode of learning

In developing educational programs variation in learning styles must be considered. There is a large body of educational literature on factors involved in learning. Table 12–4 outlines student learning styles. It is difficult to meet the variations in learning styles in any one presentation, but knowledge of these aids in evaluation. No one person fits one learning style at all times for most people use combinations.

Mode of learning varies among people. Some learn by visual means, using either pictures or written information, others by auditory or by a combination. The best programs provide opportunities for all modes of learning, by spoken presentation, visual aids, and written support material. While many can read and understand, others must have the information explained or diagrams provided. The use of workbooks and cassette tape recordings is an economical way to meet this need and provide individualized instruction.

goals

In planning nutrition education, clearly stated goals or objectives for a program are necessary (19). Stated goals allow those involved to determine if the objectives were accomplished and permit comparison with other programs. Objectives can define outcomes or processes. These should be clearly separated. End goals describe behaviors students will demonstrate at the end of a program. Means goals describe what students will do during the program.

Specific objectives are often written in behavioral terms. A behavioral objective describes certain student behaviors that indicate a skill, attitude, or knowledge and lists the necessary critical performance the student must accomplish. Student performance is the evidence of learning. Behavioral objectives are more important when a test or other attitude instrument is used and less so in situations where goals are agreed upon. Learning is changed to behavior.

selected aids

FOOD GROUPING. A food grouping system has become the standardized tool for nutrition education. Many teaching aids produced by government agencies and private organizations are based on food groups. The United States Department of Agriculture publishes a Daily Food Guide which is included in the appendix. The guide provides a simple system for food selection that can be used by people who have limited education or those who have the nutrition knowledge but little time or interest in a complicated calculation system.

The major criticism of food groups is that they have not kept pace with food technology and changing attitudes toward food. Many foods and meals eaten away from home are nutritious but difficult to fit into food groups. Regional or cultural food patterns and vegetarian diets may require special plans for using food groups. Reorganization of the food groups for the target population, and for regional and ethnic differences, is necessary for every nutrition education program. The basic food groups and servings for ages in the life cycle are shown in Appendix Table A–3.

The USDA has developed plans for various cost levels based on the use of food groupings. The income level of the family determines the appropriate level to use (see Table 12–5). Estimated cost of food for one week is shown in Table 12–6. The amount of food needed for a week and daily to provide adequate nutrition using each level of the Food Plan is shown in Tables 12–7 and 12–8.

NUTRIENT DENSITY. A nutrient density or index of nutritional quality system (INQ) has been developed as a means to teach children and adolescents to make wise food choices (20). Students are encouraged to combine foods to meet nutrient requirements based on individual taste preferences. Nutrient density or INQ is a method of measuring a food's nutritive value based on a ratio of nutrient to energy content. The equations for calculating INQ are these:

$$\%\ \text{Standard for nutrient} = \frac{\text{Amount of nutrient in food}}{\text{RDA for nutrient}} \times 100$$

$$\text{INQ} = \frac{\%\ \text{Standard for nutrient}}{\%\ \text{Standard for energy}}$$

TABLE 12-4. Overview of Student Learning Styles

learning style	description
Independent	Like to determine what is important to learn; do not like structure; like to work alone; feel their ideas are equal to those of the instructor; confident of their ability to identify and learn the most important concepts in the subject.
Avoidant	Bored with class attendance; difficulty paying attention; present only because they are required; spend little time or energy.
Collaborative	Want an open, sharing relationship with instructor and other students; opinions of others are important; feel obligation to help other students; feel students should be encouraged to work together.
Dependent	Expect the instructor to structure the course and clearly state objectives; follow instructions carefully; accept the validity of the information presented; do not like class discussion.
Competitive	Are aggressive; compete with others for attention and to promote their point; avoid helping other students; want to rank their knowledge with others.
Participant	Participate actively in class and assignments; are eager to learn; work for understanding of the material; expect to learn something important; intend to accomplish their best.

SOURCE: Dr. Anthony Grasha and Dr. Sheryl Riechmann, Department of Psychology, University of Cincinnati, Ohio. Based on research reported in *American Psychologist* 27 (1972) and *The Journal of Psychology* 87 (1974): 213–223.

NUTRITION LABELING. Nutrition labeling acknowledges the buyer's right to know about the nutritional quality of foods. Labeling informs a person that foods differ in energy value and kinds and amounts of other nutrients, and that no single food contains all the nutrients an individual needs unless it has been supplemented. This provides visual reinforcement of the need for a variety of foods in order to obtain the recommended amounts each day. Nutrition labeling is limited to foods that are canned or packaged in some way. Fresh fruits, vegetables, and meat are not labeled. Tables of food values such as those published by USDA are useful supplements for information on fresh foods.

The Food and Drug Administration developed the U.S. Recommended Daily Allowances (USRDA) based on the 1968 Recommended Dietary Allowances (RDA) of the National Academy of Sciences (see Table 12–9). The values for protein, vitamin C, and riboflavin are from the figures for the adult man; vitamin D, thiamin, niacin, and iron are from values for the adolescent boy (21). There is no value for calories.

TABLE 12–5. The Food Plan for the Family, 1979

income (before taxes)	1-person family	2-person family	3-person family	4-person family	5-person family	6-person family
$ 2,500–$ 5,000	T or LC	T or LC	T	T	T	T
$ 5,000–$10,000	MC	LC	T or LC	T	T	T
$10,000–$15,000	L	MC	LC or MC	LC	T or LC	T
$15,000–$20,000	L	L	MC	LC or MC	LC	T or LC
$20,000–$30,000	L	L	MC or L	MC	LC or MC	LC
$30,000–$40,000	L	L	L	MC or L	MC or L	MC
$40,000 or more	L	L	L	L	L	MC or L

NOTE: T Thrifty LC Low Cost MC Moderate Cost L Liberal. *To use this table:* Locate the column that corresponds to the number of persons in the family. Then move down this column to the point opposite the family income before taxes are deducted. The plan shown there costs about the amount a typical household (of similar size and income) spends for food. It is the plan a family of that size and income can usually afford.

SOURCE: *Family Food Budgeting for Good Meals and Good Nutrition.* USDA, Home and Garden Bulletin, No. 94, Washington, D.C., 1979.

Nutrition labeling is based on the USRDAs (see Figures 12–3 and 12–4). Percentages are given to the nearest 2 percent in steps of 2,4, 6, up to 10; to the nearest 5 percent in steps of 5, 10, 15, up to 50 percent; and to the nearest 10 percent in steps of 60, 70, 80, above 50 percent. An asterisk (*) indicates that the food has less of the nutrient than 1 percent of the USRDA or none.

Nutrition labeling is voluntary except when a nutrient is added to a food as a fortification or to restore nutrients, or when a nutritional claim is made through advertising. Under such circumstances, labeling is mandatory. Nutrient quantities are expressed in terms of an average serving, which is defined as a reasonable quantity of food suited for consumption as part of a meal by an adult male engaged in light physical activity. For ingredients, the amount of a food customarily used in the preparation of a meal is called a portion.

Food manufacturers may slightly understate amounts of nutrients and overstate the number of calories in the food to be reasonably sure the labeling meets regulations, which require that the food provide at least the amounts of nutrients stated on the label and no additional calories. Values may be for the ready-to-eat form, although the only values required by law for most foods are for the food as it comes from the container.

Labeling can help consumers judge the cost of protein foods. Comparisons of protein content and determination of cost per gram of protein may show a "cheap" source of protein to be expensive. A serving of lean, boneless meat may have two times the amount of protein as a serving of franks or luncheon meat (22). Nutrition education is needed to interpret the data on package labels. If people can be educated to select a combination of labeled and fresh foods to provide at least 100 percent of the USRDA for the eight nutrients specified, they should have a high-quality diet. And if these nutrients are provided in sufficient amounts by ordinary foods, the other nutrients should also be supplied.

Using the USRDA as a guide for all ages and conditions of the life cycle requires interpretation or education. Table 12–10 suggests a way to use the US

TABLE 12-6. Estimated Cost of One Week's Food at Home, United States Average, March 1979

family or family member	thrifty plan	low-cost plan	moderate-cost plan	liberal plan
Family of two:*				
20–54 years	$27.80	$36.40	$45.60	$54.70
55 years and over	25.00	32.30	40.00	48.00
Family of four: Couple with				
Children, 1–2 and 3–5 years	39.20	50.70	63.30	75.80
Children, 6–8 and 9–11 years	47.20	61.10	76.70	91.80
Family members:†				
Child:				
7 months to 1 year	5.60	6.80	8.30	9.80
1–2 years	6.30	8.00	9.90	11.80
3–5 years	7.60	9.60	11.90	14.30
6–8 years	9.70	12.40	15.60	18.70
9–11 years	12.20	15.60	19.60	23.40
Male:				
12–14 years	13.00	16.50	20.80	24.90
15–19 years	14.30	18.40	23.10	27.70
20–54 years	13.90	18.30	23.10	27.80
55 years and over	12.40	16.10	20.00	24.10
Female:				
12–19 years	11.60	14.80	18.40	22.00
20–54 years	11.40	14.80	18.40	21.90
55 years and over	10.30	13.30	16.40	19.50
Pregnant	14.30	18.20	22.40	26.70
Nursing	15.20	19.30	24.10	28.60

NOTE: Costs are for quantities of food shown in Table 12–7. They assume that food for all meals and snacks is purchased at the store and prepared at home. Food selections within groups are based on selections made by families in a nationwide food consumption survey. Current costs are available on request from the Consumer and Food Economics Institute, Science and Education Administration, U.S. Department of Agriculture, Hyattsville, Md. 20782.

*10 percent added for family-size adjustment

†Costs given are for individuals in four-person families. For individuals in other-size families, adjust costs.

TABLE 12-7. Food Plans: Amounts of Food for a Week

family member	milk, cheese, ice cream*	meat, poultry, fish†	eggs	dry beans and peas, nuts**	dark-green, deep-yellow vege-tables	citrus fruit, tomatoes	potatoes	other vege-tables, fruit	cereal	flour	bread	other bakery products	fats, oils	sugar, sweets
						THRIFTY								
Child:	Qt	Lb	No.	Lb	Lb	Lb	Lb	Lb	Lb	Lb	Lb	Lb	Lb	Lb
7 months to 1 year	5.0	0.39	1.2	0.15	0.41	0.55	0.09	2.49	1.02††	0.02	0.08	0.04	0.04	0.19
1–2 years	3.3	0.83	3.3	0.17	0.22	0.89	0.65	2.26	1.02††	0.31	0.78	0.24	0.11	0.30
3–5 years	3.5	0.95	2.5	0.28	0.20	0.92	0.88	2.28	1.03	0.37	0.94	0.53	0.38	0.74
6–8 years	4.2	1.27	2.4	0.49	0.22	1.10	1.23	2.50	1.12	0.62	1.42	0.79	0.51	0.94
9–11 years	4.9	1.61	3.4	0.53	0.28	1.52	1.48	3.38	1.34	0.81	1.82	1.10	0.60	1.20
Male:														
12–14 years	5.2	1.79	3.6	0.67	0.33	1.45	1.59	3.30	1.22	0.81	2.07	1.13	0.77	1.21
15–19 years	5.1	2.35	4.0	0.43	0.32	1.70	2.10	3.43	0.98	0.99	2.36	1.46	1.00	1.05
20–54 years	2.6	3.03	4.0	0.44	0.39	1.80	2.02	3.69	0.89	0.92	2.29	1.33	0.95	0.86
55 years and over	2.4	2.45	4.0	0.25	0.51	1.85	1.75	3.77	1.09	0.80	1.90	1.12	0.79	0.94
Female:														
12–19 years	5.4	1.80	3.8	0.28	0.42	1.74	1.22	3.61	0.72	0.76	1.49	0.84	0.51	0.74
20–54 years	2.8	2.41	4.0	0.27	0.52	1.86	1.51	3.39	0.90	0.67	1.41	0.67	0.57	0.57
55 years and over	2.8	1.84	4.0	0.19	0.60	2.02	1.26	3.73	1.12	0.68	1.30	0.58	0.37	0.45
Pregnant	5.2§	2.69	4.0	0.42	0.56	2.17	1.89	4.03	1.13	0.58	1.41	0.66	0.59	0.58
Nursing	5.2§	3.00	4.0	0.38	0.57	2.36	1.92	4.27	0.98	0.63	1.56	0.82	0.80	0.75
						LOW-COST								
Child:	Qt	Lb	No.	Lb	Lb	Lb	Lb	Lb	Lb	Lb	Lb	Lb	Lb	Lb
7 months to 1 year	5.7	0.56	2.1	0.15	0.35	0.42	0.06	3.43	0.71††	0.02	0.06	0.05	0.05	0.18
1–2 years	3.6	1.26	3.6	0.16	0.23	1.01	0.60	2.88	0.99††	0.27	0.76	0.33	0.12	0.36
3–5 years	3.9	1.52	2.7	0.25	0.25	1.20	0.85	2.95	0.90	0.30	0.91	0.57	0.38	0.71
6–8 years	4.7	2.03	2.9	0.39	0.31	1.58	1.10	3.67	1.11	0.45	1.27	0.84	0.52	0.90
9–11 years	5.5	2.57	3.9	0.44	0.38	2.13	1.41	4.81	1.24	0.62	1.65	1.20	0.61	1.15
Male:														
12–14 years	5.7	2.98	4.0	0.56	0.40	1.99	1.50	3.90	1.15	0.67	1.88	1.25	0.77	1.15
15–19 years	5.5	3.74	4.0	0.34	0.39	2.20	1.87	4.50	0.90	0.75	2.10	1.55	1.05	1.04
20–54 years	2.7	4.56	4.0	0.33	0.48	2.32	1.87	4.81	0.93	0.71	2.10	1.47	0.91	0.81
55 years and over	2.6	3.63	4.0	0.21	0.61	2.38	1.72	4.92	1.02	0.62	1.73	1.23	0.77	0.90

TABLE 12-7. (Continued)

family member	milk, cheese, ice cream*	meat, poultry, fish†	eggs	dry beans and peas, nuts**	dark-green, deep-yellow vegetables	citrus fruit, tomatoes	potatoes	other vegetables, fruit	cereal	flour	bread	other bakery products	fats, oils	sugar, sweets
Female:														
12–19 years	5.6	2.55	4.0	0.24	0.46	2.17	1.17	4.57	0.75	0.63	1.44	1.05	0.53	0.88
20–54 years	3.0	3.21	4.0	0.19	0.55	2.34	1.40	4.17	0.71	0.55	1.31	0.94	0.59	0.72
55 years and over	2.0	2.45	4.0	0.15	0.62	2.54	1.22	4.57	0.97	0.58	1.24	0.86	0.38	0.64
Pregnant	5.2§	3.68	4.0	0.29	0.67	2.80	1.65	4.99	0.95	0.66	1.52	1.06	0.55	0.78
Nursing	5.2§	4.16	4.0	0.26	0.66	2.99	1.67	5.33	0.78	0.61	1.55	1.16	0.76	0.91
MODERATE-COST														
Child:	Qt	Lb	No.	Lb	Lb	Lb	Lb	Lb	Lb	Lb	Lb	Lb	Lb	Lb
7 months to 1 year	6.5	0.80	2.2	0.13	0.41	0.49	0.06	3.98	0.64††	0.02	0.06	0.05	0.05	0.19
1–2 years	4.0	1.69	4.0	0.15	0.29	1.24	0.59	3.44	1.03††	0.26	0.81	0.33	0.12	0.28
3–5 years	4.7	1.88	3.0	0.22	0.30	1.46	0.85	3.51	0.74	0.27	0.82	0.73	0.41	0.81
6–8 years	5.8	2.60	3.3	0.34	0.37	1.94	1.17	4.39	0.84	0.39	1.14	1.11	0.56	1.03
9–11 years	6.7	3.31	4.0	0.38	0.45	2.61	1.40	5.76	1.03	0.51	1.47	1.51	0.66	1.31
Male:														
12–14 years	7.0	3.77	4.0	0.48	0.48	2.44	1.52	4.66	0.94	0.56	1.69	1.54	0.85	1.34
15–19 years	6.6	4.65	4.0	0.29	0.47	2.73	2.00	5.45	0.80	0.67	1.98	1.82	1.05	1.15
20–54 years	3.4	5.73	4.0	0.29	0.59	2.92	1.94	5.93	0.76	0.65	1.97	1.65	0.95	0.96
55 years and over	3.0	4.64	4.0	0.19	0.70	2.91	1.69	5.88	0.89	0.53	1.58	1.45	0.87	1.05
Female:														
12–19 years	6.2	3.32	4.0	0.24	0.53	2.62	1.21	5.38	0.68	0.56	1.34	1.22	0.56	0.97
20–54 years	3.4	4.12	4.0	0.19	0.62	2.84	1.35	4.94	0.54	0.49	1.28	1.08	0.65	0.81
55 years and over	3.4	3.21	4.0	0.14	0.72	3.09	1.17	5.50	0.81	0.52	1.20	0.98	0.45	0.73
Pregnant	5.4§	4.57	4.0	0.25	0.91	3.52	1.60	6.13	0.73	0.83	1.77	1.28	0.46	0.85
Nursing	5.3§	5.01	4.0	0.26	0.91	3.76	1.73	6.52	0.74	0.81	1.84	1.42	0.69	1.00

TABLE 12–7. (Continued)

family member	milk, cheese, ice cream*	meat, poultry, fish†	eggs	dry beans and peas, nuts**	dark-green, deep-yellow vegetables	citrus fruit, tomatoes	potatoes	other vegetables, fruit	cereal	flour	bread	other bakery products	fats, oils	sugar, sweets
						LIBERAL								
Child:	Qt	Lb	No.	Lb	Lb	Lb	Lb	Lb	Lb	Lb	Lb	Lb	Lb	Lb
7 months to 1 year	6.9	0.97	2.3	0.14	0.43	0.60	0.06	4.71	0.64††	0.02	0.05	0.06	0.05	0.20
1–2 years	4.3	2.07	4.0	0.17	0.31	1.50	0.59	4.10	1.07††	0.28	0.82	0.35	0.13	0.27
3–5 years	5.1	2.35	3.1	0.23	0.32	1.77	0.85	4.18	0.76	0.27	0.79	0.78	0.45	0.85
6–8 years	6.2	3.18	3.4	0.36	0.40	2.35	1.18	5.21	0.85	0.39	1.08	1.23	0.60	1.08
9–11 years	7.2	4.04	4.0	0.39	0.48	3.15	1.41	6.83	1.04	0.51	1.39	1.67	0.71	1.38
Male:														
12–14 years	7.6	4.57	4.0	0.50	0.51	2.94	1.52	5.52	0.95	0.56	1.60	1.71	0.92	1.40
15–19 years	7.2	5.59	4.0	0.31	0.50	3.29	2.01	6.45	0.84	0.69	1.92	2.05	1.07	1.20
20–54 years	3.6	6.83	4.0	0.32	0.62	3.51	1.95	6.99	0.79	0.66	1.91	1.86	0.95	1.00
55 years and over	3.2	5.54	4.0	0.19	0.76	3.52	1.68	6.97	0.89	0.54	1.49	1.57	0.94	1.09
Female:														
12–19 years	6.7	3.97	4.0	0.25	0.56	3.15	1.21	6.34	0.71	0.59	1.31	1.35	0.54	0.98
20–54 years	3.6	4.86	4.0	0.20	0.66	3.41	1.35	5.81	0.56	0.51	1.24	1.22	0.66	0.84
55 years and over	3.6	3.79	4.0	0.15	0.76	3.71	1.14	6.42	0.74	0.54	1.17	1.12	0.48	0.77
Pregnant	5.9§	5.43	4.0	0.26	0.96	4.22	1.57	7.17	0.70	0.87	1.70	1.45	0.46	9.87
Nursing	5.8§	5.97	4.0	0.28	0.97	4.51	1.72	7.66	0.75	0.84	1.76	1.58	0.68	1.02

NOTE: Amounts are for food as purchased or brought into the kitchen from garden or farm. Amounts allow for a discard of about one-fourth of the *edible* food as plate waste, spoilage, etc. For general use, round the total amount of food groups for the family to the nearest tenth or quarter of a pound. In addition to groups shown, most families use some other foods: coffee, tea, cocoa, soft drinks, punches, ades, leavening agents, and seasonings.

*Fluid milk and beverage made from dry or evaporated milk. Cheese and ice cream may replace some milk. Count as equivalent to a quart of fluid milk: natural or processed Cheddar-type cheese, 6 ounces; cottage cheese, 2 1/2 pounds; ice cream or ice milk, 1 1/2 quarts; unflavored yogurt, 4 cups.

† Bacon and salt pork should not exceed 1/3 pound for each 5 pounds of this group.

**Weight in terms of dry beans and peas, shelled nuts, and peanut butter. Count 1 pound of canned dry beans, such as pork and beans or kidney beans, as 0.33 pound.

†† Cereal fortified with iron is recommended.

§ For pregnant and nursing teenagers, 7 quarts is recommended.

TABLE 12-8. Food Plans at Four Costs: Food to Serve Each Day

food plan and family member	milk* (cup)	cooked lean meat or alternate† (ounce)	vegetables and fruit (½ cup)**	cereal and bakery products (portion)††
THRIFTY PLAN				
Child:				
1–5 years	2	1½ to 2	2	3 or more
6–11 years	2 to 3	2½ to 3	2½ to 3½	6 or more
Male:				
12–19 years	3	3 to 4	3 to 4	7 or more
20–54 years	1½	4 to 5	3 to 4	7 or more
55 years and over	1½	4	3 to 4	7 or more
Female:				
12–19 years	3	3	3 to 4	5 or more
20–54 years	1½	4	3 to 4	5 or more
55 years and over	1½	3	3 to 4	5 or more
LOW-COST PLAN				
Child:				
1–5 years	2 to 3	2 to 3	2 to 3	3 or more
6–11 years	2 to 3	3 to 4	3 to 4	5 or more
Male:				
12–19 years	3 to 4	5 to 6	4 to 5	6 or more
20–54 years	1½ to 2	6 to 7	4 to 5	6 or more
55 years and over	1½ to 2	5	4 to 5	6 or more
Female:				
12–19 years	3 to 4	4	4	5 or more
20–54 years	1½ to 2	4 to 5	4	5 or more
55 years and over	1½ to 2	3 to 4	4	5 or more
MODERATE-COST PLAN				
Child:				
1–5 years	2 to 3	2½ to 3	2 to 3	3 or more
6–11 years	3 to 4	4 to 5	4 to 5	4 or more
Male:				
12–19 years	4	5 to 7	4½ to 5½	6 or more
20–54 years	2	7 to 8	5 to 6	6 or more
55 years and over	2	6 to 7	5 to 6	5 or more
Female:				
12–19 years	3½ to 4	4 to 5	4 to 5	4 or more
20–54 years	2	5 to 6	4 to 5	4 or more
55 years and over	2	4 to 5	5	4 or more

TABLE 12-8. Continued

LIBERAL PLAN				
Child:				
1–5 years	2½ to 3	3 to 3½	3 to 4	3 or more
6–11 years	3½ to 4½	5 to 6	5 to 6	4 or more
Male:				
12–19 years	4 to 4½	6 to 8	5 to 6	5 or more
20–54 years	2	9	6 to 7	5 or more
55 years and over	2	7 to 8	6 to 7	5 or more
Female:				
12–19 years	4	5 to 6	5 to 6	4 or more
20–54 years	2	6 to 7	5 to 6	4 or more
55 years and over	2	5 to 6	5 to 6	4 or more

*As alternates: ¾ ounce of hard cheese or ¾ cup of cottage cheese, ice cream, or ice milk or ½ cup of unflavored yogurt may replace ½ cup of fluid milk.

†As alternates: 1 ounce of cooked poultry or fish, one egg, ½ cup of cooked dry beans or peas, or 2 tablespoons of peanut butter may replace 1 ounce of cooked lean meat.

**One-half cup of vegetable or fruit or a portion—one medium apple, banana, or half a medium grapefruit or cantaloupe. Smaller portions may be served, especially to young children.

††A portion is two slices of bread, one hamburger bun, one large muffin or cupcake, 1 ounce ready-to-eat cereal, or ¾ cup cooked cereal, such as oatmeal, rice, spaghetti, macaroni, or noodles. Smaller servings may be given, especially to young children, girls, and women; but the total daily amounts on the average should add up to portions listed.

RDA for various ages. Special consideration should be given to adolescents and pregnant or lactating women in relation to calcium. The figures are useful for consumers to compare the nutritive value of foods. Labeling provides information about the nutritive value of many foods previously given little attention. Nutrition labeling is useful for the many foods on the market that are difficult to classify using a four-food group system.

ANIMAL FEEDING DEMONSTRATIONS. Well-designed and carefully conducted animal feeding demonstrations using white rats or other small laboratory animals can be an effective device for stimulating awareness of food in relation to growth and health. The effects of dietary intake can be seen quickly in a weanling animal that requires specific nutrients for growth. Using foods eaten by people and charting the growth of an animal can make an immediate impact.

Careful plans must be made for a feeding demonstration. Cages for the animals must be large enough, feeding procedures and sanitation must be planned, the diet should be dried to prevent spoilage, and the objectives must

TABLE 12–9. United States Recommended Daily Allowance

nutrient	amount
MANDATORY	
Protein	65 g
Vitamin A	5000 IU
Vitamin C	60 mg
Thiamin	1.5 mg
Riboflavin	1.7 mg
Niacin	20 mg
Calcium	1.0 mg
Iron	18 mg
OPTIONAL	
Vitamin D	400 IU
Vitamin E	30 IU
Vitamin B_6	2.0 mg
Folic acid	2.0 mg
Vitamin B_{12}	6 μg
Phosphorus	1.0 g
Iodine	150 μg
Magnesium	400 mg
Zinc	15 mg
Copper	2 mg
Biotin	0.3 mg
Pantothenic acid	10 mg

SOURCE: B. Peterkin, J. Nichols, and C. Cromwell, *Nutrition Labeling, Tools for Its Use.* U.S. Department of Agriculture, Agriculture Information Bulletin No. 382, Washington, D.C., 1975.

be understood. Only some animal experiments relate to humans. Observations and measurements of nutritional status must be established. Table 12–11 shows some characteristics of rats. Young people must understand that weight gain is an excellent measure of nutritional status during growth, but may not be desirable in adults. The National Dairy Council suggests the following comparison between rat and human ages:

Human age (years)   2½ 3 3½ 4 4½ 5 5½ 6 6½ 7

ages of humans compared with ages of rats

Rat age (weeks)   1 4 5 6 7 8 9 10 11 12 13

Albino rats are clean and safe, require small amounts of food, little space, and grow rapidly. Rats eat about the same food as humans. A large body of research

US. Recommended Daily Allowances

The U.S. Recommended Daily Allowances (U.S. RDA's) are the amounts of protein, vitamins, and minerals used as standards in nutrition labeling.

These allowances were derived from the Recommended Dietary Allowances (RDA's) set by the Food and Nutrition Board of the National Research Council. The RDA's are judged by the National Research Council to be adequate for nearly all healthy persons and generous for most persons.

The U.S. RDA for most nutrients is the highest RDA of all sex-age categories. Therefore, a diet that furnishes the U.S. RDA for a nutrient will furnish the RDA for most people and more than the RDA for many.

Special U.S. RDA's for infants and young children may be used for baby and junior-type food.

Percentage

The amounts of protein, vitamins, and minerals in a serving are shown on the nutrition information panel as percentages of the U.S. Recommended Dietary Allowances (U.S. RDA's).

Percentages of the U.S. RDA are given in increments of 2 percent (2, 4, 6, etc.) up to 10 percent; of 5 percent (10, 15, 20, etc.) up to 50 percent; and of 10 percent (50, 60, 70, etc.) above 50 percent.

Vitamin A

Vitamin A is needed for normal growth and for normal vision in dim light. It also helps maintain the skin and the inner linings of the body. Some foods you can get it from are liver, eggs, butter, margarine, whole milk, and some kinds of cheese. You get carotene, which the body can change to vitamin A, from some vegetables and fruits, particularly dark-green and deep-yellow vegetables and some deep-yellow fruits.

NUTRITION INFORMATION

(PER SERVING)

SERVING SIZE=1 CUP*

SERVINGS PER CONTAINER=24

	FLAKES	FLAKES+BUTTER, MILK, WATER, SALT*
CALORIES	140	280
PROTEIN, GRAMS	4	6
CARBOHYDRATE, GRAMS	30	32
FAT, GRAMS	0	14
PERCENTAGE OF U.S. RECOMMENDED DAILY ALLOWANCES (U.S. RDA)		
PROTEIN	4	8
VITAMIN A	2	10
VITAMIN C	80	80
THIAMIN	10	15
RIBOFLAVIN	2	8
NIACIN	10	10
CALCIUM	2	4
IRON	4	4

*PREPARED ACCORDING TO RECIPE ON BACK OF PACKAGE.

Vitamin C

Vitamin C, or ascorbic acid, helps to keep blood vessels strong and to develop connective tissues. It has a number of other roles, from tooth and bone formation to wound healing. You can get the amount of vitamin C you need in a day from a serving of a rich food source such as citrus fruit or juice, or strawberries. Other important sources include melons, tomatoes, cabbage, certain dark-green leafy vegetables, and potatoes and sweetpotatoes, especially when cooked in the jacket.

Calcium

Calcium is the most abundant mineral element in the body. Teamed up with phosphorus, it is largely responsible for the hardness of bones and teeth. Milk is an outstanding source of calcium. Cheese, ice cream, and certain dark-green leafy vegetables also contribute valuable amounts of calcium to the diet.

Iron

The body requires iron for making hemoglobin, the red part of blood that carries oxygen to the cells and carbon dioxide away from them. Iron also helps the cells get energy from food. Only a few foods are good sources of iron: lean meats, liver, and other organ meats, shellfish, dry beans and peas, dark-green vegetables, dried fruit, egg yolk, and molasses are some of them. Whole-grain and enriched breads and cereals contain small amounts, but are important sources when eaten frequently.

Thiamin, riboflavin, niacin

These B vitamins play a central role in the release of energy from food. They also help with proper functioning of nerves, normal appetite, good digestion, and healthy skin. Generally, foods in the meat group are leading sources of these vitamins. Whole-grain and enriched breads and cereals supply smaller, but important, amounts. A few foods are outstanding sources—milk for riboflavin, lean pork for thiamin, and organ meats for all three.

FIG. 12–3. Source: B. Peterkin, J. Nichols, and C. Cromwell, "Nutrition Labeling, Tools for Its use," Agriculture Information Bulletin No. 382, Washington, D.C.: U.S. Department of Agriculture, 1975.

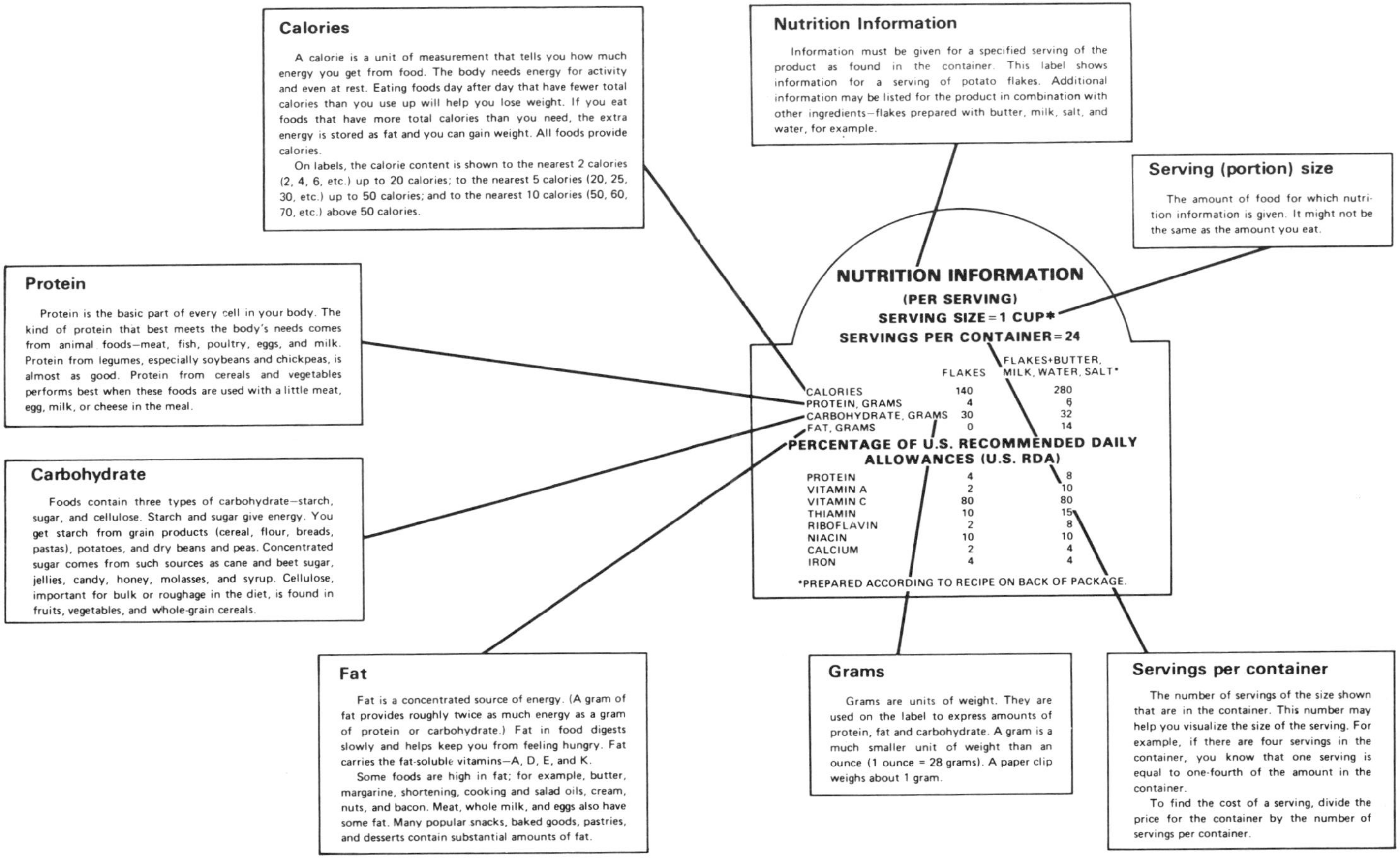

FIG. 12–4. Source: B. Peterkin, J. Nichols, and C. Cromwell, "Nutrition Labeling, Tools for Its Use," Agriculture Information Bulletin No. 382, Washington, D.C.: U.S. Department of Agriculture, 1975.

TABLE 12–10. Allowances for Food Energy and Percentages of the U.S. Recommended Daily Allowances Needed to Meet the Recommended Dietary Allowances for Children, Men, and Women of Different Ages

age (yr)	food energy* (calorie)	protein† (%)	vitamin A (%)	vitamin C (%)	thiamin (%)	riboflavin (%)	niacin** (%)	calcium (%)	iron (%)
Child									
1–3	1300	35%	40%	70%	50%	50%	30%	80%	85%
4–6	1800	50	50	70	60	65	35	80	60
7–10	2400	55	70	70	80	75	50	80	60
Male									
11–14	2800	70	100	75	95	90	55	120	100
15–18	3000	85	100	75	100	110	55	120	100
19–22	3000	85	100	75	100	110	60	80	60
23–50	2700	90	100	75	95	95	45	80	60
51 +	2400	90	100	75	80	90	35	80	60
Female									
11–14	2400	70	80	75	80	80	45	120	100
15–18	2100	75	80	75	75	85	30	120	100
19–22	2100	75	80	75	75	85	35	80	100
23–50	2000	75	80	75	70	75	30	80	100
51 +	1800	75	80	75	70	65	25	80	60
Pregnant	+300††	+50††	100	100	+20††	+20††	35	120	100+
Nursing	+500††	+35††	120	135	+20††	+30††	35	120	100

*Calorie needs differ depending on body composition and size, age, and activity of the person.

†U.S. RDA of 65 grams is used for this table. In labeling, a U.S. RDA of 45 grams is used for foods providing high-quality protein, such as milk, meat, and eggs.

**The percentage of the U.S. RDA shown for niacin will provide the RDA for niacin if the RDA for protein is met. Some niacin is derived in the body from tryptophan, an amino acid present in protein.

††To be added to the percentage for the girl or woman of the appropriate age.

SOURCE: U.S. Recommended Daily Allowance, "Food Labeling," *Federal Register*, 33 (March 14, 1973): part II. *Recommended Dietary Allowances*. 8th ed. 1974, National Academy of Sciences, National Research Council.

TABLE 12–11. Characteristics of Albino Rats

well-nourished	poorly nourished
Fur—Clean, smooth, glossy	Shaggy, dull and possibly thin
Tail—Smooth, no roughness	Rough, dry, scaly
Ears—Pinkish	Scaly, dry, rough
Feet—Smooth, pinkish	Rough, dry, scaly
Eyes—Bright pink, clear	Not clear, dull
Whiskers—Long, sharp	Short, possibly dirty
Nails—Firm	Possibly soft
Behavior—Easily handled, good natured, quick, alert movements, good muscle tone	Restless, irritable, cross
Health—Good	Breathing difficulty

information is available on the physiological and nutritional needs of rats. Eppright and others describe demonstrations for classroom use (23). For some demonstrations, chicks can be used instead of rats. Information is readily available on avian nutritional needs and chick feed can be purchased from poultry supply sources.

life cycle emphasis

Long-term changes in dietary intake can reduce risks for some chronic diseases in the United States. The most pressing need is to promote increased consumption of fruits, vegetables, and whole grains. There is a need to eat only enough calories to maintain body weight at desirable levels. This requires reduced intake of fats, sugar, and alcoholic beverages for many people. For some with family tendencies toward certain chronic diseases, reduced intakes of salt, cholesterol, and saturated fats are indicated. Guidance in making wise choices for the individual is important. Careful segmentation of the target group is also important in designing education programs.

Effective nutrition education uses a variety of sites for learning and transmitting information—not only schools, clinics, hospitals, and clubs, but also stores, streets, and the mass media. Long-term programs covering months and years are more effective than short-term approaches. Information should be consistent but not dogmatic. Family, friends and associates, or peers who influence the target population must be educated as well. Each generation must be taught to use the existing food supply intelligently (24).

PREGNANCY. In the United States, most prenatal nutrition education is focused on low-income clients enrolled in public health programs. Obstetricians and professional organizations have emphasized nutrition as a necessary component of maternity care. Nutrition education in parenting education programs varies in content and intensity.

One of the more effective federal programs is the Women's, Infant's and Children's program (WIC). Vouchers for specific foods and nutrition education are provided. Evaluations demonstrate improved nutrition knowledge, reduced incidence of anemia, and weight normalization in underweight infants and children.

Discussions should include physiological changes in pregnancy, desirable weight gain (22 to 27 lb), the extra nutritional needs of the mother and fetus, and how to obtain the correct nutrients in the correct amounts. Special problems related to drugs, alcohol, and weight control must be emphasized. A counseling format has been used effectively.

LACTATION. Nursing mothers need information on the process of lactation and the benefits and problems of breast feeding. The effect of the mother's diet and activities on the quantity and quality of the milk supply needs emphasis. Nutritional status during pregnancy, life style, and other factors will affect the kinds and amounts of food needed for successful breast feeding.

INFANCY. Information should emphasize the health advantages of breast feeding but introduce bottle feeding as an alternative when indicated or preferred. Education for this group must focus on the parents or caregivers. With more children being cared for outside the home, broader nutrition education is necessary. Information available to child care workers should be evaluated carefully for validity. Parents serve as role models, structure the environment of children, and mediate what children learn at home and elsewhere. Parents and caregivers need assistance in providing a comfortable environment conducive to adequate food intake for infants.

CHILDHOOD. Nursery schools and child care centers provide excellent opportunities for nutrition education. Nutrition has been incorporated effectively into the federal Head Start program. The educational process is accomplished through the development of good habits and exposure of children to a wide variety of foods. The preschool child has the ability to comprehend that food is good, and that there are many good foods in a variety of shapes, colors, textures, and tastes. Many activities can be planned using food.

School-age children can classify food into groups. Younger children are not ready to understand the concept of nutrients. In the upper elementary grades nutrients can be introduced on a limited basis. Several curriculum guides have been developed for nutrition education in the classroom. In grade school, children begin to develop eating habits that differ from family patterns. Many older children prepare some meals for themselves and other family members.

Nutrition education for school-age children has become more systematic and comprehensive. Emphasis should be placed on the changing nature of the food supply and individualization of curriculums. The most effective programs involve a comprehensive plan implemented in a stepwise fashion and related to the developmental levels of the children. Such a plan must support and interact with the overall educational goals. The integration of nutrition education with school feeding programs is vital to effective teaching. Under these circumstances, the school lunch and breakfast become a learning laboratory. The relationship and attitude between teachers and food service personnel is an important factor. Positive interaction of food service personnel with children improves acceptance of food.

In October 1977, Congress passed legislation funding nutrition education as a part of the National School Lunch Act. Funds were made available to each state for a nutrition education coordinator, a needs assessment, and for implementing a state plan for nutrition education. Because these programs are state based, the needs and activities have varied among the states.

ADOLESCENCE. Motivating adolescents must take into consideration the fact that at this age individuals are very absorbed with self. For the adolescent, the benefits of nutrition must be tangible and as immediate as possible. Information needs to be directed to such benefits as changes in appearance, effects on skin or body weight; and improved athletic performance. Long-term plans for a healthy adult life, children, or reduced rate of degeneration in aging are unacceptable goals.

The interest in self, growth, development, and the functioning of the body can be used by nutrition educators. Nutrition as a part of the process of maturation is relevant, vital and urgent to young people. Food is a part of the social process for teenagers. Eating together for snacks and meals has an influence on the foods selected. Many young people work and go to school, thus altering their childhood meal patterns.

ADULTHOOD. During the adult period, life styles vary and may change markedly from those of earlier years. Soon after the completion of formal education, many adults become uninterested in taking classes; thus, informal methods or mass media may be useful. Adult participation is almost always voluntary, and motivation is necessary. Currently, the interest in the health benefits of good nutrition may be useful. Planning with adults rather than for them may improve motivation. Adults should be encouraged to diagnose their own needs. Assumptions about prior knowledge and experience is difficult with adults, and educational backgrounds vary widely.

The many responsibilities of the adult for work, career advancement, social life, and family result in numerous tensions. Effective nutrition education must provide a substantial reward for a limited expenditure of energy. Some companies provide health seminars that include nutrition for employees.

OLD AGE. For the elderly with a lifetime of food preferences, good nutrition is dependent upon conditions from earlier years. Individuality is important in developing plans. Some foods have deep significance or emotional meaning (6). Elderly people may have desires for specific foods prepared and served in certain ways.

Preferences for such foods should be determined and incorporated into individual dietary plans whenever possible. Limiting a popular food in the diet of an elderly person requires a good physiological reason.

Good nutrition is important in keeping the elderly happier, more fit, and more independent (25). For the elderly, nutrition education may be new, since it was not a part of their training in youth. The first vitamin was discovered in 1912, so nutrition is younger than some of our elderly. Many elderly need the same basic information provided for children. Small-scale recipes to prepare nutritious foods for one or two are useful. Teaching selection of food for simple preparation techniques may improve acceptance. An emergency store of food that has a long shelf life is a good idea for bad weather, illness, or other times when the person is homebound. Some elderly need assistance in storing food without refrigeration. Nutrition education for this group involves motivation to consider one's nutritional needs seriously, management of the costs and waste in cooking for one, substituting acceptable foods on a restricted diet, or strategies for coping with increased food prices on a static income (26). Group feeding programs are another possibility: they expose the elderly to a variety of healthy foods in pleasant circumstances.

Nutrition educators must be sensitive to the needs of the elderly. The process of education is general for the entire adult life span; however, certain factors should be taken into consideration when working with elderly adults. The process of education for the elderly must be approached in a manner that maintains self-esteem. The ability to learn remains intact throughout the life cycle, although the ability to respond rapidly may decrease. Timed materials requiring a rapid response may not be effective with older adults. Those who are old now learned with printed material and the spoken word, rather than television and movies. Utilize patterns of teaching that the elderly will accept. Changes in visual acuity or hearing ability may reduce the response of older adults. It is important to use microphones, large print, and large writing. It is also wise to investigate the psychological factors and situations that are most conducive to learning, as well as the background knowledge of the group so that the information presented will be meaningful in view of previous experiences.

Future Work

Research into nutrition education raises many questions. Knowledge of the factors motivating changes in behavior is important. A national nutrition education program is needed, but it should be a broad-based effort distinct from food assistance programs. The greatest research need is in evaluation methods for nutrition education. Evaluation is in a developing stage, and the outcomes of nutrition education are complex and often separated by many years from the teaching-learning environment. There is a lack of consensus on desirable outcomes. Evaluation criteria are different for knowledge, behavioral, and physiological outcomes.

Goals and priorities for human nutrition education research must be mutually agreeable to consumers, educators, legislators, and food suppliers (27). The federal government is the largest supporter of nutrition education and intervention programs. Many programs are directed toward the lower socioeconomic groups. One important aspect that is needed in federal programs relates to research on behavior and nutrition. From a theoretical framework of nutritional behavior, methods for studying nutritional behavior must be developed. In the future we must identify the factors that affect lifetime eating habits and determine when education is most effective. Simplified tools for providing consumer information are also needed.

The nutrition programs of the future should meet specific needs at various stages of the life cycle, rather than be geared to eliminating agricultural surpluses. In addition, the guidelines should be based on nutrition surveillance of the population so that program changes can be made as needed, and the programs' effectiveness measured and evaluated to be sure the proper goals are reached.

Summary

The object of nutrition education is to change the behavior of the learners so that they improve their nutritional status. The food we eat is determined by the available supply, the culture, how much time we have, and our value system. Programs of nutrition education must take all these factors into account, along with stages of the life cycle, educational level, and income. Some other considerations are the effects of faddism, the fact that humans do not "instinctively" eat the right foods, and changing life styles in the United States.

Nutrition education began nearly a hundred years ago with a focus on low-income groups and special diets for those suffering from disease. Today, with TV and mass marketing techniques, plus increased popular interest, nutrition education and behavior change are more complex processes.

Approaches to education programs therefore vary, although most make use of basic concepts and curriculum guidelines developed over the past two decades by government and private agencies working together. Successful programs make use of multidisciplinary and multimedia techniques. Specific objectives are often written in behavioral terms. Some standard tools are food groupings, the index of nutritional quality system, nutrition labeling, and the US Recommended Daily Allowances. Animal feeding demonstrations are another.

Most programs have a life cycle emphasis and are designed for specific target groups—pregnant or nursing women, mothers of infants and young children, school-age children, adolescents, adults, older people. They are implemented in government facilities, in schools, and in community centers, for the aim is to bring as much nutrition information as possible to as wide a range of the population as possible.

TABLE 12-12. National Conference on Nutrition Education, Directions for the 80's

specific recommendations

THE GENERAL PUBLIC

The recommendations of the Task Force on the General Public are as follows:

1. New goals for nutrition education of the general public are needed.
   a. Federally funded nutrition education programs aimed at the general public should concentrate on informing the public about the dietary guidelines and the relationship between diet, exercise, and health and on motivating the public to adapt their diets to these guidelines.
   b. Priority in federal funding for nutrition education aimed at the general public should be given to programs which will concentrate on the dietary guidelines.
   c. The federal government should develop food labels which permit the selection of foods in conformity with sound dietary recommendations, including the dietary guidelines.
   d. Food production, marketing, and distribution should reflect the guidelines to ensure that the entire population has access to such foods.
2. A national strategy to implement these goals is required.
   a. The present federal Interagency Nutrition Coordination Committee should establish a subcommittee devoted exclusively to nutrition education. Areas the subcommittee might address include establishing a nutrition education policy, including concentration on the dietary guidelines; providing a forum in which representatives of various sectors could present their views about nutrition education policy; establishing a clearinghouse of current government and private programs and resources in nutrition education; creating a resource bank of people involved in nutrition education; and providing public access to accurate and timely nutrition information.
   b. In addition, existing federal, state, local, and private-sector resources should be expanded, integrated, and coordinated to support the implementation of nutrition education programs.
3. More careful targeting of messages to specific groups within the general public is needed.
   a. Funds for research should be provided for investigations to gather pertinent information from specific segments of the general public. This research should focus on the food habits, beliefs, related behaviors, and other issues associated with designing programs to promote the dietary guidelines.
   b. Funds for research should not be limited to universities and other conventional sources of nutrition education studies. The private sector, especially marketing, has developed sophisticated tools for understanding consumer groups. Nutrition education should take advantage of these resources.
4. More effective methods for bringing about behavior change must be employed.
   a. The time and space available for delivering nutrition information through the mass media should be expanded. It should be proportional, though not necessarily equal to, the amount and frequency of food advertisements during each part of the day.
   b. A media campaign should be undertaken to inform the public of the surgeon general's dietary recommendations including information on how to implement the recommendations through food selection and preparation.
5. Nutrition education efforts need more careful evaluation.
   a. Evaluation expectations should be brought into line with the limitations of evaluation techniques.
   b. Federal funding agencies should consider seriously whether grant application requirements which call for overly elaborate and ambitious evaluation plans for nutrition education programs are necessary.
   c. Additional funds should be invested in development of evaluation designs which are practical and low cost so that state and local agencies, together with federal agencies, will build up a body of comparable data about program effectiveness.

TABLE 12–12. Continued

PREGNANT WOMEN, CHILDREN, AND ADOLESCENTS

The recommendations of the Task Force on Pregnant Women, Children, and Adolescents are as follows:

1. Nutrition education needs a new goal orientation, both for the message and its delivery.
   a. Nutritionists and others responsible for nutrition education must reach consensus on the basic messages which are relevant to each of these target groups and acknowledge those areas in which controversy exists so that consensus is not yet possible. Scientific groups such as the Food and Nutrition Board, National Academy of Sciences, should take the leadership in defining valid messages.
   b. The messages in nutrition education should recognize nutrition's role in total health and lifestyle and the individual's responsibility for promotion and maintenance of health.
   c. The promotion of attitudinal and behavioral change when it is necessary and reinforcement of sound existing practices must be stressed. This implies a focus upon consumer needs and wants for nutrition education.
   d. Nutrition educators should use findings derived from market research studies and apply social marketing techniques to promote attitudinal and behavioral change.
   e. A federally supported National Nutrition Education Council of diverse membership should be established for a three-year period and be capable of receiving contributions from the private sector. Its functions will be to provide leadership, serve as an advocate for nutrition education, advise federal programs, provide a forum for exchange of information, establish policy, facilitate coordination of nutrition education, provide follow-up for the National Conference on Nutrition Education, and monitor progress in implementing recommendations.
2. Nutrition messages must be matched with the desires and special developmental characteristics of the target groups as well as with their cultural, social, and economic orientations and needs.
   a. Appropriate nutrition messages should be developed for all groups of the population—all income groups, sexes, ethnic groups, sociocultural patterns and lifestyles.
   b. The specific nutrition messages should recognize existing social support systems (such as the family) and interactions which occur relative to nutrition.
3. Nutrition education curricula for preschools through secondary schools must be evaluated and, if necessary, designed and refocused to the target group's level of understanding.
   a. Criteria for assessing the scientific content and message of food and nutrition curricula and training guides must be established, periodically reviewed, and disseminated by appropriate professional groups. These will furnish the basis for evaluation of the content of nutrition education and training.
   b. A federal focus for evaluating nutrition education materials and curricula and for sharing the results with state and local groups is needed.
   c. A common core of objectives should be addressed in addition to program-specific activities. For each specific program, behavioral objectives and performance standards must be established under the direction of competent nutritionists and those in other appropriate disciplines.
   d. Desirable characterisitcs of nutrition programs, which should be included in model or demonstration projects and in planning and evaluating other projects, include these:
      - Logical progression of subject matter and learning experiences in the overall sequence and structure of the program
      - Acknowledgement of individuality and differences in learning styles and physiological needs
      - Emphasis on the importance of individual responsibility for self care via nutrition in both achieving optimal health and preventing disease
      - Provision of practical information which is useful to individuals as they evaluate information about diet in making their own decisions about what they will eat

TABLE 12–12. Continued

PREGNANT WOMEN, CHILDREN, AND ADOLESCENTS (CONTINUED)

- Self-involvement in learning
- Enhancement of development of sensory, motor, and psychosocial skills
- Consideration of different cultural or ethnic orientations and lifestyles and situations involving specific dietary prescriptions and restrictions
- Relationship to other curricula and the aims of general education in a meaningful way
- Inclusion of nonformal learning environments outside of the school as well as formal environments within it
- Explorations of associations between food and energy from the context of the world food supply and ecology as well as in relationship to personal diets
- Utilization of resources from the wide variety of public and private agencies presently involved in nutrition education
- Support of the family as the basic institution of society.

e. Funding and support must be provided for the development, testing, and dissemination of materials for programs which are designed taking the above objectives into account. Support is also necessary for adequate training of those who will use the materials.

4. The nutrition educator's role must be recognized, and all providers of nutrition and food education must be well trained.

a. Professional health and education organizations should identify and publicize nutrition education competencies which professionals and paraprofessionals are expected to demonstrate. These competencies should be used as a basis for curriculum development and institutional program review.

b. Certification requirements must be established for nutrition education and/or training specialists as well as supervisory specialists.

c. Grants to develop multiple centers of academic excellence in both research and training in nutrition education should be provided.

d. These professionals and paraprofessionals who function incidentally as nutrition educators must be trained more systematically so that they will recognize and clarify their activities in this area and assume greater responsibility for them.

e. Nutrition education should be a requisite for teacher certification or recertification in some if not all specialty areas.

f. All professionals and paraprofessionals involved in nutrition education should have access to in-service and continuing education. In part, this can be accomplished by encouraging voluntary and professional associations to develop and promote continuing education programs in nutrition education using nutrition experts as teachers.

g. More emphasis needs to be paid in training nutrition educators on processes other than solely the distribution of informational materials for helping people to make informed decisions about choices of food.

5. Ways to reach out and provide nutrition education in different settings should be explored.

a. More innovative use must be made of informal and nonformal settings such as waiting rooms in health care facilities, correctional institutions, recreational centers and libraries, food markets, laundromats, and beauty salons to reach children and parents with nutrition education.

b. The workplace also offers great potential for nutrition education of parents which is sponsored by labor and management organizations.

c. The Department of Health, Education, and Welfare (DHEW) should assure that standards and criteria for health care programs include specific requirements for nutrition services, including nutrition counseling and education.

TABLE 12–12. Continued

PREGNANT WOMEN, CHILDREN, AND ADOLESCENTS (CONTINUED)

d. DHEW and the Department of Agriculture (USDA) cooperatively should promote more effective use of school lunch programs as a learning laboratory for all students regardless of economic levels.

e. Greater emphasis on community participation and self-help in developing nutrition education programs is needed.

6. The mass media and other new technology should be used more effectively to improve the image of nutrition and to initiate large-scale change in attitudes about healthy eating.

a. Programs to support general nutrition education efforts as well as special nutrition messages targeted to particular concerns or issues should be developed by both commercial as well as public service and educational television.

b. Priority should be given to developing high quality nutrition messages with a specific focus.

c. Government and industry should cooperate to develop nutrition education programs which utilize the mass media and other new techniques.

d. Programmers should be trained in nutrition and encouraged to work with nutritionists in considering the images they portray.

e. Greater use of role models and stories to illustrate the solution of nutrition problems encountered in everyday life should be stressed.

f. The Stanford Heart Disease Prevention Project model should be tested in four regions of the country for its ability to reach pregnant teenagers, obese children, and young, single adults.

g. A study of the feasibility of utilizing new technology for nutrition education should be undertaken by the communications industry, and the findings shared with persons in the nutrition and education fields.

7. Evaluation of nutrition education should receive more emphasis.

a. Support services for evaluating nutrition education efforts should be developed and expanded in collaboration with professional groups in both nutrition and education.

b. Evaluators must be trained in the conduct of both formative and summative evaluation methodologies. Nutritionists should receive training in evaluation during their formal education.

c. All federal food and nutrition assistance programs should require and fund evaluation efforts. These include School Feeding, Head Start, Public Health Nutrition Services, and Nutrition Education and Training programs. Evaluations should also be expected from grantees, and appropriate guidelines and priorities established to inform them of their obligations in this regard.

d. Funding agencies should develop self-assessment tools which grantees can use to assess and improve the quality of nutrition education programs.

8. Research in nutrition education must be expanded.

a. Both DHEW and USDA must give priority to research which will provide baseline data and other information about target populations.

b. Other areas of nutrition education research which need attention by these and other public and private agencies include the following:

- Effective delivery methods and techniques
- Approaches to learning and learner characteristics
- Systematization of nutrition knowledge for specific target audiences
- Validation of techniques for evaluating curricular and reinforcement materials
- Studies which relate the developmental levels of young children to their perceptions of the relationships between food, nutrition, and health
- The effects of dissemination of nutrition messages through alternative delivery systems and of affording educators with an opportunity to obtain feedback for recipients

TABLE 12–12. Continued

PREGNANT WOMEN, CHILDREN, AND ADOLESCENTS (CONTINUED)

- Surveys on the food habits of ethnic groups
- Epidemiological surveys to identify the nature, magnitude, and location of nutritional problems so that appropriate nutrition education can be developed.

c. DHEW and USDA should give high priority to implementing a cooperative National Nutrition Status Monitoring System.

d. DHEW and USDA should strive to assure that effective mechanisms exist for obtaining input from and feedback between the constituent agencies responsible for research on the one hand and service delivery on the other.

e. All of the federal agencies involved in nutrition education must review their requirements for funding of grant applications. The objective should be to modify requirements which prohibit or negate a comprehensive approach to the development, implementation, and evaluation of nutrition education research and programs.

9. The coordination of nutrition education needs to be improved.

a. DHEW and USDA along with other federal agencies and organizations should demonstrate a coordinated approach to nutrition education. The National Academy of Sciences or some other such agency could serve as a focal point for an interdepartmental task force with the mission of identifying priorities in nutrition education, obtaining agreement on the message, and coordinating agency responses.

b. At the state and local level, more attention also needs to be paid to the need for coordinated community plans for nutrition education. Nutrition councils may be able to furnish support and leadership for such efforts.

c. DHEW and USDA, as well as other agencies if appropriate, should support two or three model programs of coordinated community nutrition education. These could then be disseminated to other communities for replication.

d. Federal agencies administering service delivery programs in health, education, food assistance, income maintenance, and social services should give more attention to the coordination and integration of nutrition education into their programs.

10. Nutrition education needs more financial support.

a. Federal agencies responsible for nutrition education programs or services should give priority to obtaining sound cost-effectiveness data.

b. If program funds are inadequate to support implementation of all regulations relating to nutrition education, program administrators should establish priorities for the guidance of grantees.

c. Reimbursement for nutrition counseling provided as a health care service should be available, and federal legislation and regulations should provide for such reimbursement.

LOW-INCOME AND ELDERLY POPULATIONS

The recommendations of the Task Force on Low-Income and Elderly Populations are as follows:

1. Adequate incomes, nutrition education, and access to food for all Americans must be assured.

There must be a national commitment to job and income supplements to ensure a level of income that allows for the purchase of a nutritionally adequate diet for all Americans. In conjunction with this, there should be an active, continual nutrition education program for the entire population.

2. A national nutrition education policy must be developed.

A new national nutrition education program must be established, and a wide variety of possible funding sources for this program must be explored. The nutrition education components of the federal feeding programs should be integrated into this broader based effort, with funding for these programs kept distinct from funding for any food assistance programs.

TABLE 12–12. Continued

LOW-INCOME AND ELDERLY POPULATIONS (CONTINUED)

3. Programs must be targeted to nutritionally vulnerable individuals.

Specific provisions must be made to direct nutrition education activities to nutritionally vulnerable individuals who, because of unique circumstances, require nutrition education on special topics and with special approaches.

4. A holistic, multidisciplinary focus for nutrition education programs is needed.

Nutrition education for low-income and elderly populations, as well as for the general public, must be conducted from a perspective which includes consumerism, food management, food preparation, and human relations. The changing lifestyles and food consumption patterns of the American public must be recognized in developing programs which are integrated with these related home economics skills.

5. Involvement of target groups in program development is necessary.

Nutrition education activities must be developed in collaboration with the low-income and elderly consumer audience in order to reflect needs and interests as perceived by the community.

6. Nutrition education should be a reimbursable component of health care.

The cost of these services needs to be reimbursable by Medicaid, Medicare, and private health insurance and/or deductible from gross income for income tax purposes.

7. Preparation of nutrition educators must be strengthened.

Nutrition educators must be better prepared for working with low-income or elderly populations. Such preparation includes the principles of community development, program development (content and methodologies), nutrition and its related sociological and physiological aspects, evaluation to determine program effectiveness, and mass communications.

8. The mass media must be a major component of programs.

Mass media must be incorporated into many of the nutrition education programs designed for low-income and elderly populations. This incorporation must reflect the cultural and physical environments of the target audience for the particular program and the ways in which the target populations use television, radio, and print media.

9. Thorough evaluation of nutrition education programs is required.

Programs must be better evaluated at local, state, and federal levels. Priority concerns for improvement are:

- Research to develop methodologies
- Evaluation designs which focus on appropriate goals and objectives
- Evaluation designs which consider both the continuous study of the education process and its products
- Programs for upgrading the evaluation skills of nutrition educators and program administrators
- Recognition in program planning and execution of evaluation as a necessary component needing time and funding
- Understanding of the political aspects of evaluation of nutrition education programs.

PERSONS WITH DIET-RELATED DISEASES

The Task Force on Persons with Diet-Related Diseases concur on the following recommendations:

1. The content and goals of nutrition education for persons with diet-related diseases need to be specified.

   a. The ultimate objective of nutrition education of such persons is lifelong dietary behavior changes.

   b. Nutrition education for such persons must be tailored to the disease and factors unique to each patient.

   c. Nutrition education for such persons must be in the context of the total clinical management of the patient.

TABLE 12–12. Continued

PERSONS WITH DIET-RELATED DISEASES (CONTINUED)

d. The patient and the health care professional should be involved in planning and implementing the dietary compliance procedures.

e. A three-level model for integrating the expertise of various persons on the health team should be considered in nutrition education planning.

f. Available nutrition personnel, such as registered dietitians, should be fully utilized in educating health care personnel and in planning and providing nutritional care to patients. If insufficient personnel exist, priority should be placed on increasing their numbers.

g. Statewide referral systems for identifying health care providers of both nutritional care and nutrition counseling should be established.

h. A system should be developed to ensure that health care professionals acquire both knowledge of nutrition and ability to use existing nutrition education resources as well as to be able to communicate this information.

i. Standards that will enhance the quality of nutrition education for persons with diet-related diseases should be developed by certification and licensing boards in cooperation with curriculum committees and specialty societies. The regulatory process should be used to raise standards, and to that end, standards need to be developed for ambulatory settings.

j. People improving the quality of nutrition education for persons with diet-related diseases must consider critically current sources and channels of nutrition education. Inadequacies in the sources should be corrected.

k. A clearinghouse for nutrition education resources should be established for use by health care professionals, and its availability should be widely publicized.

l. A conference should be held for those who supervise and operate existing nutrition education information exchange programs and clearinghouses to increase communication and decrease duplication of tasks. A concise pamphlet should be compiled which describes what is available, and it should be widely disseminated.

m. Various types of nutrition education systems, e.g., audiovisuals, media, and personalized counseling, must be considered, depending upon the availability and expertise of health care personnel.

n. Developers of nutrition education programs for persons with diet-related diseases should explore and evaluate advances in technology related to behavior change, patients' education, and communication research.

o. There is a need for continuing research into the effects of disease and therapy on nutritional needs.

2. Factors affecting food choices of persons with diet-related diseases must be identified and means for influencing them found.

a. Investigate and document the relationship between the level of adherence to dietary recommendations and physical, psychological and cultural, and immediate environmental factors.

b. Study the various dietary counseling methods, and identify practitioners to deliver them.

c. Validate and disseminate advances in technology related to nutrition science, education, and communication research which could improve nutrition education.

d. Study ways to use advertising more effectively.

e. Study the effects of disease and therapy on nutrient needs.

f. Investigate ways of assuring that existing nutrition education materials and programs incorporate environmental considerations.

g. Investigate communication models based on the behavior of persons with diet-related diseases.

h. Identify present patterns of use of dietary counseling services and how they vary by disease, medical specialties, type of medical care facility, and so on.

TABLE 12–12. Continued

PERSONS WITH DIET-RELATED DISEASES (CONTINUED)

3. Professional education systems need improvement.
   a. Physicians
      1) In order to improve the training of medical students, a system must be developed which permits, encourages, and requires that physicians are taught applied clinical nutrition during their medical education at the basic science, clinical clerkship, residency, and continuing education levels; that they are taught to use professional support systems; and that they are trained to establish and use a system to incorporate effectively and efficiently client nutrition education into their practice.
      2) Applied clinical nutrition knowledge and positive attitudes toward its application must be integrated or reinforced in the residencies and postgraduate programs of physicians. Residency review committees for each specialty should establish requirements for nutrition training programs. Certifying boards of medical specialties should incorporate nutrition questions. Medical board qualifying examinations at the federal and state level should do likewise.
   b. Dietitians and nutritionists
      1) More registered dietitians should be certified to disseminate effectively nutrition information for persons with diet-related diseases. Training should emphasize both skills for communicating with patients and for ensuring compliance.
      2) In order to ensure that dietitians are adequately trained, the qualifying examination and continuing education of registered dietitians should include assessment of patients' education and communication skills as well as the biomedical aspects of nutrition.
      3) The Commission on Registration of the American Dietetic Association should be strongly urged to reconsider its criteria for qualification examinations so that they are less allied to qualifications for membership in the American Dietetic Association.
      4) The possibility of a specialization in nutrition education within the profession should be investigated, and the ways of increasing the number of internships and Coordinated Undergraduate Programs must be studied.
   c. Allied health professionals
      1) Patients, medical professionals, and allied health workers should be educated to distinguish between health professionals with credentials in nutrition versus those who deliver nutrition information but lack such expertise.
      2) Professional and specialty societies should encourage emphasis on nutrition education through a wide variety of activities.
      3) Such professionals should be included in conferences on nutrition education.
   d. Professional education research
      1) Investigate outcomes of early nutrition education interventions on diet-related diseases.
      2) Document cost-effectiveness of training programs on future medical practices which include applied clinical and preventive nutrition education.
      3) Develop criteria for evaluating and implementing a patient's short-term adherence versus sustained adherence.
      4) Develop model systems for nutrition education for use at a variety of levels in the health care system before large-scale efforts are begun.
      5) Document the cost-effectiveness of counseling in relation to ameliorating outcomes of various disease states.
      6) Identify and validate methods of locating existing community services, and establish such services where they do not exist.
      7) Evaluate programs for appropriateness, effectiveness, efficiency, adequacy, and side effects.

TABLE 12–12. Continued

PERSONS WITH DIET-RELATED DISEASES (CONTINUED)

4. Nutrition education systems for patients need coordination and improvement.
   a. Methods of dissemination
      1) Develop new or identify existing ways to disseminate valid information to persons with diet-related diseases.
      2) Increase the use of interactive and self-instructional materials to extend the professional's time.
      3) Use the food industry or retail food outlets as potential vehicles for dissemination of nutrition information.
      4) Prepare guidelines on adopting the presentation and content of general materials to the specific environmental, cultural, or economic factors relevant to each patient. The use of other languages and special ethnic foods must also be given consideration.
      5) Integrate materials into existing health care delivery programs with adequate support and follow-up.
      6) Increase publicity about and the dissemination of such materials.
      7) Critical evaluations of old materials are necessary prior to establishing the need for new materials.
      8) When possible, existing materials should be reevaluated and modified.
      9) Patients should be involved in the presentation and evaluation of materials.
      10) Diet-related disease clubs composed of health professionals and individuals with specific disorders should be encouraged.
   b. Resource centers
      1) Resource centers should be established across the country where professionals can easily locate the materials they need for themselves and for their patients.
      2) Nutrition clinics should be established in areas of high population concentration, such as public housing projects.
   c. Delivery systems
      1) Those who are trained to disseminate diet-related information should receive education which includes emphasis on the most effective communication concepts and skills.
      2) Ambulatory and acute care nutrition counseling need to be better coordinated.
      3) Practical methodologies need to be developed and implemented to evaluate the effectiveness of existing programs, disseminate validated procedures, and document the cost-effectiveness of nutritional counseling.
5. Nutrition concerns must be more fully integrated into the health care delivery system.
   a. Statewide programs to identify the risks of diet-related diseases need to be developed. Those people found to be at risk can then be referred for qualified help.
   b. Adequate and appropriate reimbursement mechanisms for nutrition education for persons with diet-related diseases must be investigated.
   c. Pilot projects of the three-level health care delivery system for nutrition education and evaluations of their effectiveness should be mounted.
   d. The use of nutrition aides and nurse aides trained in nutrition as extenders of nutrition education should be evaluated.
   e. Local and regional needs and resources should be inventoried and better cooperation between them developed, especially in providing continuing education on nutrition education for professionals who deal with persons suffering from diet-related diseases.

TABLE 12–12. Continued

PERSONS WITH DIET-RELATED DISEASES (CONTINUED)

f. Examine the potential of integrating nutrition into preventive medicine or nonhospital-based programs, such as school health, industry-based efforts, and private-practice clinics.

g. Develop measurable standards for assessing the effectiveness of nutrition evaluation and instruction programs for persons with diet-related diseases.

h. Evaluate the economic impacts of diet-related diseases.

i. Expand research on the cost-effectiveness of nutritional treatment.

j. Develop criteria and parameters for professional nutrition services in acute and ambulatory settings, including staffing patterns and ratios according to the characteristics of the client population.

k. Expand research on individual requirements and sensitivities to specific nutrients.

references

1. Knowles, J. H. *Nutritive Value of American Foods.* Agriculture Handbook No. 456. Washington, D.C.: United States Department of Agriculture, 1975.
2. Olsen, R. E. "Are Professionals Jumping the Gun in the Fight against Chronic Disease?" *Journal of the American Dietetic Association* 74 (1979): 543.
3. Fusillo, A. F., and A. M. Beloian. "Consumer Nutrition Knowledge and Self-Reported Food Shopping Behavior." *American Journal of Public Health* 67 (1977): 846.
4. Cummings, R. O. *The American and His Food.* Chicago: University of Chicago Press, 1939.
5. Burk, C. *Influences of Economic and Social Factors on U.S. Food Consumption.* Minneapolis: Burgess,1961.
6. Boykin, L. S. "Soul Food for Some Older Americans." *Journal of the American Geriatric Society* 23 (1975): 380.
7. Gifft, H., M. B. Washbon, and G. G. Harrison. *Nutrition, Behavior and Change.* Englewood Cliffs, N.J.: Prentice-Hall, 1972.
8. Mead, M. *Food Habits Research: Problems of the 1960's.* Pub. 1225, National Academy of Sciences, National Research Council, Washington, D.C., 1964.
9. Le Gros Clark, F. "Food Habits as a Practical Nutrition Problem." *World Review of Nutrition and Dietetics* 9 (1968): 56.
10. Aherns, R. A. *Nutrition for Health.* Belmont, Calif.: Wadsworth, 1979.
11. Todhunter, E. N. "Food Habits, Food Faddism and Nutrition." *World Review of Nutrition and Dietetics* 16 (1973): 286.
12. Whitehead, F. E. "Nutrition Education for Children in the U.S. since 1900." *Journal of the American Dietetic Association* 33 (1957): 880.
13. *Education and Training in Nutrition.* FAO Basic Study, No. 6. Rome, Italy, 1962.
14. McKenzie, J. C., and P. Mumford. "The Evaluation of Nutrition Education Programs: A Review of the Present Situation." *World Review of Nutrition and Dietetics* 5 (1965): 21.
15. Harper, A. E. "Nutrition: Where Are We? Where Are We Going?" *American Journal of Clinical Nutrition* 22 (1969): 87.
16. "Position Paper on Nutrition Education for the Public." *Journal of the American Dietetic Association* 62 (1973): 429.

17. "National Nutrition Education Conference: Directions for the 1980's." *Journal of Nutrition Education* 13 (1980): suppl. 1.

18. Holmes, A. C. *Visual Aids in Nutrition Education.* Rome: Food and Agriculture Organization of the United Nations, 1968.

19. Morris, L. L., and C. T. Fitz-Gibbon. *How to Deal with Goals and Objectives.* Beverly Hills: Sage Publications, 1978.

20. *Nutrient Density Nutrition Education Curriculum Materials, Department of Nutrition and Food Sciences.* Logan, Utah: Utah State University, 1979.

21. *Nutrition Labeling.* Fed. Reg. 37: 6493, March 31, 1972.

22. *Nutrition Labeling: How It Can Work For You.* Bethesda, Md.: Nutrition Consortium, Inc., 1976.

23. Eppright, E., M. Pattison, and H. Barbour. *Teaching Nutrition,* 2nd ed. Ames: Iowa State University Press, 1963.

24. Whitehead, F. E. *Nutrition Education Research Project, Report Phase 1.* Office of Nutrition, Technical Assistance Bureau, Agency for International Development, Washington, D.C., 1970

25. Davies, L. "Nutrition Education for the Elderly." *Proceedings of the Nutrition Society* 35 (1976): 125.

26. Parham, E. S. "Nutrition Education for the Elderly." *Journal of Home Economics* 72 (1980): 24.

27. Woteki, C. E. "Building Consensus for Nutrition Education Research." *Journal of Nutrition Education* 11 (1979): 7.

APPENDIX

TABLE A-1. 1980 Revised Recommended Dietary Allowances

The following tables have been approved by the National Academy of Sciences for distribution. They included tables on (a) Recommended energy intakes, together with mean heights and weights; (b) the Recommended Dietary Allowances for protein, fat-soluble vitamins, water-soluble vitamins, and minerals; and (c) estimates of adequate and safe intakes of selected vitamins, trace elements, and electrolytes.

Reproduced from: Recommended Dietary Allowances, Ninth Revised Edition (1980), with the permission of the National Academy of Sciences, Washington, D.C.

For further information, write or call: Myrtle L. Brown, PH.D., Executive Secretary, Food and Nutrition Board, 2101 Constitution Avenue, Washington, D.C. 20418; 202—389-6366.

MEAN HEIGHTS AND WEIGHTS AND RECOMMENDED ENERGY INTAKE*

age and sex group	weight		height		energy NEEDS		
	kg.	lb.	cm.	in.	MJ	kcal	Range in kcal
infants							
0.0–0.5 yr.	6	13	60	24	kg. × 0.48	kg. × 115	95– 145
0.5–1.0 yr.	9	20	71	28	kg. × 0.44	kg. × 105	80– 135
children							
1–3 yr.	13	29	90	35	5.5	1,300	900–1,800
4–6 yr.	20	44	112	44	7.1	1,700	1,300–2,300
7–10 yr.	28	62	132	52	10.1	2,400	1,650–3,300
males							
11–14 yr.	45	99	157	62	11.3	2,700	2,000–3,700
15–18 yr.	66	145	176	69	11.8	2,800	2,100–3,900
19–22 yr.	70	154	177	70	12.2	2,900	2,500–3,300
23–50 yr.	70	154	178	70	11.3	2,700	2,300–3,100
51–75 yr.	70	154	178	70	10.1	2,400	2,000–2,800
76+ yr.	70	154	178	70	8.6	2,050	1,650–2,450
females							
11–14 yr.	46	101	157	62	9.2	2,200	1,500–3,000
15–18 yr.	55	120	163	64	8.8	2,100	1,200–3,000
19–22 yr.	55	120	163	64	8.8	2,100	1,700–2,500
23–50 yr.	55	120	163	64	8.4	2,000	1,600–2,400
51–75 yr.	55	120	163	64	7.6	1,800	1,400–2,200
76+ yr.	55	120	163	64	6.7	1,600	1,200–2,000
pregnancy						+300	
lactation						+500	

*From Recommended Dietary Allowances, Revised 1980, Food and Nutrition Board, National Academy of Sciences—National Research Council, Washington, D.C. The data in this table have been assembled from the observed median heights and weights of children, together with desirable weights for adults for mean heights of men (70 in.) and women (64 in.) between the ages of eighteen and thirty-four years as surveyed in the U.S. population (DHEW/NCHS data).

Energy allowances for the young adults are for men and women doing light work. The allowances for the two older age groups represent mean energy needs over these age spans, allowing for a 2 per cent decrease in basal (resting) metabolic rate per decade and a reduction in activity of 200 kcal per day for men and women between fifty-one and seventy-five years; 500 kcal for men over seventy-five years; and 400 kcal for women over seventy-five. The customary range of daily energy output is shown for adults in the range column and is based on a variation in energy needs of ±400 kcal at any one age, emphasizing the wide range of energy intakes appropriate for any group of people.

Energy allowances for children through age eighteen are based on median energy intakes of children of these ages followed in longitudinal growth studies. Ranges are the 10th and 90th percentiles of energy intake, to indicate range of energy consumption among children of these ages.

TABLE A–1. (Continued)

RECOMMENDED DIETARY ALLOWANCES, REVISED 1980[a]
DESIGNED FOR THE MAINTENANCE OF GOOD NUTRITION OF PRACTICALLY ALL HEALTHY PEOPLE IN THE U.S.A.
FOOD AND NUTRITION BOARD, NATIONAL ACADEMY OF SCIENCES-NATIONAL RESEARCH COUNCIL

age and sex group	weight kg.	weight lb.	height cm.	height in.	protein gm.	fat-soluble vitamins: Vitamin A μg. R.E.[b]	Vitamin D μg.[c]	Vitamin E mg. αT.E.[d]	water-soluble vitamins: Vitamin C mg.	Thiamin mg.	Riboflavin mg.	Niacin mg. N.E.[e]	Vitamin B_6 mg.	Folacin[f] μg.	Vitamin B_{12} μg.	minerals: Calcium mg.	Phosphorus mg.	Magnesium mg.	Iron mg.	Zinc mg.	Iodine μg.
infants																					
0.0–0.5 yr.	6	13	60	24	kg. × 2.2	420	10	3	35	0.3	0.4	6	0.3	30	0.5[g]	360	240	50	10	3	40
0.5–1.0 yr.	9	20	71	28	kg. × 2.0	400	10	4	35	0.5	0.6	8	0.6	45	1.5	540	360	70	15	5	50
children																					
1–3 yr.	13	29	90	35	23	400	10	5	45	0.7	0.8	9	0.9	100	2.0	800	800	150	15	10	70
4–6 yr.	20	44	112	44	30	500	10	6	45	0.9	1.0	11	1.3	200	2.5	800	800	200	10	10	90
7–10 yr.	28	62	132	52	34	700	10	7	45	1.2	1.4	16	1.6	300	3.0	800	800	250	10	10	120
males																					
11–14 yr.	45	99	157	62	45	1,000	10	8	50	1.4	1.6	18	1.8	400	3.0	1,200	1,200	350	18	15	150
15–18 yr.	66	145	176	69	56	1,000	10	10	60	1.4	1.7	18	2.0	400	3.0	1,200	1,200	400	18	15	150
19–22 yr.	70	154	177	70	56	1,000	7.5	10	60	1.5	1.7	19	2.2	400	3.0	800	800	350	10	15	150
23–50 yr.	70	154	178	70	56	1,000	5	10	60	1.4	1.6	18	2.2	400	3.0	800	800	350	10	15	150
51+ yr.	70	154	178	70	56	1,000	5	10	60	1.2	1.4	16	2.2	400	3.0	800	800	350	10	15	150
females																					
11–14 yr.	46	101	157	62	46	800	10	8	50	1.1	1.3	15	1.8	400	3.0	1,200	1,200	300	18	15	150
15–18 yr.	55	120	163	64	46	800	10	8	60	1.1	1.3	14	2.0	400	3.0	1,200	1,200	300	18	15	150
19–22 yr.	55	120	163	64	44	800	7.5	8	60	1.1	1.3	14	2.0	400	3.0	800	800	300	18	15	150
23–50 yr.	55	120	163	64	44	800	5	8	60	1.0	1.2	13	2.0	400	3.0	800	800	300	18	15	150
51+ yr.	55	120	163	64	44	800	5	8	60	1.0	1.2	13	2.0	400	3.0	800	800	300	10	15	150
pregnancy					+30	+200	+5	+2	+20	+0.4	+0.3	+2	+0.6	+400	+1.0	+400	+400	+150	*h*	+ 5	+25
lactation					+20	+400	+5	+3	+40	+0.5	+0.5	+5	+0.5	+100	+1.0	+400	+400	+150	*h*	+10	+50

[a] The allowances are intended to provide for individual variations among most normal persons as they live in the United States under usual environmental stresses. Diets should be based on a variety of common foods in order to provide other nutrients for which human requirements have been less well defined. See preceding table for weights and heights by individual year of age and for suggested average energy intakes.

[b] Retinol equivalents: 1 retinol equivalent = 1 μg. retinol or 6 μg. β-carotene.

[c] As cholecalciferol: 10 μg. cholecalciferol = 400 I.U. vitamin D.

[d] α tocopherol equivalents: 1 mg. d-α-tocopherol = 1αT.E.

[e] 1 N.E. (niacin equivalent) = 1 mg. niacin or 60 mg. dietary tryptophan.

[f] The folacin allowances refer to dietary sources as determined by *Lactobacillus casei* assay after treatment with enzymes ("conjugases") to make polyglutamyl forms of the vitamin available to the test organism.

[g] The RDA for vitamin B_{12} in infants is based on average concentration of the vitamin in human milk. The allowances after weaning are based on energy intake (as recommended by the American Academy of Pediatrics) and consideration of other factors, such as intestinal absorption.

[h] The increased requirement during pregnancy cannot be met by the iron content of habitual American Diets or by the existing iron store of many women; therefore, the use of 30 to 60 mg. supplemental iron is recommended. Iron needs during lactation are not substantially different from those of non-pregnant women, but continued supplementation of the mother for two to three months after parturition is advisable in order to replenish store depleted by pregnancy.

TABLE A–1. (Continued)

ESTIMATED SAFE AND ADEQUATE DAILY DIETARY INTAKES OF ADDITIONAL SELECTED VITAMINS AND MINERALS[a]

	vitamins			trace elements[b]						electrolytes		
age group	Vitamin K	Biotin	Pantothenic Acid	Copper	Manganese	Fluoride	Chromium	Selenium	Molybdenum	Sodium	Potassium	Chloride
	← μg.	→	←					mg.				→
infants												
0.0–0.5 yr.	12	35	2	0.5–0.7	0.5–0.7	0.1–0.5	0.01–0.04	0.01–0.04	0.03–0.06	115– 350	350– 925	275– 700
0.5–1.0 yr.	10– 20	50	3	0.7–1.0	0.7–1.0	0.2–1.0	0.02–0.06	0.02–0.06	0.04–0.08	250– 750	425–1,275	400–1,200
children and adolescents												
1–3 yr	15– 30	65	3	1.0–1.5	1.0–1.5	0.5–1.5	0.02–0.08	0.02–0.08	0.05–0.1	325– 975	550–1,650	500–1,500
4–6 yr.	20– 40	85	3–4	1.5–2.0	1.5–2.0	1.0–2.5	0.03–0.12	0.03–0.12	0.06–0.15	450–1,350	775–2,325	700–2,100
7–10 yr.	30– 60	120	4–5	2.0–2.5	2.0–3.0	1.5–2.5	0.05–0.2	0.05–0.2	0.1 –0.3	600–1,800	1,000–3,000	925–2,775
11+ yr.	50–100	100–200	4–7	2.0–3.0	2.5–5.0	1.5–2.5	0.05–0.2	0.05–0.2	0.15–0.5	900–2,700	1,525–4,575	1,400–4,200
adults	70–140	100–200	4–7	2.0–3.0	2.5–5.0	1.5–4.0	0.05–0.2	0.05–0.2	0.15–0.5	1,100–3,300	1,875–5,625	1,700–5,100

[a]From Recommended Dietary Allowances. Revised 1980. Food and Nutrition Board, National Academy of Sciences—National Research Council. Because there is less information on which to base allowances, these figures are not given in the main table of the RDAs and are provided here in the form of ranges of recommended intakes.

[b]Since the toxic levels for many trace elements may be only several times usual intakes, the upper levels for the trace elements given in this table should not be habitually exceeded.

TABLE A–2. Recommended Intakes of Nutrients

Age	Body Weight	Energy[1]		Protein[1,2]	Vitamin A[3,4]	Vitamin D[5,6]	Thiamin[3]	Riboflavin[3]	Niacin[3]	Folic Acid[5]	Vitamin B_{12}[5]	Ascorbic Acid[5]	Calcium[7]	Iron[5,8]
	kilograms	kilocalories	megajoules	grams	micrograms	micrograms	milligrams	milligrams	milligrams	micrograms	micrograms	milligrams	grams	milligrams
Children														
< 1	7.3	820	3.4	14	300	10.0	0.3	0.5	5.4	60	0.3	20	0.5–0.6	5–10
1–3	13.4	1,360	5.7	16	250	10.0	0.5	0.8	9.0	100	0.9	20	0.4–0.5	5–10
4–6	20.2	1,830	7.6	20	300	10.0	0.7	1.1	12.1	100	1.5	20	0.4–0.5	5–10
7–9	28.1	2,190	9.2	25	400	2.5	0.9	1.3	14.5	100	1.5	20	0.4–0.5	5–10
Male adolescents														
10–12	36.9	2,600	10.9	30	575	2.5	1.0	1.6	17.2	100	2.0	20	0.6–0.7	5–10
13–15	51.3	2,900	12.1	37	725	2.5	1.2	1.7	19.1	200	2.0	30	0.6–0.7	9–18
16–19	62.9	3,070	12.8	38	750	2.5	1.2	1.8	20.3	200	2.0	30	0.5–0.6	5–9
Female adolescents														
10–12	38.0	2,350	9.8	29	575	2.5	0.9	1.4	15.5	100	2.0	20	0.6–0.7	5–10
13–15	49.9	2,490	10.4	31	725	2.5	1.0	1.5	16.4	200	2.0	30	0.6–0.7	12–24
16–19	54.4	2,310	9.7	30	750	2.5	0.9	1.4	15.2	200	2.0	30	0.5–0.6	14–28
Adult man (moderately active)	65.0	3,000	12.6	37	750	2.5	1.2	1.8	19.8	200	2.0	30	0.4–0.5	5–9
Adult woman (moderately active)	55.0	2,200	9.2	29	750	2.5	0.9	1.3	14.5	200	2.0	30	0.4–0.5	14–28
Pregnancy (later half)		+350	+1.5	38	750	10.0	+0.1	+0.2	+2.3	400	3.0	50	1.0–1.2	(9)
Lactation (first 6 months)		+550	+2.3	46	1,200	10.0	+0.2	+0.4	+3.7	300	2.5	50	1.0–1.2	(9)

[1] Energy and Protein Requirements. Report of a Joint FAO/WHO Expert Group, FAO, Rome, 1972.

[2] As egg or milk protein.

[3] Requirements of Vitamin A, Thiamin, Riboflavin and Niacin. Report of a Joint FAO/WHO Expert Group, FAO, Rome, 1965.

[4] As retinol.

[5] Requirements of Ascorbic Acid, Vitamin D, Vitamin B_{12}, Folate and Iron. Report of a Joint FAO/WHO Expert Group, FAO, Rome, 1970.

[6] As cholecalciferol.

[7] Calcium Requirements. Report of a FAO/WHO Expert Group, FAO, Rome, 1961.

[8] On each line the lower value applies when over 25 percent of calories in the diet come from animal foods, and the higher value when animal foods represent less than 10 percent of calories.

[9] For women whose iron intake throughout life has been at the level recommended in this table, the daily intake of iron during pregnancy and lactation should be the same as that recommended for nonpregnant, nonlactating women of childbearing age. For women whose iron status is not satisfactory at the beginning of pregnancy, the requirement is increased, and in the extreme situation of women with no iron stores, the requirement can probably not be met without supplementation.

TABLE A–3. Daily Food Guide

VEGETABLE/FRUIT GROUP

Four Basic Servings Daily: Include one good vitamin C source each day. Also frequently include deep-yellow or dark-green vegetables (for vitamin A) and unpeeled fruits and vegetables and those with edible seeds, such as berries (for fiber).

What's a Serving?

Includes all fruits and vegetables.

Count 1/2 cup as a serving, or a typical portion—one orange, half a medium grapefruit or cantaloupe, juice of one lemon, a wedge of lettuce, a bowl of salad, and one medium potato.

What's in It for You?

This group is important for its contribution of vitamins A and C and fiber, although individual foods in this group vary widely in how much of these they provide. Dark-green and deep-yellow vegetables are good sources of vitamin A. Most dark-green vegetables, if not overcooked, are also reliable sources of vitamin C, as are citrus fruits (oranges, grapefruit, tangerines, lemons) melons, berries, and tomatoes. Dark-green vegetables are valued for riboflavin, folacin, iron, and magnesium, as well. Certain greens—collards, kale, mustard, turnip, and dandelion—provide calcium. Nearly all vegetables and fruits are low in fat, and none contains cholesterol.

BREAD/CEREAL GROUP

Four Basic Servings Daily: Select only whole-grain and enriched or fortified products. (But include some whole-grain bread or cereals for sure!) Check labels.

What's a Serving?

Includes all products made with whole grains or enriched flour or meal; bread, biscuits, muffins, waffles, pancakes, cooked or ready-to-eat cereals, cornmeal, flour, grits, macaroni and spaghetti, noodles, rice, rolled oats, barley, and bulgur.

Count as a serving 1 slice of bread; 1/2 cup to 3/4 cup cooked cereal, cornmeal, grits, macaroni, noodles, rice, or spaghetti; or 1 oz. ready-to-eat cereal.

What's in It for You?

These whole-grain or enriched foods are important sources of B vitamins and iron. They also provide protein and are a major source of this nutrient in vegetarian diets. Whole-grain products contribute magnesium, folacin, and fiber, in addition.

Most breakfast cereals are fortified at nutrient levels higher than those occurring in natural whole grain. In fact, some fortification adds vitamins not normally found in cereals (vitamins A, B_{12}, C, and D). However, even these cereals, if refined, and other refined products (enriched or not), may be low in some other vitamins and trace minerals, which are partially removed from the whole grain in the milling process and are not added. For this reason, it's a good idea to include some less refined or whole-grain products in your diet.

TABLE A-3. (Continued)

MILK/CHEESE GROUP

Basic Servings Daily (based on servings of fluid milk; for milk product equivalents see below): Children under 9, 2 to 3 servings; Children 9 to 12, 3 servings; Teens, 4 servings; Adults, 2 servings; Pregnant Women, 3 servings; Nursing Mothers, 4 servings.

What's a Serving?

Includes milk in any form: whole, skim, lowfat, evaporated, buttermilk, and nonfat dry milk; also yogurt, ice cream, ice milk, and cheese, including cottage cheese.

Count one 8-ounce cup of milk as a serving.

Common portions of some dairy products and their milk equivalents in calcium are:

1 cup plain yogurt	=	1 cup milk
1 ounce Cheddar or Swiss cheese (natural or process)	=	3/4 cup milk
1-inch cube cheddar or Swiss cheese (natural or process)	=	1/2 cup milk
1 ounce process cheese food	=	1/2 cup milk
1/2 cup ice cream or ice milk	=	1/3 cup milk
1 tablespoon or 1/2 ounce process cheese spread; or 1 tablespoon Parmesan cheese	=	1/4 cup milk
1/2 cup cottage cheese	=	1/4 cup milk

Note: You'll get about the same amount of calcium in each of these portions, but varying amounts of calories.

Milk used in cooked foods—such as in creamed soups, sauces, puddings—can count toward filling your daily quota in this group.

What's in It for You?

Milk and most milk products are relied on to provide calcium (they're the major source of this mineral in the American diet) and riboflavin and to contribute protein and vitamins A, B_6, and B_{12}. They also provide vitamin D, when fortified with this vitamin.

Fortified (with vitamins A and D) lowfat or skim-milk products have essentially the same nutrients as whole-milk products but fewer calories.

MEAT/POULTRY/FISH/BEANS GROUP

Two Basic Servings Daily

What's a Serving?

Includes beef, veal, lamb, pork, poultry, fish, shellfish (shrimp, oysters, crabs, etc.), organ meats (liver, kidneys, etc.), dry beans or peas, soybeans, lentils, eggs, seeds, nuts, peanuts, and peanut butter.

Count 2 to 3 ounces of lean, cooked meat, poultry, or fish without bone as a serving. One egg, 1/2 to 3/4 cup cooked dry beans, dry peas, soybeans or lentils, 2 tablespoons peanut butter, and 1/4 to 1/2 cup nuts, sesame seeds, or sunflower seeds count as 1 ounce of meat, poultry, or fish.

MEAT/POULTRY/FISH/BEANS GROUP (Continued)

What's in It for You?

These foods are valued for the protein, phosphorus, vitamins B_6, B_{12}, and other vitamins and minerals they provide. However, only foods of animal origin contain vitamin B_{12} naturally.

It's a good idea to vary your choices among these foods as each has distinct nutritional advantages. For example, red meats and oysters are good sources of zinc. Liver and egg yolks are valuable sources of vitamin A. Dry beans, dry peas, soybeans and nuts are worthwhile sources of magnesium. The flesh of fish and poultry is relatively low in calories and saturated fat. Seeds (sunflower, sesame, for example) contribute polyunsaturated fatty acids which are an essential part of a balanced diet.

Cholesterol, like vitamin B_{12}, occurs naturally only in foods of animal origin. All meats contain cholesterol, which is present in both the lean and fat. The highest concentration is found in organ meats and in egg yolks. Fish and shellfish, except for shrimp, are relatively low in cholesterol. (Dairy products also supply cholesterol.)

Is Getting Enough Iron a Problem?

It can be, particularly for young children, teenage girls, and women of childbearing age.

Remember—meats are reliable sources of iron. So are whole-grain and enriched breads and cereals, dry beans, and dry peas, but the body can make better use of the iron these foods provide if they are eaten at the same time as a good source of vitamin C (orange juice, for example) or along with meat.

FATS/SWEETS/ALCOHOL GROUP

What's a Serving?

Includes foods like butter, margarine, mayonnaise and other salad dressings, and other fats and oils; candy, sugar, jams, jellies, sirups, sweet toppings, and other sweets; soft drinks and other highly sugared beverages; and alcoholic beverages such as wine, beer, and liquor. Also included are refined but unenriched breads, pastries, and flour products. Some of these foods are used as ingredients in prepared foods or are added to other foods at the table. Others are just "extras."

No serving sizes are defined because a basic number of servings is not suggested for this group.

What's in It for You?

These products, with some exceptions such as vegetable oils, provide mainly calories. Vegetable oils generally supply vitamin E and essential fatty acids.

Fats and oils have more than twice the calories, ounce for ounce, as protein, starches, or sugars, but keep hunger pangs away longer.

Pure alcohol has almost twice the calories per ounce as protein, starches, or sugars. However, few alcoholic beverages are 100 percent alcohol. Generally, the higher the alcohol content, the higher the calories, ounce for ounce.

Unenriched, refined bakery products are included here because, like other foods and beverages in this group, they usually provide relatively low levels of vitamins, minerals, and protein compared with calories.

TABLE A–3. (Continued)

USDA'S DAILY FOOD GUIDE TO THE RESCUE!

This Guide tells you the kinds and amounts of foods that make up a nutritious diet. But it lets you make choices to fit your eating style and needs. The guidelines we offer you today are based on what we know today. But—be prepared. In the future, the Guide may change! Nutrition science is in a growth phase. At another time, we may offer you new guidelines based on new understandings of the relationship of nutrition and health.

Calories are a measure of the energy food provides. The extra calories that you get and your body does not use up are stored as fat.

The Guide divides commonly eaten foods into five groups according to the nutritional contributions they make. By following the Guide, you'll be able to choose foods for their vitamins, minerals, and protein—as well as calorie content.

The suggested number of servings in the Guide average about 1,200 calories, provide adequate protein, and supply most of the vitamins and minerals you need daily. Plan your day's food around this foundation to keep you on the right track to a better diet.

Making the Guide Work for You

You can personalize the Guide by fitting it to your calorie needs. All foods, except water and non-caloric drinks, have calories. There are no "good calories" or "bad calories" nutritionally, but there are foods which give you little but calories, and others which give you calories plus nutrients.

How many calories you need depends on how much energy you use up. Generally, older people need fewer calories than younger people, women fewer than men, and bridge players and bookkeepers fewer than tennis players and construction workers.

If you are gaining unwanted weight, cut down first on portions from the fifth group (Fats–Sweets–Alcohol). If you are still gaining weight, cut down next on portion sizes from the other groups . . . cut down, but don't cut out . . . and select the lower calorie foods within each group.

On the other hand, if you want to gain weight, eat larger or additional portions from the first four groups and include some foods from the fifth group.

Remember, the Guide gives you only the basics. You have to choose foods which meet your special needs. But you're usually better off by eating a wide assortment of foods from the first four food groups.

One Last Thought

It gets a little complicated when you run into foods that span several groups. Eat a beef taco, for example, and you'll be eating cheese from the Milk–Cheese group, ground beef from the Meat–Poultry–Fish–Beans group, shredded lettuce and tomato from the Fruit–Vegetable group, and a taco shell from the Bread–Cereal group. There is no way to determine "portions" of these different food groups for a taco—it all depends on how many tacos you eat and how much of each food is used in the recipe. You'll just have to estimate for yourself.

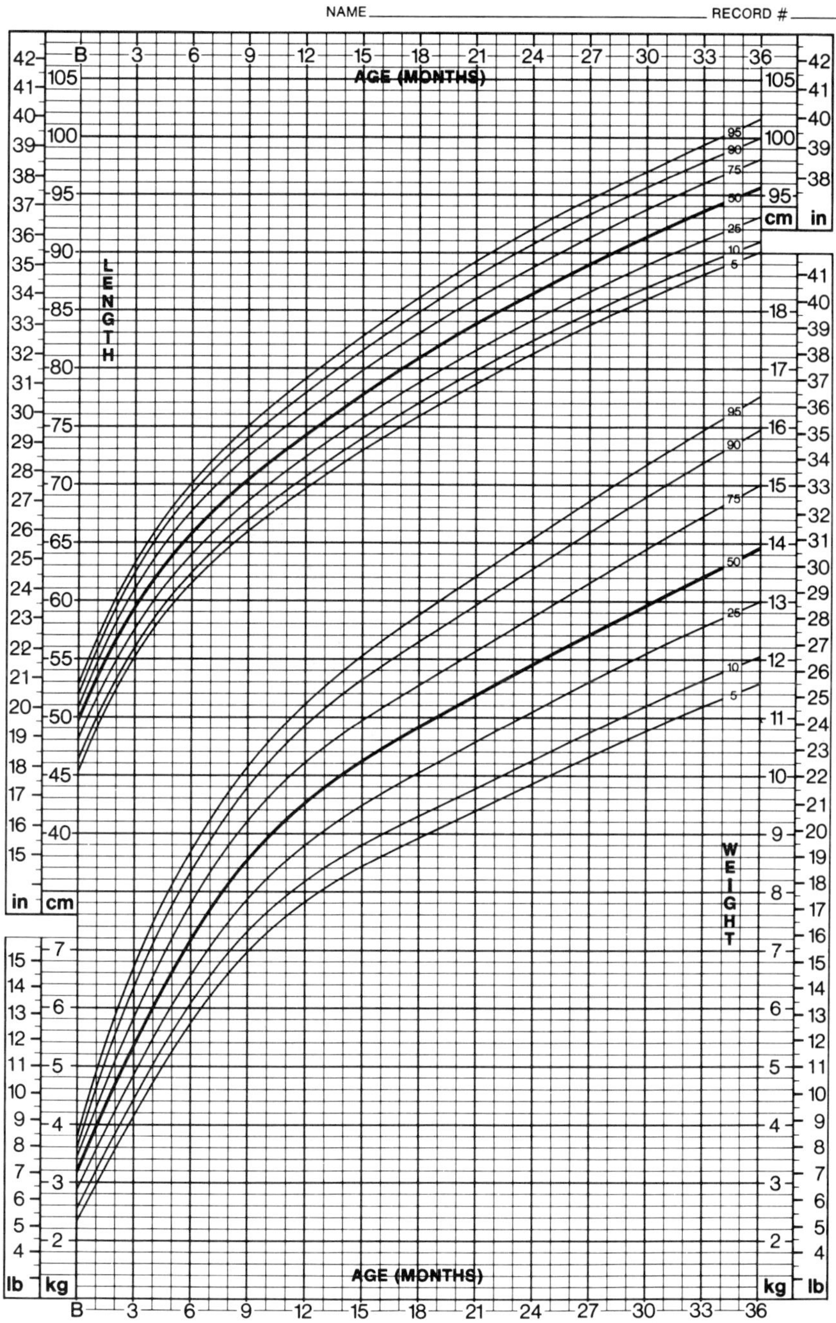

Adapted from: Hamill PVV, Drizd TA, Johnson CL, Reed RB, Roche AF, Moore WM: Physical growth: National Center for Health Statistics percentiles. AM J CLIN NUTR 32:607-629,1979. Data from the Fels Research Institute, Wright State University School of Medicine, Yellow Springs, Ohio.

FIG. A–1. Girls (birth to 36 months): Physical Growth NCHS Percentiles.

NAME ______________________ RECORD # ____________

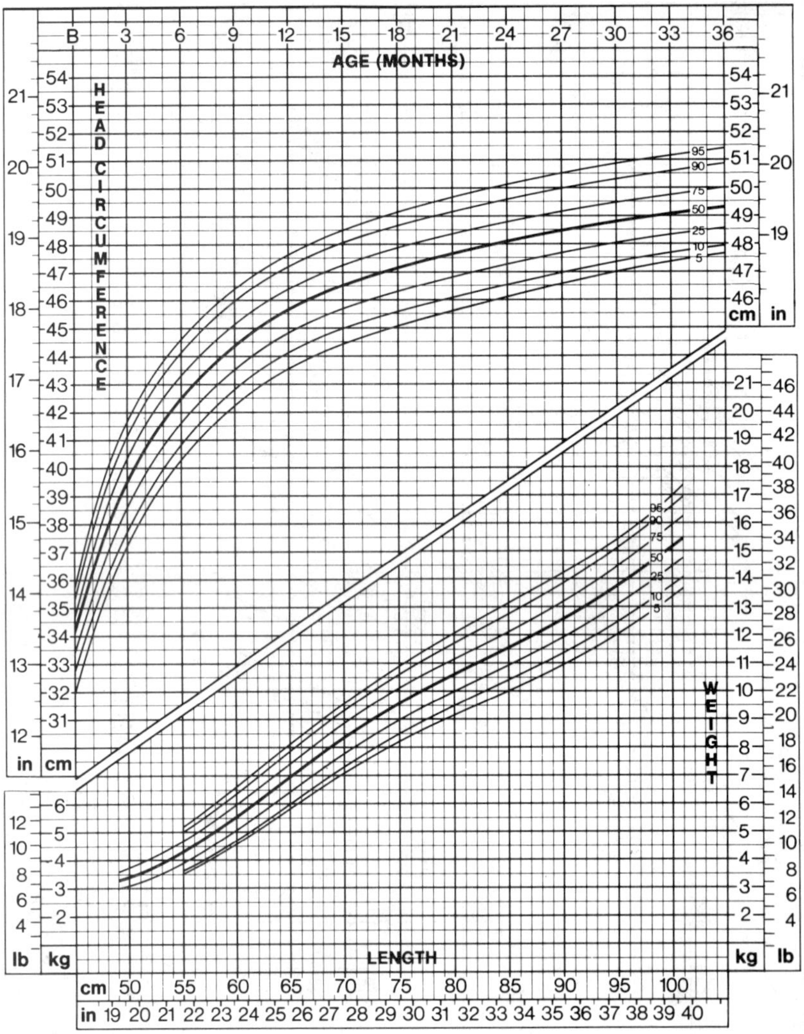

Adapted from: Hamill PVV, Drizd TA, Johnson CL, Reed RB, Roche AF, Moore WM: Physical growth: National Center for Health Statistics percentiles. AM J CLIN NUTR 32:607-629,1979. Data from the Fels Research Institute, Wright State University School of Medicine, Yellow Springs, Ohio.

DATE	AGE	LENGTH	WEIGHT	HEAD C.
	BIRTH			

DATE	AGE	LENGTH	WEIGHT	HEAD C.

FIG. A–2. Girls (birth to 36 months): Physical Growth NCHS Percentiles.

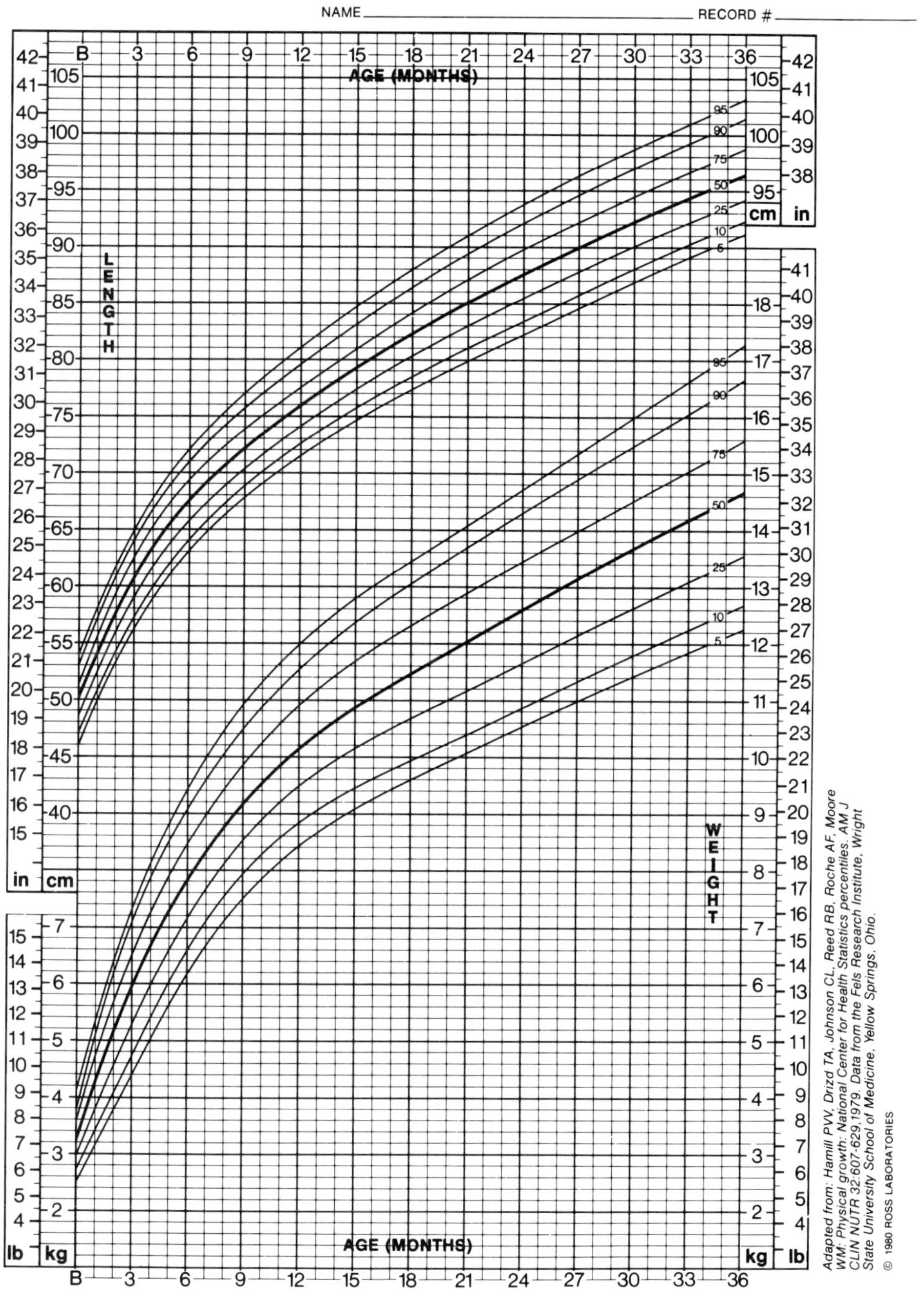

FIG. A–3. Boys (birth to 36 months): Physical Growth NCHS Percentiles.

NAME ____________________ RECORD # ____________

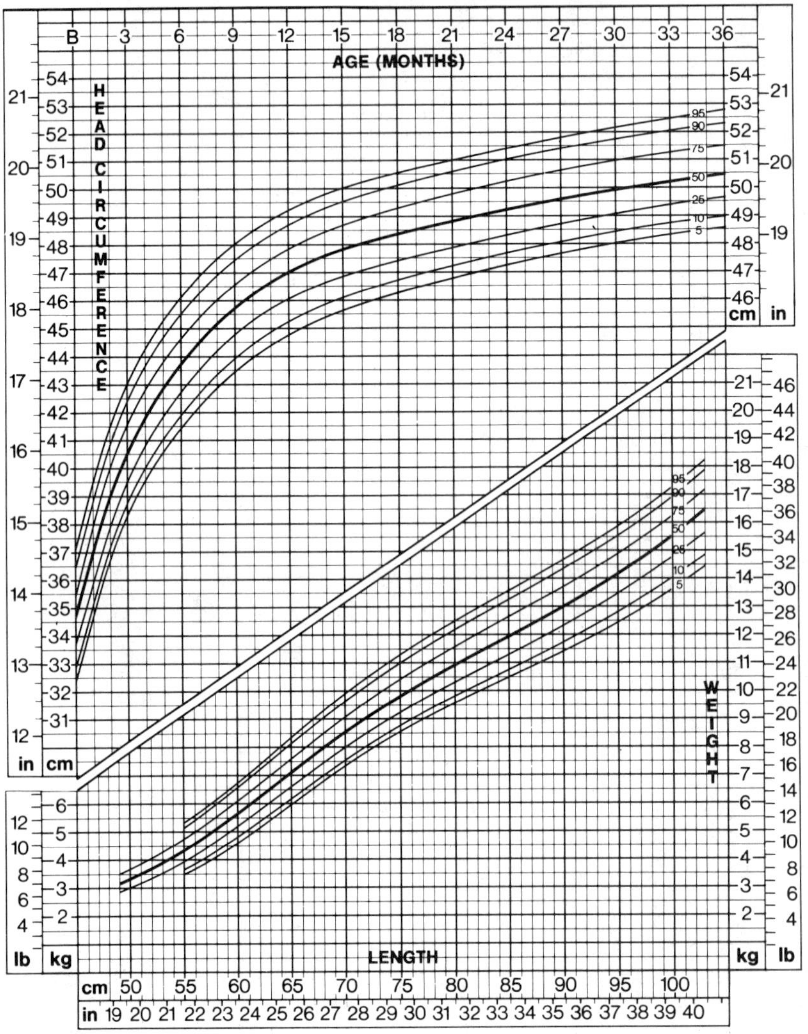

Adapted from: Hamill PVV, Drizd TA, Johnson CL, Reed RB, Roche AF, Moore WM: Physical growth: National Center for Health Statistics percentiles. AM J CLIN NUTR 32:607-629,1979. Data from the Fels Research Institute, Wright State University School of Medicine, Yellow Springs, Ohio.

DATE	AGE	LENGTH	WEIGHT	HEAD C.
	BIRTH			

DATE	AGE	LENGTH	WEIGHT	HEAD C.

FIG. A–4. Boys (birth to 36 months): Physical Growth NCHS Percentiles.

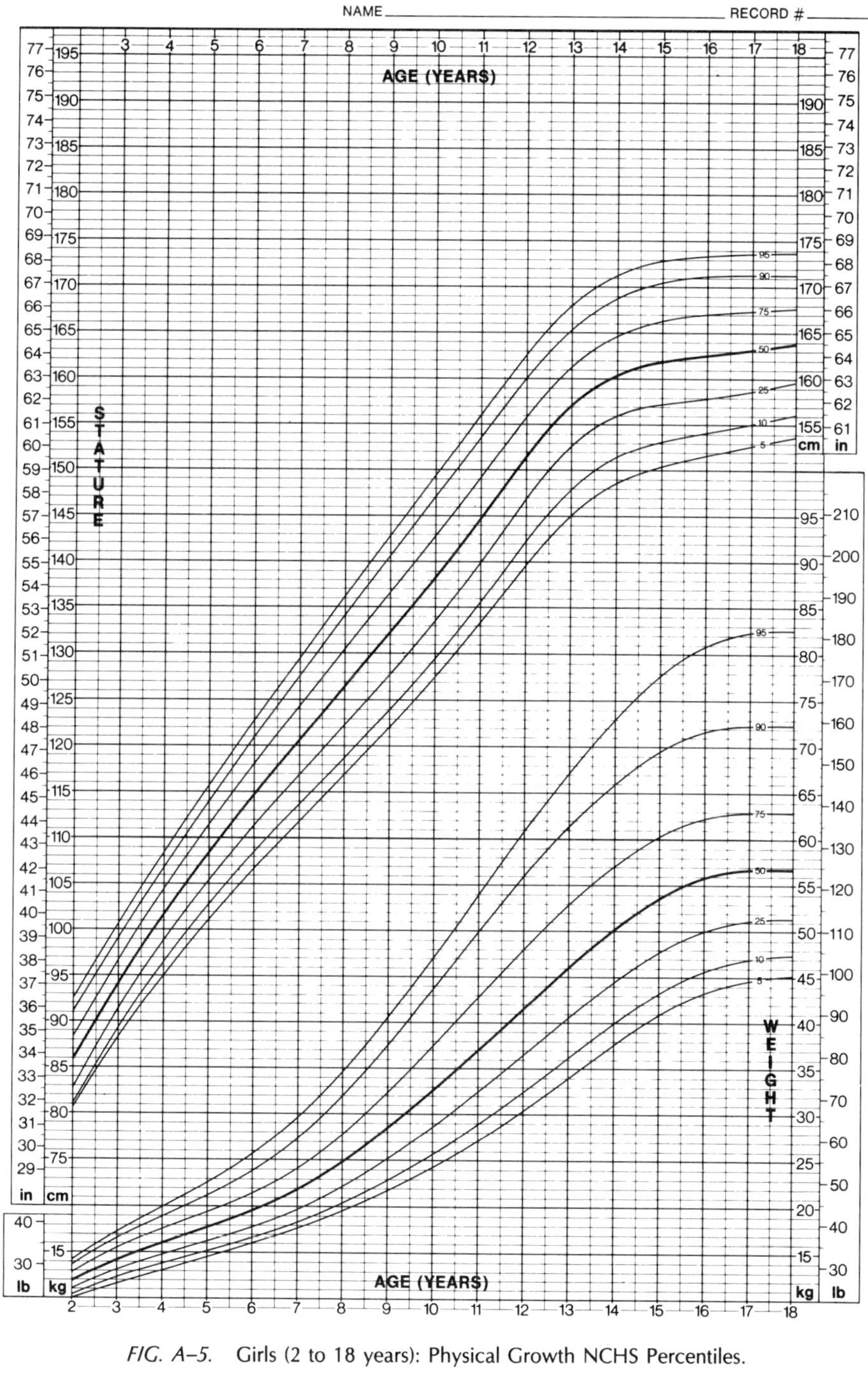

Adapted from: Hamill PVV, Drizd TA, Johnson CL, Reed RB, Roche AF, Moore WM: Physical growth: National Center for Health Statistics percentiles. AM J CLIN NUTR 32:607-629,1979. Data from the National Center for Health Statistics (NCHS) Hyattsville, Maryland

FIG. A–5. Girls (2 to 18 years): Physical Growth NCHS Percentiles.

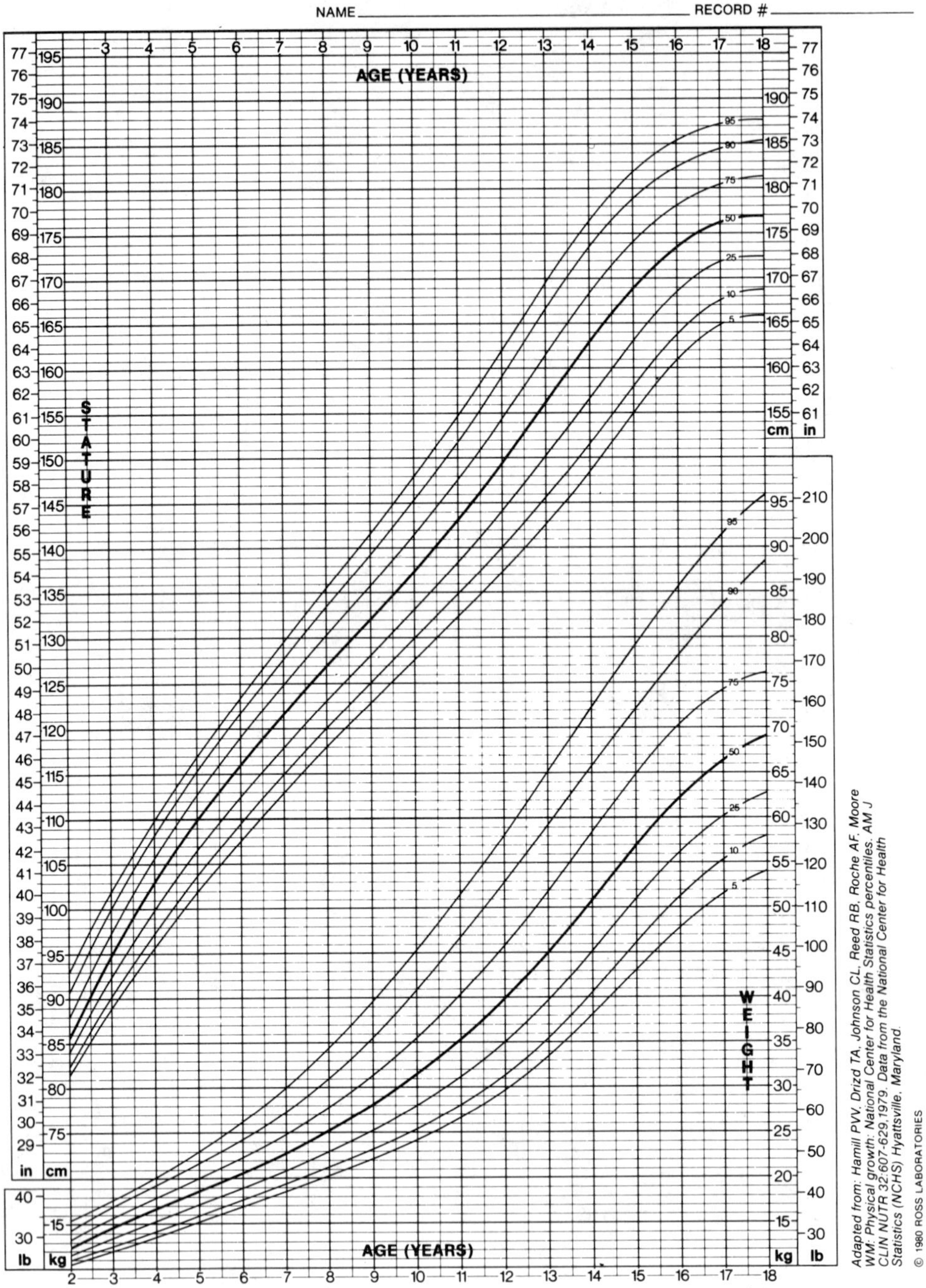

Adapted from: Hamill PVV, Drizd TA, Johnson CL, Reed RB, Roche AF, Moore WM: Physical growth: National Center for Health Statistics percentiles. AM J CLIN NUTR 32:607-629,1979. Data from the National Center for Health Statistics (NCHS) Hyattsville, Maryland.

FIG. A–6. Boys (2 to 18 years): Physical Growth NCHS Percentiles.

NAME ______________________ RECORD # ____________

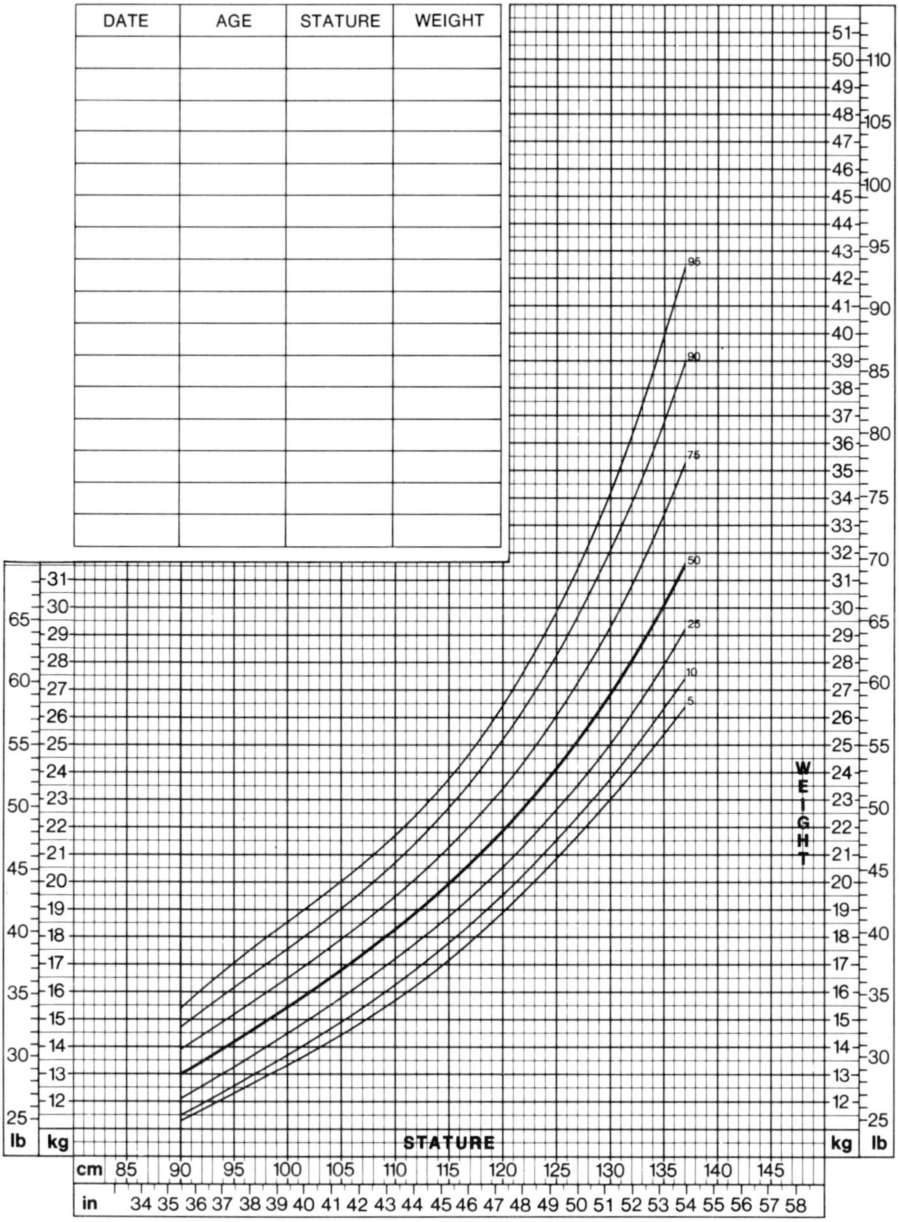

Adapted from: Hamill PVV, Drizd TA, Johnson CL, Reed RB, Roche AF, Moore WM: Physical growth: National Center for Health Statistics percentiles. AM J CLIN NUTR 32:607-629,1979. Data from the National Center for Health Statistics (NCHS) Hyattsville, Maryland.

FIG. A–7. Prepubescent Girls: Physical Growth NCHS Percentiles.

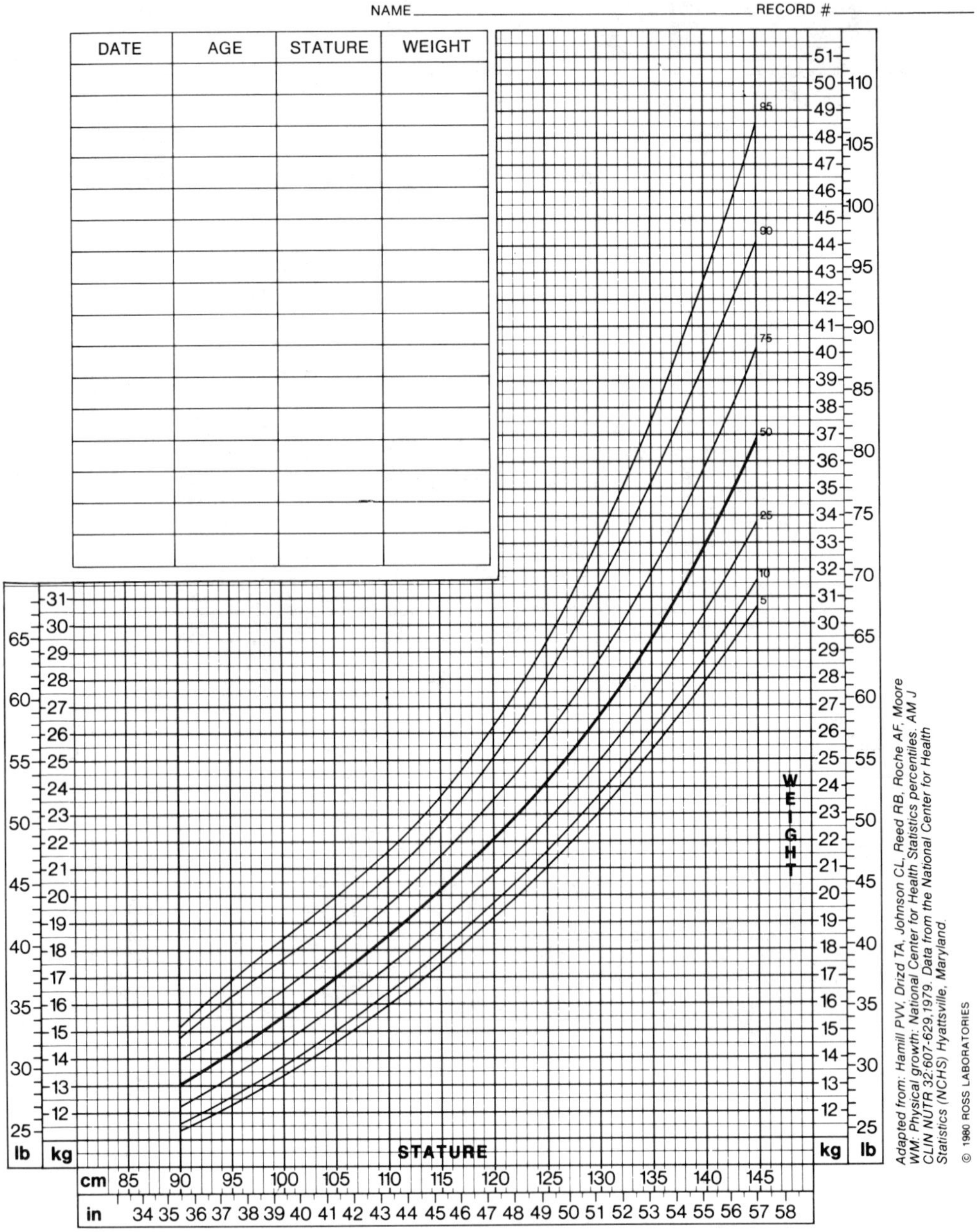

FIG. A–8. Prepubescent Boys: Physical Growth NCHS Percentiles.

TABLE A–4. Table of Desirable Weights, with Three Frame Categories

women 25 years of age and over

HEIGHT WITH SHOES ON (2-INCH HEELS)		SMALL FRAME	MEDIUM FRAME	LARGE FRAME
4 ft.	10 in.	92–98	96–107	104–119
4	11	94–101	98–110	106–122
5	0	96–104	101–113	109–125
5	1	99–107	104–116	112–128
5	2	102–110	107–119	115–131
5	3	105–113	110–122	118–134
5	4	108–116	113–126	121–138
5	5	111–119	116–130	125–142
5	6	114–123	120–135	129–146
5	7	118–127	124–139	133–150
5	8	122–131	128–143	137–154
5	9	126–135	132–147	141–158
5	10	130–140	136–151	145–163
5	11	134–144	140–155	149–168
6	0	138–148	144–159	153–173

men 25 years of age and over

HEIGHT WITH SHOES ON (1-INCH HEELS)		SMALL FRAME	MEDIUM FRAME	LARGE FRAME
5 ft.	2 in.	112–120	118–129	126–141
5	3	115–123	121–133	129–144
5	4	118–126	124–136	132–148
5	5	121–129	127–139	135–152
5	6	124–133	130–143	138–156
5	7	128–137	134–147	142–161
5	8	132–141	138–152	147–166
5	9	136–145	142–156	151–170
5	10	140–150	146–160	155–174
5	11	144–154	150–165	159–179
6	0	148–158	154–170	164–184
6	1	152–162	158–175	168–189
6	2	156–167	162–180	173–194
6	3	160–171	167–185	178–199
6	4	164–175	172–190	182–204

NOTE: Courtesy Metropolitan Life Insurance Co., Four Steps to Weight Control, 1969. Based on 1959 Build and blood pressure study. Weight in pounds, according to frame (in indoor clothing).

TABLE A–4a. Table of Desirable Weights with Three Frame Categories

HEIGHT	SMALL FRAME	MEDIUM FRAME	LARGE FRAME
	women—weight in kg		
147	41.8–44.55	43.6–48.6	47.5–54.0
150	42.7–45.9	44.5–50.0	48.2–55.4
152	43.6–47.3	45.9–51.4	49.5–56.8
155	45.0–48.6	47.3–52.7	50.0–58.2
157	46.4–50.0	48.6–54.1	52.3–59.5
160	47.7–51.4	50.0–55.4	53.6–60.7
163	49.1–52.7	51.4–57.3	55.0–62.7
165	50.5–54.1	52.7–59.0	56.8–64.5
168	51.8–55.9	54.5–61.4	58.6–66.4
170	53.6–57.7	56.4–63.2	60.4–68.2
172	55.4–59.5	58.2–65.0	62.3–70.0
175	57.3–61.4	60.0–66.8	64.1–71.8
178	59.1–63.3	61.8–68.6	65.9–74.1
180	60.9–65.4	63.6–70.4	67.7–76.4
183	67.2–67.3	65.4–72.3	69.5–78.6
	men—weight in kg in indoor clothing		
157	50.9–54.5	53.6–58.6	57.3–64.0
160	52.3–55.9	55.0–60.4	58.6–65.4
163	53.6–57.3	56.4–61.8	60.0–67.3
165	55.0–58.6	57.7–63.2	61.4–69.0
168	56.4–60.4	59.0–65.0	62.7–70.9
170	58.2–62.3	60.9–66.8	64.5–73.2
172	60.0–64.0	62.7–69.0	66.8–75.4
175	61.8–65.9	64.5–70.9	68.6–77.3
178	63.6–68.2	66.3–72.7	70.4–79.0
180	65.4–70.0	68.1–75.0	72.3–81.4
183	67.3–71.8	70.0–77.3	74.5–83.6
185	69.0–73.6	71.8–79.5	76.4–85.9
188	70.9–75.9	73.6–81.8	78.6–88.2
190	72.9–77.7	75.9–84.1	80.9–90.4
193	74.5–79.5	77.7–86.4	82.7–92.7

NOTE: Conversion to metric from Metropolitan Life Insurance Co.

TABLE A-5. Food Sources of Nutrients, Standards for Dietary Intake, and Classification Guidelines and Methodology for Biochemical Determinations

Food sources of selected nutrients, functions, and problems associated with nutrient deficiency

nutrient	major function	problems associated with deficiency	major food sources
Calories	Supply energy for growth and development, basal metabolism, and physical activity.	Inadequate caloric intake in children is evidenced by lack of growth and energy, loss of weight in all age groups.	All foods. Starchy, sweet, and fat foods are concentrated sources.
Protein	Essential for normal growth and development; for maintenance and repair of all body tissue.	A severe or prolonged deficiency results in retarded growth; symptoms may include edema, lassitude, and decreased resistance to infections.	Eggs, milk and milk products, meats, fish, poultry, soybeans, dry beans, peas, and nuts.
Vitamin A	Essential for the maintenance of healthy skin and mucous membranes, for normal night vision; aids in maintaining resistance to infections.	Deficiency signs: night blindness and skin changes characterized by dry, rough skin. Prolonged deficiency can lead to permanent blindness.	Liver, whole milk and whole milk products, and dark green leafy and deep yellow vegetables.
Vitamin C	Production of intercellular cementing substance; wound healing. Plays a role in normal resistance to infections.	Deficiency results in soft, spongy gums, prolonged wound healing, and in the advanced deficiency state, the classical disease scurvy.	Citrus fruits, tomatoes, strawberries, cantaloupe, raw cabbage, and green peppers.
Calcium	Necessary for formation of bones and teeth. Plays a role in blood coagulation and normal reactions of nerve and muscle tissue.	Deficiency in children may be associated with rickets; in adults, calcium may be lost from the bones (osteoporosis).	Milk and milk products, certain green leafy vegetables, oysters, clams, and shrimp.
Iron	Necessary for formation of hemoglobin, the oxygen-carrying pigment of red blood cells.	Weakness and fatigability. Advanced deficiency leads to anemia.	Liver and other organ meats, dark green leafy vegetables, dried fruits, whole grain and enriched cereals and cereal products, and molasses.

TABLE A–6. Guides for Nutritional Assessment of the Mentally Retarded and Developmentally Disabled

I. Anthropometric
   A. Purpose: To collect data related to growth and body composition
   B. Levels of assessment
      1. Minimal
         a. Weight[a]
            (1) Conditions: no shoes light clothing
            (2) Suggested standard: reference data assembled by National Center for Health Statistics
         b. Height[a]
            (1) Conditions: recumbent length[b]
            (2) Suggested standard: reference data assembled by National Center for Health Statistics
         c. Head circumference
            (1) Conditions: up to age 6 years
            (2) Suggested standard: reference data assembled by National Center for Health Statistics
      2. In-depth
         a. Skin fold: triceps and subscapular desirable[a]
            (1) Conditions: obtain duplicate readings
            (2) Suggested standard: reference data assembled by Fomon and National Center for Health Statistics
         b. Arm circumference[a]
            (1) Conditions: desirable, if possible
            (2) Suggested standard: Gurney and Jelliffe nomogram
   C. Equipment specification and maintenance
      1. Calibrated weight scale (balance-type)
      2. Measuring board (stadiometer) for measuring recumbent length or vertical surface with leveler for measuring standing height
      3. Narrow flexible steel or plastic coated tape measure for measuring circumference of head and arm
      4. Calibrated calipers

II. Clinical
   A. Purpose: To observe clinical signs of chronic or subacute disease
   B. Levels of assessment
      1. Minimal: review of past and present records of medical and dental examinations for signs suggestive of poor nutritional status
      2. In-depth
         a. Collection of health history with special attention to areas of nutritional risk, e.g.
            (1) Prenatal; pattern and total amount of maternal weight gain, complications of pregnancy, etc.
            (2) Postnatal; client or family history of diabetes, coronary heart disease, infections, anemia, constipation, diarrhea, hyperactivity, food intolerances, pica, inborn errors of metabolism, malabsorption syndromes, etc.
         b. Observation
            (1) General appearance
            (2) Speech
            (3) Oral hygiene
   C. Suggested standards
      1. Fomon
      2. Christakis
      3. Goldsmith

TABLE A-6. (Continued)

III. Biochemical
- A. Purpose: To obtain objective data related to present nutrition status or recent dietary intake
- B. Levels of assessment
  1. Minimal
     - a. Complete blood count
     - b. Routine urinalysis including microscopic
     - c. Semi-quantitative amino acid screening[c]
  2. In-depth
     - a. Serum total protein and albumin
     - b. Fasting blood glucose
     - c. Serum urea nitrogen
     - d. Transferrin saturation
     - e. Organic acids as primary screening for metabolic disorders
     - f. Quantitative urinary and plasma amino acid screening
  3. Other tests to respond to special conditions or problems (examples only)

Condition/problem	Tests[d]
a. anticonvulsants	Folic acid, ascorbic acid, calcium, vitamin D, alkaline phosphatase, phosphorus, vitamin B_6
b. Prader-Willi Syndrome	Glucose tolerance test
c. Pica	Lead, hemoglobin

- C. Suggested standards
  1. Foman
  2. Christakis

IV. Dietary
- A. Purpose: To determine a usual dietary pattern and/or nutrient intake
- B. Criteria for dietary assessment
  1. Family income
  2. Mechanical feeding problems
  3. Growth deviations
  4. Age
  5. Specific nutritional disorders or inborn errors of metabolism
  6. Feeding behavior problems
  7. Response to parents' or other professionals' concerns
- C. Levels of assessment
  1. Minimal
     - a. Twenty-four hour recall using food models and/or measures and food frequency with verbal questioning
     - b. Feeding history questionnaire to include parents' concerns regarding nutrition status
  2. In-depth
     - a. Three-day dietary intake kept by parent
       - (1) Verbal instruction in dietary record keeping
       - (2) Kept during two week days and week-end day
       - (3) Dietary supplements and/or medications included
       - (4) Occurrences affecting validity recorded, i.e., illness or holidays
       - (5) Quantity, preparation and brand names of food included
       - (6) Where, when and with whom client eats included

TABLE A-6. (Continued)

IV. Dietary (Continued)

- C. Levels of assessment (continued)
  - 2. In-depth (continued)
    - b. Activity record (as needed)
    - c. Pertinent historical information related to feeding
    - d. Present influences on dietary intake
  - 3. Other

    Certain conditions (i.e., inborn errors of metabolism or syndromes) may require further dietary investigation necessitating more detailed data collection
- D. Suggested standards
  - 1. Recommended Dietary Allowances
  - 2. Fomon
  - 3. FAO

V. Behavioral and Feeding Skill Development

- A. Purpose: To determine the influence of level of feeding development and behavior on nutritional status
- B. Levels of assessment
  - 1. Minimal
    - a. Parental perception of feeding skills and behavior
    - b. Professional perception of feeding skills and behavior
  - 2. In-depth
    - a. Review of past history and interview to determine feeding skill development and present level of functioning
    - b. Observations[e]
      - (1) Physical
        - (a) Oral structure and function including primitive reflexes, sucking, swallowing, biting, chewing, occlusion and caries
        - (b) Neuromuscular development including gross and fine motor skills, head and trunk control, eye-hand coordination and position for feeding
      - (2) Behavioral
        - (a) Parent (care-giver)-child interaction
        - (b) Reinforcement patterns (positive and negative)
        - (c) Environmental influences
- C. Suggested standards
  - 1. Gesell and Amatruda
  - 2. Vineland Social Maturity Scale

---

[a] Measurement to be made by well-trained, motivated personnel

[b] Standards for recumbent length for normal children are available only up to 2 years of age; however, this method yields more accurate measurement of physically handicapped children over 2 years, especially when they are unable to stand without support

[c] Screening with multiple Guthrie tests and/or thin layer chromatography or chomatography alone

[d] Professional judgment is warranted and a current search of literature should be done to determine appropriateness of tests before they are used

[e] Observations both at home and outside home with and without primary care-giver and/or conjoint professional assessments are valuable

SOURCE: Reprinted from M. H. S. Smith, *Guides for Nutritional Assessment of the Mentally Retarded and the Developmentally Disabled.* Child Development Center, University of Tennessee Center for the Health Sciences, Memphis, Tennessee and the Maternal and Child Health Service, Title V, Social Security Act, Bureau of Community Health Services, Health Services Administration, U.S. Department of Health, Education and Welfare, Rockville, Maryland, 1976.

TABLE A–7. Food Exchange Lists*

milk exchanges—list 1

One Exchange of Milk contains 12 gm of carbohydrate, 8 gm of protein, a trace of fat and 80 kcal.

NONFAT FORTIFIED MILK

Skim or nonfat milk†	1 cup
Powdered (nonfat dry, before adding liquid)	1/3 cup
Canned, evaporated skim milk	1/2 cup
Buttermilk made from skim milk	1 cup
Yogurt made from skim milk (plain, unflavored)	1 cup

Low-fat Fortified Milk

1% fat fortified milk (omit 1/2 Fat Exchange)	1 cup
2% fat fortified milk (omit 1 Fat Exchange)	1 cup
Yogurt made from 2% fortified milk (plain, unflavored) (omit 1 Fat Exchange)	1 cup

Whole Milk (Omit 2 Fat Exchanges)

Whole milk	1 cup
Canned, evaporated whole milk	1/2 cup
Buttermilk made from whole milk	1 cup
Yogurt made from whole milk (plain, unflavored)	1 cup

vegetable exchanges—list 2

One Exchange of Vegetables contains about 5 gm of carbohydrate, 2 gm of protein and 25 kcal. The list shows the kinds of vegetables to use for one Vegetable Exchange. One Exchange is 1/2 cup.

Asparagus
Bean sprouts
Beets
Broccoli
Brussels sprouts
Cabbage
Carrots
Cauliflower
Celery
Cucumbers
Eggplant
Green pepper
Beet Greens
Chard Greens
Collard Greens
Dandelion Greens
Kale Greens
Mustard Greens
Spinach Greens
Turnip Greens
Mushrooms
Okra
Onions
Rhubarb
Rutabaga
Sauerkraut
String beans, green/yellow
Summer squash
Tomatoes
Tomato juice
Turnips
Vegetable juice cocktail
Zucchini

The following raw vegetables may be used as desired:

Chicory
Chinese cabbage
Lettuce
Parsley

*The exchange lists are based on material in the *Exchange Lists for Meal Planning* prepared by Committees of the American Diabetes Association, Inc., and The American Dietetic Association in cooperation with the National Institute of Arthritis, Metabolism and Digestive Diseases and the National Heart and Lung Institute, National Institutes of Health, Public Health Service, U.S. Department of Health, Education and Welfare.

†**Bold Type indicates low-fat or nonfat item.** To plan a diet low in saturated fat and cholesterol, choose only those exchanges in **bold type.**

TABLE A–7. (Continued)

Endive	**Radishes**
Escarole	**Watercress**

Starchy vegetables are found in the Bread Exchange List.

fruit exchanges—list 3

One Exchange of Fruit contains 10 gm of carbohydrate and 40 kcal. The list shows the kinds and amounts of fruit to use for one Fruit Exchange.

Apple	1 small	**Mango**	1/2 small
Apple juice	1/3 cup	**Melon**	
Applesauce (unsweetened)	1/2 cup	**Cantaloupe**	1/4 small
Apricots, fresh	2 medium	**Honeydew**	1/8 medium
Apricots, dried	4 halves	**Watermelon**	1 cup
Banana	1/2 small	**Nectarine**	1 small
Berries		**Orange**	1 small
Blackberries	1/2 cup	**Orange juice**	1/2 cup
Blueberries	1/2 cup	**Papaya**	3/4 cup
Raspberries	1/2 cup	**Peach**	1 medium
Strawberries	3/4 cup	**Pear**	1 small
Cherries	10 large	**Persimmon, native**	1 medium
Cider	1/3 cup	**Pineapple**	1/2 cup
Dates	2	**Pineapple juice**	1/3 cup
Figs, fresh	1	**Plums**	2 medium
Figs, dried	1	**Prunes**	2 medium
Grapefruit	1/2	**Prune juice**	1/4 cup
Grapefruit juice	1/2 cup	**Raisins**	2 tbsp
Grapes	12	**Tangerine**	1 medium
Grape juice	1/4 cup		

Cranberries may be used as desired if no sugar is added.

bread exchanges—list 4

One Exchange of Bread contains 15 gm of carbohydrate, 2 gm of protein and 70 kcal. The list shows the kinds and amounts of breads, cereals, starchy vegetables and prepared foods to use for one Bread Exchange.

BREAD

White (including French & Italian)	1 slice
Whole wheat	1 slice
Rye or pumpernickel	1 slice
Raisin	1 slice
Bagel, small	1/2
English muffin, small	1/2
Plain roll, bread	1
Frankfurter roll	1/2
Hamburger bun	1/2
Dried bread crumbs	3 tbsp
Tortilla, 6″	1

CEREAL

Bran flakes	1/2 cup
Other ready-to-eat unsweetened cereal	3/4 cup
Puffed cereal (unfrosted)	1 cup
Cereal (cooked)	1/2 cup
Grits (cooked)	1/2 cup
Rice or barley (cooked)	1/2 cup
Pasta (cooked)	1/2 cup
Spaghetti, noodles, macaroni	
Popcorn (popped, no fat added)	3 cups
Cornmeal (dry)	2 tbsp
Flour	2 1/2 tbsp
Wheat germ	1/4 cup

bread exchanges—list 4 (continued)

CRACKERS

Arrowroot	3
Graham, 2 1/2″ sq.	2
Matzoth 4″ × 6″	1/2
Oyster	20
Pretzels, 3 1/8″ long × 1/8″ dia	25
Rye wafers, 2″ × 3 1/2″	3
Saltines	6
Soda, 2 1/2″ sq.	4

DRIED BEANS, PEAS AND LENTILS

Beans, peas, lentils (dried and cooked)	1/2 cup
Baked beans, no pork (canned)	1/4 cup

STARCHY VEGETABLES

Corn	1/3 cup
Corn on cob	1 small
Lima beans	1/2 cup
Parsnips	2/3 cup
Peas, green (canned or frozen)	1/2 cup
Potato, white	1 small
Potato (mashed)	1/2 cup
Pumpkin	3/4 cup
Winter squash, acorn or butternut	1/2 cup
Yam or sweet potato	1/4 cup

PREPARED FOODS

Biscuit 2″ dia (omit 1 Fat Exchange)	1
Corn bread, 2″ × 2″ × 1″ (omit 1 Fat Exchange)	1
Corn muffin, 2″ dia (omit 1 Fat Exchange)	1
Crackers, round butter type (omit 1 Fat Exchange)	5
Muffin, plain small (omit 1 Fat Exchange)	1
Potatoes, French fried, length 2″ to 3 1/2″ (omit 1 Fat Exchange)	8
Potato or corn chips (omit 2 Fat Exchanges)	15

Pancake, 5″ × 1/2″ (omit 1 Fat Exchange)	1
Waffle, 5″ × 1/2″ (omit 1 Fat Exchange)	1

meat exchanges lean meat—list 5

One Exchange of Lean Meat (1 oz) contains 7 gm of protein, 3 gm of fat and 55 kcal. This list shows the kinds and amounts of lean meat and other protein-rich foods to use for one low-fat Meat Exchange.

Beef: Baby beef (very lean, chipped beef, chuck, flank steak, tenderloin, plate ribs, plate skirt steak, round (bottom, top), all cuts rump, spare ribs, tripe	1 oz
Lamb: Leg, rib, sirloin, loin (roast and chops), shank, shoulder	1 oz
Pork: Leg (whole rump, center shank), ham, smoked (center slices)	1 oz
Veal: Leg, loin, rib, shank, shoulder, cutlets	1 oz
Poultry: Meat without skin of chicken, turkey, Cornish hen, guinea hen, pheasant	1 oz
Fish: Any fresh or frozen	1 oz
Canned salmon, tuna, mackerel, crab and lobster	1/4 cup
Clams, oysters, scallops, shrimp	5 or 1 oz
Sardines, drained	3
Cheeses containing less than 5% butterfat	1 oz
Cottage cheese, dry and 2% butterfat	1/4 cup
Dried beans and peas (omit 1 Bread Exchange)	1/2 cup

meat exchanges medium-fat meat

For each Exchange of Medium-fat Meat omit 1/2 Fat Exchange. The list shows the kinds and amounts of medium-fat meat and other protein-rich foods to use for one medium-fat Meat Exchange.

Beef: Ground (15% fat), corned beef (canned), rib eye, round (ground commercial)	1 oz
Pork: Loin (all cuts tenderloin), shoulder arm (picnic), shoulder blade, Boston butt, Canadian bacon, boiled ham	1 oz
Liver, heart, kidney and sweetbreads (these are high in cholesterol)	1 oz
Cottage cheese, creamed	1/4 cup
Cheese: Mozzarella, ricotta, farmer's cheese, Neufchatel,	1 oz
Parmesan	3 tbsp
Egg (high in cholesterol)	1
Peanut butter (omit 2 additional Fat Exchanges)	2 tbsp

meat exchanges high-fat meat

For each Exchange of High-fat Meat omit 1 Fat Exchange. This list shows the kinds and amounts of high-fat meat and other protein-rich foods to use for one High-fat Meat Exchange.

Beef: Brisket, corned beef (brisket), ground beef (more than 20% fat), hamburger (commercial), chuck (ground commercial), roasts (rib), steaks (club and rib)	1 oz
Lamb: Breast	1 oz
Pork: Spare ribs, loin (back ribs), pork (ground), country-style ham, deviled ham	1 oz
Veal: Breast	1 oz
Poultry: Capon, duck (domestic), goose	1 oz
Cheese: Cheddar types	1 oz
Cold Cuts:	4 1/2″ × 1/8″ slice
Frankfurter:	1 small

fat exchanges—list 6‡

One Exchange of Fat contains 5 gm of fat and 45 kcal. This list shows the kinds and amounts of fat-containing foods to use for one Fat Exchange.

Margarine, soft, tub or stick[a]	1 tsp
Avocado (4″ dia)	1/8
Oil, corn, cottonseed, safflower, soy, sunflower	1 tsp
Oil, olive[b]	1 tsp
Oil, peanut[b]	1 tsp
Olives[b]	5 small
Almonds[b]	10 whole
Pecans[b]	2 large whole
Peanuts[b]	
Spanish	20 whole
Virginia	10 whole
Walnuts	6 small
Nuts, other[b]	6 small
Margarine, regular stick	1 tsp
Butter	1 tsp
Bacon fat	1 tsp
Bacon, crisp	1 strip
Cream, light	2 tbsp
Cream, sour	2 tbsp
Cream, heavy	1 tbsp
Cream cheese	1 tbsp
French dressing[c]	1 tbsp
Italian dressing[c]	1 tbsp
Lard	1 tsp
Mayonnaise[c]	1 tsp
Salad dressing, mayonnaise type[c]	2 tsp
Salt pork	3/4″ cube

[a] Made with corn, cottonseed, safflower, soy or sunflower oil only.

[b] Fat content is primarily monounsaturated.

[c] If made with corn, cottonseed, safflower, soy or sunflower oil can be used on fat-modified diet.

‡ To plan a diet low in saturated fat select only those Exchanges which appear in **bold type**; they are polyunsaturated.

TABLE A–8. Diet Exchanges for a Vegetarian Diet*

list 1—milk exchanges

Kefir	1 cup (omit 2 Fat Exchanges)
Soy milk (fortified)	1 cup (add 1/2 Bread Exchange)

list 2—vegetable exchanges

Bamboo shoots	3/4 cup
Bean sprouts: raw or cooked	
Alfalfa	1 cup
Mung	1 cup
Soy	1 cup
Water chestnuts	4

list 3—fruit exchanges

Carrot juice	1/2 cup

list 4—bread exchanges

Brown rice (cooked)	1/3 cup
Buckwheat flour (dark)	3 tbsp
Bulgur wheat	2 tbsp
Millet (cooked)	1/2 cup
Miso	3 tbsp
Oats, dry	1/4 cup
Pita (Syrian) bread	1/2 of a 2 1/2-oz loaf
Rye flour	3 tbsp
Wheat berries (cooked)	1/3 cup
Wild rice (cooked)	1/2 cup

list 5—"lean meat" exchanges†

Dried beans and peas	1/2 cup cooked
Black-eyed peas	(omit 1 Bread Exchange)
Broad beans	(omit 1 Bread Exchange)
Garbanzo	(omit 1 Bread Exchange)
Kidney	(omit 1 Bread Exchange)
Lentils	(omit 1 Bread Exchange)
Lima	(omit 1 Bread Exchange)
Mung	(omit 1 Bread Exchange)
Navy	(omit 1 Bread Exchange)
Pinto	(omit 1 Bread Exchange)
Soy flour	1/4 cup (omit 1/2 Bread Exchange)

"medium-fat meat" exchanges†

Cheeses:	
Camembert	1 oz
Edam	1 oz
Liederkranz	1 oz
Soybeans	1/3 cup
Tofu	2 1/2" × 2 3/4" × 1"

"high-fat meat" exchanges†

Cheeses:	
Blue, Roquefort	1 oz
Brick	1 oz
Gorgonzola	1 oz
Gouda	1 oz
Gruyere	1 oz
Limburger	1 oz
Muenster	1 oz
Parmesan	1 oz
Swiss	1 oz
Hummus	4 tbsp (omit 1 Bread Exchange)
Peanuts §	4 tbsp (omit 1/2 Bread and 2 Fat Exchanges)
Pignolia nuts §	6 tbsp (omit 1/2 Vegetable and 1 Fat Exchange)
Pumpkin seeds §	4 tbsp (omit 1/2 Bread and 1 1/2 Fat Exchanges)
Sesame seeds §	4 tbsp (omit 1/2 Bread and 2 Fat Exchanges)
Sunflower seeds §	4 tbsp (omit 1/2 Bread and 2 Fat Exchanges)

list 6—fat exchanges

Tahini	1 tsp

Foods containing complementary proteins may be eaten together, thereby increasing protein quality. Examples of foods that may be complemented to yield high-quality protein are listed below.

Food	*Complementary Protein*
Grains	Combine rice with: cheese, legumes, sesame
	Combine wheat with: legumes, peanuts and milk, sesame and soybean
	Combine corn with: legumes
Legumes	Combine beans with: wheat, corn
	Combine soybeans with: rice and wheat, corn and milk, wheat and sesame, peanuts and sesame, peanuts and wheat and rice
Nuts and Seeds	Combine sesame with: beans, peanuts and soybeans, soybeans and wheat
	Combine peanuts with: sunflower seeds

diet patterns

LACTO-OVOVEGETARIAN

Calories: 1500
CH_2O—190 gm 50%
Pro—75 gm 20%
Fat—47 gm 30%

daily food allowance

3 Skim Milk Exchanges
2 Vegetable Exchanges
4 Fruit Exchanges
7 Bread Exchanges

STRICT VEGETARIAN

Calories: 1500
CH_2O—190 gm 50%
Pro—75 gm 20%
Fat—47 gm 30%

daily food allowance

3 Soybean Milk Exchanges (Note: Add 1/2 bread for each cup)
2 Vegetable Exchanges
4 Fruit Exchanges
7 Bread Exchanges

TABLE A-8. (Continued)

4 "Lean-meat" Exchanges	4 "Lean-meat" Exchanges
1 "Medium-fat Meat" Exchange	1 "Medium-fat Meat" Exchange
6 Fat Exchanges	6 Fat Exchanges
Meal Pattern	Meal Pattern
breakfast	breakfast
1 Fruit Exchange	1 Fruit Exchange
2 Bread Exchanges	2 Bread Exchanges
1 "Medium-fat Meat" Exchange	1 "Medium-fat Meat" Exchange
2 Fat Exchanges	2 Fat Exchanges
1 Skim Milk Exchange	1 Milk Exchange
lunch	lunch
2 "Lean-meat" Exchanges	2 "Lean-meat" Exchanges
2 Bread Exchanges	2 Bread Exchanges
1 Vegetable Exchange	1 Vegetable Exchange
2 Fruit Exchanges	2 Fruit Exchanges
2 Fat Exchanges	2 Fat Exchanges
dinner	dinner
2 "Lean-meat" Exchanges	2 "Lean-meat" Exchanges
2 Bread Exchanges	2 Bread Exchanges
1 Vegetable Exchange	1 Vegetable Exchange
1 Fruit Exchange	1 Fruit Exchange
2 Fat Exchanges	2 Fat Exchanges
1 Skim Milk Exchange	1 Milk Exchange
bedtime snack	bedtime snack
1 Skim Milk Exchange	1 Milk Exchange
1 Bread Exchange	1 Bread Exchange

guidelines for the professional

You may want to revise the patient's meal plan to allow more calories from carbohydrate (50 to 60 per cent) because of the high consumption of complex carbohydrates by vegetarians.

Many vegetarians use butter instead of margarine because it is considered a natural food.

The commercial meat analogs are very high in sodium, ranging in values from 300 mg to 3000 mg per 100 gm edible portion. Nutritional analyses of these products are available upon request from Loma Linda Foods, Riverside, California 92505, and Worthington Foods, Miles Laboratories, Worthington, Ohio 43085.

Some vegetarians use diet supplements such as wheat germ and brewer's yeast. Include these in the diet as follows:

Brewer's yeast, powder: 1 level tbsp = 1/2 "Lean-meat" Exchange
Wheat germ: 1/4 cup = 1 Bread Exchange

Vegetarian diets, unless fortified, could be deficient in iron. Iron absorption is enhanced by the inclusion of a vitamin C-rich food at each meal.

TABLE A–8. (Continued)

Vegetarian diets excluding dairy products may be inadequate in riboflavin and calcium. Two cups daily of fortified soybean milk or appropriate supplements should prevent deficiency.

For the strict vegetarian, vitamin B_{12} is also required as a vitamin supplement if 2 cups of fortified soybean milk are not consumed daily.

suggested reading for vegetarians

1. Lappe: *Diet for a Small Planet.* New York, Ballantine Books, 1975.
2. Robertson, Flinders and Godfrey: *Laurel's Kitchen, A Handbook for Vegetarian Cookery and Nutrition.* Berkeley, Nilgiri Press, 1976.
3. National Academy of Sciences, National Research Council, Food and Nutrition Board. Committee on Nutritional Misinformation, Vegetarian Diets. J. Am. Diet. Assoc., *65,* 121, 1974.
4. Williams: Making vegetarian diets nutritious. Am. J. Nurs., *75,* 12, 1975.
5. Erhard: The new vegetarians, Part 1. Vegetarianism and its medical consequences. Nutr. Today, *8,* 4, 1973. Part 2. The Zen macrobiotic movement and other cults based on vegetarianism. Nutr. Today, *9,* 20, 1974.
6. Beckner, et al.: *Diet Manual Utilizing a Vegetarian Diet Plan.* Loma Linda, The Seventh Day Adventist Dietetic Association, 1975.
7. Smith: A guide to good eating the vegetarian way. J. Nutr. Educ., *7,* 109, 1975.

* Supplement to Exchange Lists for Meal Planning Vegetarian Cookery. American Diabetes Association, Washington, D.C. Area Affiliate, Inc., Food and Nutrition Committee, 1978. See Table A–7 for Standard Exchange lists.

† Meat analogs: Vegetable protein foods which closely duplicate the flavor, texture and appearance of meat—"meatless" meats. See company information in the Guidelines for the Professional given below.

§ Seeds and nuts can be considered a "High-fat Meat" exchange and a complete protein only when they are complemented.

TABLE A–9. Nutritive Values of the Edible Part of Foods

Item No. (a)	Foods, Approximate Measures, Units, and Weight (edible part unless footnotes indicate otherwise) (b)			Water (c)	Food Energy (d)	Protein (e)	Fat (f)	Fatty Acids: Saturated (total) (g)	Fatty Acids: Unsaturated: Oleic (h)	Fatty Acids: Unsaturated: Linoleic (i)	Carbohydrate (j)	Calcium (k)	Phosphorus (l)	Iron (m)	Potassium (n)	Vitamin A Value (o)	Thiamin (p)	Riboflavin (q)	Niacin (r)	Ascorbic Acid (s)
			grams	per-cent	Cal-ories	grams	grams	grams	grams	grams	grams	milli-grams	milli-grams	milli-grams	milli-grams	inter-national units	milli-grams	milli-grams	milli-grams	milli-grams
	dairy products (cheese, cream, imitation cream, milk; related products)																			
	Butter. See Fats, oils; related products, items 103–108.																			
	Cheese:																			
	Natural:																			
1	Blue	1 oz	28	42	100	6	8	5.3	1.9	0.2	1	150	110	0.1	73	200	0.01	0.11	0.3	0
2	Camembert (3 wedges per 4-oz container).	1 wedge	38	52	115	8	9	5.8	2.2	0.2	Tr	147	132	0.1	71	350	0.01	0.19	0.2	0
	Cheddar:																			
3	Cut pieces	1 oz	28	37	115	7	9	6.1	2.1	0.2	Tr	204	145	0.2	28	300	0.01	0.11	Tr	0
4		1 cu in	17.2	37	70	4	6	3.7	1.3	0.1	Tr	124	88	0.1	17	180	Tr	0.06	Tr	0
5	Shredded	1 cup	113	37	455	28	37	24.2	8.5	0.7	1	815	579	0.8	111	1,200	0.03	0.42	0.1	0
	Cottage (curd not pressed down):																			
	Creamed (cottage cheese, 4% fat):																			
6	Large curd	1 cup	225	79	235	28	10	6.4	2.4	0.2	6	135	297	0.3	190	370	0.05	0.37	0.3	Tr
7	Small curd	1 cup	210	79	220	26	9	6.0	2.2	0.2	6	126	277	0.3	177	340	0.04	0.34	0.3	Tr
8	Low fat (2%)	1 cup	226	79	205	31	4	2.8	1.0	0.1	8	155	340	0.4	217	160	0.05	0.42	0.3	Tr
9	Low fat (1%)	1 cup	226	82	165	28	2	1.5	0.5	0.1	6	138	302	0.3	193	80	0.05	0.37	0.3	Tr
10	Uncreamed (cottage cheese dry curd, less than 1/2% fat).	1 cup	145	80	125	25	1	0.4	0.1	Tr	3	46	151	0.3	47	40	0.04	0.21	0.2	0
11	Cream	1 oz	28	54	100	2	10	6.2	2.4	0.2	1	23	30	0.3	34	400	Tr	0.06	Tr	0
	Mozzarella, made with–																			
12	Whole milk	1 oz	28	48	90	6	7	4.4	1.7	0.2	1	163	117	0.1	21	260	Tr	0.08	Tr	0
13	Part skim milk	1 oz	28	49	80	8	5	3.1	1.2	0.1	1	207	149	0.1	27	180	0.01	0.10	Tr	0
	Parmesan, grated:																			
14	Cup, not pressed down	1 cup	100	18	455	42	30	19.1	7.7	0.3	4	1,376	807	1.0	107	700	0.05	0.39	0.3	0

Nutrients in indicated quantity (columns c–s).

TABLE A–9. (Continued)

Item No. (a)	Foods, Approximate Measures, Units, and Weight (edible part unless footnotes indicate otherwise) (b)			Water (c)	Food Energy (d)	Protein (e)	Fat (f)	Fatty Acids: Saturated (total) (g)	Fatty Acids: Unsaturated: Oleic (h)	Fatty Acids: Unsaturated: Linoleic (i)	Carbohydrate (j)	Calcium (k)	Phosphorus (l)	Iron (m)	Potassium (n)	Vitamin A Value (o)	Thiamin (p)	Riboflavin (q)	Niacin (r)	Ascorbic Acid (s)
			grams	per-cent	Cal-ories	grams	grams	grams	grams	grams	grams	milli-grams	milli-grams	milli-grams	milli-grams	inter-national units	milli-grams	milli-grams	milli-grams	milli-grams
15	Tablespoon	1 tbsp	5	18	25	2	2	1.0	0.4	Tr	Tr	69	40	Tr	5	40	Tr	0.02	Tr	0
16	Ounce	1 oz	28	18	130	12	9	5.4	2.2	0.1	1	390	229	0.3	30	200	0.01	0.11	0.1	0
17	Provolone	1 oz	28	41	100	7	8	4.8	1.7	0.1	1	214	141	0.1	39	230	0.01	0.09	Tr	0
	Ricotta, made with–																			
18	Whole milk	1 cup	246	72	1,790	28	32	20.4	7.1	0.7	7	509	389	0.9	257	1,210	0.03	0.48	0.3	0
19	Part skim milk	1 cup	246	74	340	28	19	12.1	4.7	0.5	13	669	449	1.1	308	1,060	0.05	0.46	0.2	0
20	Romano	1 oz	28	31	110	9	8	—	—	—	1	302	215	—	—	160	—	0.11	Tr	0
21	Swiss	1 oz	28	37	105	8	8	5.0	1.7	0.2	1	272	171	Tr	31	240	0.01	0.10	Tr	0
	Pasteurized process cheese:																			
22	American	1 oz	28	39	105	6	9	5.6	2.1	0.2	Tr	174	211	0.1	46	340	0.01	0.10	Tr	0
23	Swiss	1 oz	28	42	95	7	7	4.5	1.7	0.1	1	219	216	0.2	61	230	Tr	0.08	Tr	0
24	Pasteurized process cheese food, American.	1 oz	28	43	95	6	7	4.4	1.7	0.1	2	163	130	0.2	79	260	0.01	0.13	Tr	0
25	Pasteurized process cheese spread, American.	1 oz	28	48	82	5	6	3.8	1.5	0.1	2	159	202	0.1	69	220	0.01	0.12	Tr	0
	Cream, sweet:																			
26	Half-and-half (cream and	1 cup	242	81	315	7	28	17.3	7.0	0.6	10	254	230	0.2	314	260	0.08	0.36	0.2	2
27	milk)–	1 tbsp	15	81	20	Tr	2	1.1	0.4	Tr	1	16	14	Tr	19	20	0.01	0.02	Tr	Tr
28	Light, coffee, or table	1 cup	240	74	470	6	46	28.8	11.7	1.0	9	231	192	0.1	292	1,730	0.08	0.36	0.1	2
29		1 tbsp	15	74	30	Tr	3	1.8	0.7	0.1	1	14	12	Tr	18	110	Tr	0.02	Tr	Tr
	Whipping, unwhipped (volume about double when whipped):																			
30	Light	1 cup	239	64	700	5	74	46.2	18.3	1.5	7	166	146	0.1	231	2,690	0.06	0.30	0.1	1
31		1 tbsp	15	64	45	Tr	5	2.9	1.1	0.1	Tr	10	9	Tr	15	170	Tr	0.02	Tr	Tr
32	Heavy	1 cup	238	58	820	5	88	54.8	22.2	2.0	7	154	149	0.1	179	3,500	0.05	0.26	0.1	1
33		1 tbsp	15	58	80	Tr	6	3.5	1.4	0.1	Tr	10	9	Tr	11	220	Tr	0.02	Tr	Tr
34	Whipped topping,	1 cup	60	61	155	2	13	8.3	3.4	0.3	7	61	54	Tr	88	550	0.02	0.04	Tr	0
35	(pressurized)–	1 tbsp	3	61	10	Tr	1	0.4	0.2	Tr	Tr	3	3	Tr	4	30	Tr	Tr	Tr	0
36	Cream, sour	1 cup	230	71	495	7	48	30.0	12.1	1.1	10	268	195	0.1	331	1,820	0.08	0.34	0.2	2
37		1 tbsp	12	71	25	Tr	3	1.6	0.6	0.1	1	14	10	Tr	17	90	Tr	0.02	Tr	Tr

Columns (c) through (s): nutrients in indicated quantity

TABLE A-9. (Continued)

Item No. (a)	Foods, Approximate Measures, Units, and Weight (edible part unless footnotes indicate otherwise) (b)			Water (c)	Food Energy (d)	Protein (e)	Fat (f)	Fatty Acids: Saturated (total) (g)	Fatty Acids: Unsaturated: Oleic (h)	Fatty Acids: Unsaturated: Linoleic (i)	Carbohydrate (j)	Calcium (k)	Phosphorus (l)	Iron (m)	Potassium (n)	Vitamin A Value (o)	Thiamin (p)	Riboflavin (q)	Niacin (r)	Ascorbic Acid (s)
			grams	per-cent	Cal-ories	grams	grams	grams	grams	grams	grams	milli-grams	milli-grams	milli-grams	milli-grams	inter-national units	milli-grams	milli-grams	milli-grams	milli-grams
	Cream products, imitation (made with vegetable fat):																			
	Sweet:																			
	Creamers:																			
38	Liquid (frozen)	1 cup	245	77	335	2	24	22.8	0.3	Tr	28	23	157	0.1	467	220[1]	0	0	0	0
39		1 tbsp	15	77	20	Tr	1	1.4	Tr	0	2	1	10	Tr	29	10[1]	0	0	0	0
40	Powdered	1 cup	94	2	515	5	33	30.6	0.9	Tr	52	21	397	0.1	763	190[1]	0	0.16[1]	0	0
41		1 tsp	2	2	10	Tr	1	0.7	Tr	0	1	Tr	8	Tr	16	Tr[1]	0	Tr[1]	0	0
	Whipped topping:																			
42	Frozen	1 cup	75	50	240	1	19	16.3	1.0	0.2	17	5	6	0.1	14	650[1]	0	0	0	0
43		1 tbsp	4	50	15	Tr	1	0.9	0.1	Tr	1	Tr	Tr	Tr	1	30[1]	0	0	0	0
44	Powdered, made with	1 cup	80	67	150	3	10	8.5	0.6	0.1	13	72	69	Tr	121	290[1]	0.02	0.09	Tr	1
45	whole milk.	1 tbsp	4	67	10	Tr	Tr	0.4	Tr	Tr	1	4	3	Tr	6	10[1]	Tr	Tr	Tr	Tr
46	Pressurized	1 cup	70	60	185	1	16	13.2	1.4	0.2	11	4	13	Tr	13	330[1]	0	0	0	0
47		1 tbsp	4	60	10	Tr	1	0.8	0.1	Tr	1	Tr	1	Tr	1	20[1]	0	0	0	0
48	Sour dressing (imitation sour cream) made with	1 cup	235	75	415	8	39	31.2	4.4	1.1	11	266	205	0.1	380	20[1]	0.09	0.38	0.2	2
49	nonfat dry milk.	1 tbsp	12	75	20	Tr	2	1.6	0.2	0.1	1	14	10	Tr	19	Tr[1]	0.01	0.02	Tr	Tr
	Ice cream. See Milk desserts, frozen (items 75–80).																			
	Ice milk. See Milk desserts, frozen (items 81–83).																			
	Milk:																			
	Fluid:																			
50	Whole (3.3% fat)	1 cup	244	88	150	8	8	5.1	2.1	0.2	11	291	228	0.1	370	310[2]	0.09	0.40	0.2	2
	Lowfat (2%):																			
51	No milk solids added	1 cup	244	89	120	8	5	2.9	1.2	0.1	12	297	232	0.1	377	500	0.10	0.40	0.2	2
	Milk solids added:																			
52	Label claim less than 10g of protein per cup.	1 cup	245	89	125	9	5	2.9	1.2	0.1	12	313	245	0.1	397	500	0.10	0.42	0.2	2

TABLE A-9. (Continued)

Item No. (a)	Foods, Approximate Measures, Units, and Weight (edible part unless footnotes indicate otherwise) (b)			Water (c)	Food Energy (d)	Protein (e)	Fat (f)	Fatty Acids: Saturated (total) (g)	Fatty Acids: Unsaturated: Oleic (h)	Fatty Acids: Unsaturated: Linoleic (i)	Carbohydrate (j)	Calcium (k)	Phosphorus (l)	Iron (m)	Potassium (n)	Vitamin A Value (o)	Thiamin (p)	Riboflavin (q)	Niacin (r)	Ascorbic Acid (s)
			grams	per-cent	Cal-ories	grams	grams	grams	grams	grams	grams	milli-grams	milli-grams	milli-grams	milli-grams	inter-national units	milli-grams	milli-grams	milli-grams	milli-grams
53	Label claim 10 or more grams of protein per cup (protein fortified).	1 cup	246	88	135	10	5	3.0	1.2	0.1	14	352	276	0.1	447	500	0.11	0.48	0.2	3
	Lowfat (1%):																			
54	No milk solids added	1 cup	244	90	100	8	3	1.6	0.7	0.1	12	300	235	0.1	381	500	0.10	0.41	0.2	2
	Milk solids added:																			
55	Label claim less than 10g of protein per cup.	1 cup	245	90	105	9	2	1.5	0.6	0.1	12	313	245	0.1	397	500	0.10	0.42	0.2	2
56	Label claim 10 or more grams of protein per cup (protein fortified)	1 cup	246	89	120	10	3	1.8	0.7	0.1	14	349	273	0.1	444	500	0.11	0.47	0.2	3
	Nonfat (skim):																			
57	No milk solids added	1 cup	245	91	85	8	Tr	0.3	0.1	Tr	12	302	247	0.1	406	500	0.09	0.37	0.2	2
	Milk solids added:																			
58	Label claim less than 10g of protein per cup.	1 cup	245	90	90	9	1	0.4	0.1	Tr	12	316	255	0.1	418	500	0.10	0.43	0.2	2
59	Label claim 10 or more grams of protein per cup (protein fortified).	1 cup	246	89	100	10	1	0.4	0.1	Tr	14	352	275	0.1	446	500	0.11	0.48	0.2	3
60	Buttermilk	1 cup	245	90	100	8	2	1.3	0.5	Tr	12	285	219	0.1	371	80[3]	0.08	0.38	0.1	2
	Canned:																			
	Evaporated, unsweetened:																			
61	Whole milk	1 cup	252	74	340	17	19	11.6	5.3	0.4	25	657	510	0.5	764	610[3]	0.12	0.80	0.5	5
62	Skim milk	1 cup	255	79	200	19	1	0.3	0.1	Tr	29	738	497	0.7	845	1,000[4]	0.11	0.79	0.4	3
63	Sweetened, condensed	1 cup	306	27	980	24	27	16.8	6.7	0.7	166	868	775	0.6	1,136	1,000[3]	0.28	1.27	0.6	8
	Dried:																			
64	Buttermilk	1 cup	120	3	465	41	7	4.3	1.7	0.2	59	1,421	1,119	0.4	1,910	260[3]	0.47	1.90	1.1	7
	Nonfat instant:																			
65	Envelope, net wt., 3.2 oz[5]	1 envelope	91	4	325	32	1	0.4	0.1	Tr	47	1,120	896	0.3	1,552	2,160[6]	0.38	1.59	0.8	5
66	Cup[7]	1 cup	68	4	245	24	Tr	0.3	0.1	Tr	35	837	670	0.2	1,160	1,610[6]	0.28	1.19	0.6	4

nutrients in indicated quantity

TABLE A-9. (Continued)

Item No. (a)	Foods, Approximate Measures, Units, and Weight (edible part unless footnotes indicate otherwise) (b)			Water (c)	Food Energy (d)	Protein (e)	Fat (f)	Fatty Acids: Saturated (total) (g)	Fatty Acids: Unsaturated: Oleic (h)	Fatty Acids: Unsaturated: Linoleic (i)	Carbohydrate (j)	Calcium (k)	Phosphorus (l)	Iron (m)	Potassium (n)	Vitamin A Value (o)	Thiamin (p)	Riboflavin (q)	Niacin (r)	Ascorbic Acid (s)
			grams	per-cent	Cal-ories	grams	grams	grams	grams	grams	grams	milli-grams	milli-grams	milli-grams	milli-grams	inter-national units	milli-grams	milli-grams	milli-grams	milli-grams
	Milk beverages:																			
	Chocolate milk (commercial):																			
67	Regular	1 cup	250	82	210	8	8	5.3	2.2	0.2	26	280	251	0.6	417	300[3]	0.09	0.41	0.3	2
68	Lowfat (2%)	1 cup	250	84	180	8	5	3.1	1.3	0.1	26	284	254	0.6	422	500	0.10	0.42	0.3	2
69	Lowfat (1%)	1 cup	250	85	160	8	3	1.5	0.7	0.1	26	287	257	0.6	426	500	0.10	0.40	0.2	2
70	Eggnog (commercial)	1 cup	254	74	340	10	19	11.3	5.0	0.6	34	330	278	0.5	420	890	0.09	0.48	0.3	4
	Malted milk, home-prepared with 1 cup of whole milk and 2 to 3 heaping tsp of malted milk powder (about 3/4 oz):																			
71	Chocolate	1 cup of milk plus 3/4 oz of powder.	265	81	235	9	9	5.5	—	—	29	304	265	0.5	500	330	0.14	0.43	0.7	2
72	Natural	1 cup of milk plus 3/4 oz of powder.	265	81	235	11	10	6.0	—	—	27	347	307	0.3	529	380	0.20	0.54	1.3	2
	Shakes, thick:[8]																			
73	Chocolate, container, net wt., 10.6 oz.	1 container	300	72	355	9	8	5.0	2.0	0.2	63	396	378	0.9	672	260	0.14	0.67	0.4	0
74	Vanilla, container, net wt., 11 oz.	1 container	313	74	350	12	9	5.9	2.4	0.2	56	457	361	0.3	572	360	0.09	0.61	0.5	0
	Milk desserts, frozen:																			
	Ice cream:																			
	Regular (about 11% fat):																			
75	Hardened	1/2 gal	1,064	61	2,155	38	115	71.3	28.8	2.6	254	1,406	1,075	1.0	2,052	4,340	0.42	2.63	1.1	6
76		1 cup	133	61	270	5	14	8.9	3.6	0.3	32	176	134	0.1	257	540	0.05	0.33	0.1	1
77		3-fl oz container	50	61	100	2	5	3.4	1.4	0.1	12	66	51	Tr	96	200	0.02	0.12	0.1	Tr
78	Soft serve (frozen custard)	1 cup	173	60	375	7	23	13.5	5.9	0.6	38	236	199	0.4	338	790	0.08	0.45	0.2	1
79	Rich (about 16% fat), hardened.	1/2 gal	1,188	59	2,805	33	190	118.3	47.8	4.3	256	1,213	927	0.8	1,771	7,200	0.36	2.27	0.9	5
80		1 cup	148	59	350	4	24	14.7	6.0	0.5	32	151	115	0.1	221	900	0.04	0.28	0.1	1

TABLE A–9. (Continued)

Item No. (a)	Foods, Approximate Measures, Units, and Weight (edible part unless footnotes indicate otherwise) (b)			Water (c)	Food Energy (d)	Protein (e)	Fat (f)	Fatty Acids: Saturated (total) (g)	Fatty Acids: Unsaturated: Oleic (h)	Fatty Acids: Unsaturated: Linoleic (i)	Carbohydrate (j)	Calcium (k)	Phosphorus (l)	Iron (m)	Potassium (n)	Vitamin A Value (o)	Thiamin (p)	Riboflavin (q)	Niacin (r)	Ascorbic Acid (s)
			grams	percent	Calories	grams	grams	grams	grams	grams	grams	milligrams	milligrams	milligrams	milligrams	international units	milligrams	milligrams	milligrams	milligrams
	Ice milk:																			
81	Hardened (about 4.3% fat)	1/2 gal	1,048	69	1,470	41	45	28.1	11.3	1.0	232	1,409	1,035	1.5	2,117	1,710	0.61	2.78	0.9	6
82		1 cup	131	69	185	5	6	3.5	1.4	0.1	29	176	129	0.1	265	210	0.08	0.35	0.1	1
83	Soft serve (about 2.6% fat)	1 cup	175	70	225	8	5	2.9	1.2	0.1	38	274	202	0.3	412	180	0.12	0.54	0.2	1
84	Sherbet (about 2% fat)	1/2 gal	1,542	66	2,160	17	31	19.0	7.7	0.7	469	827	594	2.5	1,585	1,480	0.26	0.71	1.0	31
85		1 cup	193	66	270	2	4	2.4	1.0	0.1	59	103	74	0.3	198	190	0.03	0.09	0.1	4
	Milk desserts, other:																			
86	Custard, baked	1 cup	265	77	305	14	15	6.8	5.4	0.7	29	297	310	1.1	387	930	0.11	0.50	0.3	1
	Puddings:																			
	From home recipe:																			
	Starch base:																			
87	Chocolate	1 cup	260	66	385	8	12	7.6	3.3	0.3	67	250	255	1.3	445	390	0.05	0.36	0.3	1
88	Vanilla (blancmange)	1 cup	255	76	285	9	10	6.2	2.5	0.2	41	298	232	Tr	352	410	0.08	0.41	0.3	2
89	Tapioca cream	1 cup	165	72	220	8	8	4.1	2.5	0.5	28	173	180	0.7	223	480	0.07	0.30	0.2	2
	From mix (chocolate) and milk:																			
90	Regular (cooked)	1 cup	260	70	320	9	8	4.3	2.6	0.2	59	265	247	0.8	354	340	0.05	0.39	0.3	2
91	Instant	1 cup	260	69	325	8	7	3.6	2.2	0.3	63	374	237	1.3	335	340	0.08	0.39	0.3	2
	Yogurt:																			
	With added milk solids:																			
	Made with lowfat milk:																			
92	Fruit-flavored[9]	1 container, net wt., 8 oz	227	75	230	10	3	1.8	0.6	0.1	42	343	269	0.2	439	120[10]	0.08	0.40	0.2	1
93	Plain	1 container, net wt., 8 oz	227	85	145	12	4	2.3	0.8	0.1	16	415	326	0.2	531	150[10]	0.10	0.49	0.3	2
94	Made with nonfat milk:	1 container, net wt., 8 oz	227	85	125	13	Tr	0.3	0.1	Tr	17	452	355	0.2	579	20[10]	0.11	0.53	0.3	2
	Without added milk solids:																			
95	Made with whole milk	1 container, net wt., 8 oz	227	88	140	8	7	4.8	1.7	0.1	11	274	215	0.1	351	280	0.07	0.32	0.2	1

TABLE A-9. (Continued)

Item No. (a)	Foods, Approximate Measures, Units, and Weight (edible part unless footnotes indicate otherwise) (b)			Water (c)	Food Energy (d)	Protein (e)	Fat (f)	Fatty Acids: Saturated (total) (g)	Fatty Acids: Unsaturated: Oleic (h)	Fatty Acids: Unsaturated: Linoleic (i)	Carbohydrate (j)	Calcium (k)	Phosphorus (l)	Iron (m)	Potassium (n)	Vitamin A Value (o)	Thiamin (p)	Riboflavin (q)	Niacin (r)	Ascorbic Acid (s)
			grams	percent	Calories	grams	grams	grams	grams	grams	grams	milligrams	milligrams	milligrams	milligrams	international units	milligrams	milligrams	milligrams	milligrams
	eggs																			
	Eggs, large (24 oz per dozen):																			
	Raw:																			
96	Whole, without shell	1 egg	50	75	80	6	6	1.7	2.0	0.6	1	28	90	1.0	65	260	0.04	0.15	Tr	0
97	White	1 white	33	88	15	3	Tr	0	0	0	Tr	4	4	Tr	45	0	Tr	0.09	Tr	0
98	Yolk	1 yolk	17	49	65	3	6	1.7	2.1	0.6	Tr	26	86	0.9	15	310	0.04	0.07	Tr	0
	Cooked:																			
99	Fried in butter	1 egg	46	72	85	5	6	2.4	2.2	0.6	1	26	80	0.9	58	290	0.03	0.13	Tr	0
100	Hard-cooked, shell removed	1 egg	50	75	80	6	6	1.7	2.0	0.6	1	28	90	1.0	65	260	0.04	0.14	Tr	0
101	Poached	1 egg	50	74	80	6	6	1.7	2.0	0.6	1	28	90	1.0	65	260	0.04	0.13	Tr	0
102	Scrambled (milk added) in butter. Also omelet.	1 egg	64	76	95	6	7	2.8	2.3	0.6	1	47	97	0.9	85	310	0.04	0.16	Tr	0
	fats, oils; related products																			
	Butter:																			
	Regular (1 brick or 4 sticks per lb):																			
103	Stick (1/2 cup)	1 stick	113	16	815	1	92	57.3	23.1	2.1	Tr	27	26	0.2	29	3,470[11]	0.01	0.04	Tr	0
104	Tablespoon (about 1/8 stick).	1 tbsp	14	16	100	Tr	12	7.2	2.9	0.3	Tr	3	3	Tr	4	430[11]	Tr	Tr	Tr	0
105	Pat (1 in. square, 1/3 in. high; 90 per lb).	1 pat	5	16	35	Tr	4	2.5	1.0	0.1	Tr	1	1	Tr	1	150[11]	Tr	Tr	Tr	0
	Whipped (6 sticks or two 8-oz containers per lb).																			
106	Stick (1/2 cup)	1 stick	76	16	540	1	61	38.2	15.4	1.4	Tr	18	17	0.1	20	2,310[11]	Tr	0.03	Tr	0
107	Tablespoon (about 1/8 stick).	1 tbsp	9	16	65	Tr	8	4.7	1.9	0.2	Tr	2	2	Tr	2	290[11]	Tr	Tr	Tr	0
108	Pat (1 1/4 in. square, 1/3 in. high; 120 per lb).	1 pat	4	16	25	Tr	3	1.9	0.8	0.1	Tr	1	1	Tr	1	120[11]	0	Tr	Tr	0
109	Fats, cooking (vegetable shortenings).	1 cup	200	0	1,770	0	200	48.8	88.2	48.4	0	0	0	0	0	—	0	0	0	0

TABLE A–9. (Continued)

Item No. (a)	Foods, Approximate Measures, Units, and Weight (edible part unless footnotes indicate otherwise) (b)			Water (c)	Food Energy (d)	Protein (e)	Fat (f)	Fatty Acids: Saturated (total) (g)	Fatty Acids: Unsaturated: Oleic (h)	Fatty Acids: Unsaturated: Linoleic (i)	Carbohydrate (j)	Calcium (k)	Phosphorus (l)	Iron (m)	Potassium (n)	Vitamin A Value (o)	Thiamin (p)	Riboflavin (q)	Niacin (r)	Ascorbic Acid (s)
			grams	percent	Calories	grams	grams	grams	grams	grams	grams	milligrams	milligrams	milligrams	milligrams	international units	milligrams	milligrams	milligrams	milligrams
110		1 tbsp	13	0	110	0	13	3.2	5.7	3.1	0	0	0	0	0	—	0	0	0	0
111	Lard	1 cup	205	0	1,850	0	205	81.0	83.8	20.5	0	0	0	0	0	0	0	0	0	0
112		1 tbsp	13	0	115	0	13	5.1	5.3	1.3	0	0	0	0	0	0	0	0	0	0
	Margarine:																			
	Regular (1 brick or 4 sticks per lb):																			
113	Stick (1/2 cup)	1 stick	113	16	815	1	92	16.7	42.9	24.9	Tr	27	26	0.2	29	3,750[12]	0.01	0.04	Tr	0
114	Tablespoon (about 1/8 stick).	1 tbsp	14	16	100	Tr	12	2.1	5.3	3.1	Tr	3	3	Tr	4	470[12]	Tr	Tr	Tr	0
115	Pat (1 in. square, 1/3 in. high; 90 per lb).	1 pat	5	16	35	Tr	4	0.7	1.9	1.1	Tr	1	1	Tr	1	170[12]	Tr	Tr	Tr	0
116	Soft, two 8-oz containers per lb.	1 container	227	16	1,635	1	184	32.5	71.5	65.4	Tr	53	52	0.4	59	7,500[12]	0.01	0.08	0.1	0
117		1 tbsp	14	16	100	Tr	12	2.0	4.5	4.1	Tr	3	3	Tr	4	470[12]	Tr	Tr	Tr	0
	Whipped (6 sticks per lb):																			
118	Stick (1/2 cup)	1 stick	76	16	545	Tr	61	11.2	28.7	16.7	Tr	18	17	0.1	20	2,500[12]	Tr	0.03	Tr	0
119	Tablespoon (about 1/8 stick)	1 tbsp	9	16	70	Tr	8	1.4	3.6	2.1	Tr	2	2	Tr	2	310[12]	Tr	Tr	Tr	0
	Oil, salad or cooking:																			
120	Corn	1 cup	218	0	1,925	0	218	27.7	53.6	125.1	0	0	0	0	0	—	0	0	0	0
121		1 tbsp	14	0	120	0	14	1.7	3.3	7.8	0	0	0	0	0	—	0	0	0	0
122	Olive	1 cup	216	0	1,910	0	216	30.7	154.4	17.7	0	0	0	0	0	—	0	0	0	0
123		1 tbsp	14	0	120	0	14	1.9	9.7	1.1	0	0	0	0	0	—	0	0	0	0
124	Peanut	1 cup	216	0	1,910	0	216	37.4	98.5	67.0	0	0	0	0	0	—	0	0	0	0
125		1 tbsp	14	0	120	0	14	2.3	6.2	4.2	0	0	0	0	0	—	0	0	0	0
126	Safflower	1 cup	218	0	1,925	0	218	20.5	25.9	159.8	0	0	0	0	0	—	0	0	0	0
127		1 tbsp	14	0	120	0	14	1.3	1.6	10.0	0	0	0	0	0	—	0	0	0	0
128	Soybean oil, hydrogenated (partially hardened).	1 cup	218	0	1,925	0	218	31.8	93.1	75.6	0	0	0	0	0	—	0	0	0	0
129		1 tbsp	14	0	120	0	14	2.0	5.8	4.7	0	0	0	0	0	—	0	0	0	0
130	Soybean-cottonseed oil blend, hydrogenated.	1 cup	218	0	1,925	0	218	38.2	63.0	99.6	0	0	0	0	0	—	0	0	0	0

nutrients in indicated quantity

TABLE A–9. (Continued)

Item No. (a)	Foods, Approximate Measures, Units, and Weight (edible part unless footnotes indicate otherwise) (b)			Water (c)	Food Energy (d)	Protein (e)	Fat (f)	Fatty Acids: Saturated (total) (g)	Fatty Acids: Unsaturated: Oleic (h)	Fatty Acids: Unsaturated: Linoleic (i)	Carbohydrate (j)	Calcium (k)	Phosphorus (l)	Iron (m)	Potassium (n)	Vitamin A Value (o)	Thiamin (p)	Riboflavin (q)	Niacin (r)	Ascorbic Acid (s)
			grams	per-cent	Cal-ories	grams	grams	grams	grams	grams	grams	milli-grams	milli-grams	milli-grams	milli-grams	inter-national units	milli-grams	milli-grams	milli-grams	milli-grams
131		1 tbsp	14	0	120	0	14	2.4	3.9	6.2	0	0	0	0	0	—	0	0	0	0
	Salad dressings:																			
	Commercial:																			
	Blue cheese:																			
132	Regular	1 tbsp	15	32	75	1	8	1.6	1.7	3.8	1	12	11	Tr	6	30	Tr	0.02	Tr	Tr
133	Low calorie (5 Cal per tsp)	1 tbsp	16	84	10	Tr	1	0.5	0.3	Tr	1	10	8	Tr	5	30	Tr	0.01	Tr	Tr
	French:																			
134	Regular	1 tbsp	16	39	65	Tr	6	1.1	1.3	3.2	3	2	2	0.1	13	—	—	—	—	—
135	Low calorie (5 Cal per tsp)	1 tbsp	16	77	15	Tr	1	0.1	0.1	0.4	2	2	2	0.1	13	—	—	—	—	—
	Italian:																			
136	Regular	1 tbsp	15	28	85	Tr	9	1.6	1.9	4.7	1	2	1	Tr	2	Tr	Tr	Tr	Tr	—
137	Low calorie (2 Cal per tsp)	1 tbsp	15	90	10	Tr	1	0.1	0.1	0.4	Tr	Tr	1	Tr	2	Tr	Tr	Tr	Tr	—
138	Mayonnaise	1 tbsp	14	15	100	Tr	11	2.0	2.4	5.6	Tr	3	4	0.1	5	40	Tr	0.01	Tr	—
	Mayonnaise type:																			
139	Regular	1 tbsp	15	41	65	Tr	6	1.1	1.4	3.2	2	2	4	Tr	1	30	Tr	Tr	Tr	—
140	Low calorie (8 Cal per tsp)	1 tbsp	16	81	20	Tr	2	0.4	0.4	1.0	2	3	4	Tr	1	40	Tr	Tr	Tr	—
141	Tartar sauce, regular	1 tbsp	14	34	75	Tr	8	1.5	1.8	4.1	1	3	4	0.1	11	30	Tr	Tr	Tr	Tr
	Thousand Island:																			
142	Regular	1 tbsp	16	32	80	Tr	8	1.4	1.7	4.0	2	2	3	0.1	18	50	Tr	Tr	Tr	Tr
143	Low calorie (10 Cal per tsp)	1 tbsp	15	68	25	Tr	2	0.4	0.4	1.0	2	2	3	0.1	17	50	Tr	Tr	Tr	Tr
	From home recipe:																			
144	Cooked type[13]	1 tbsp	16	68	25	1	2	0.5	0.6	0.3	2	14	15	0.1	19	80	0.01	0.03	Tr	Tr
	fish, shellfish, meat, poultry; related products																			
	Fish and shellfish:																			
145	Bluefish, baked with butter or margarine.	3 oz	85	68	135	22	4	—	—	—	0	25	244	0.6	—	40	0.09	0.08	1.6	—
	Clams:																			
146	Raw, meat only	3 oz	85	82	65	11	1	—	—	—	2	59	138	5.2	154	90	0.08	0.15	1.1	8
147	Canned, solids and liquid	3 oz	85	86	45	7	1	0.2	Tr	Tr	2	47	116	3.5	119	—	0.01	0.09	0.9	—

nutrients in indicated quantity

TABLE A-9. (Continued)

Item No. (a)	Foods, Approximate Measures, Units, and Weight (edible part unless footnotes indicate otherwise) (b)		Weight	Water (c)	Food Energy (d)	Protein (e)	Fat (f)	Fatty Acids: Saturated (total) (g)	Fatty Acids: Unsaturated: Oleic (h)	Fatty Acids: Unsaturated: Linoleic (i)	Carbohydrate (j)	Calcium (k)	Phosphorus (l)	Iron (m)	Potassium (n)	Vitamin A Value (o)	Thiamin (p)	Riboflavin (q)	Niacin (r)	Ascorbic Acid (s)
			grams	percent	Calories	grams	grams	grams	grams	grams	grams	milligrams	milligrams	milligrams	milligrams	international units	milligrams	milligrams	milligrams	milligrams
148	Crabmeat (white or king), canned, not pressed down.	1 cup	135	77	135	24	3	0.6	0.4	0.1	1	61	246	1.1	149	—	0.11	0.11	2.6	—
149	Fish sticks, breaded, cooked, frozen (stick, 4 by 1 by 1/2 in.).	1 fish stick or 1 oz	28	66	50	5	3	—	—	—	2	3	47	0.1	—	0	0.01	0.02	0.5	—
150	Haddock, breaded, fried[14]	3 oz	85	66	140	17	5	1.4	2.2	1.2	5	34	210	1.0	296	—	0.03	0.06	2.7	2
151	Ocean perch, breaded, fried[14]	1 fillet	85	59	195	16	11	2.7	4.4	2.3	6	28	192	1.1	242	—	0.10	0.10	1.6	—
152	Oysters, raw, meat only (13–19 medium Selects).	1 cup	240	85	160	20	4	1.3	0.2	0.1	8	226	343	13.2	290	740	0.34	0.43	6.0	—
153	Salmon, pink, canned, solids and liquid.	3 oz	85	71	120	17	5	0.9	0.8	0.1	0	167[15]	243	0.7	307	60	0.03	0.16	6.8	—
154	Sardines, Atlantic, canned in oil, drained solids.	3 oz	85	62	175	20	9	3.0	2.5	0.5	0	372	424	2.5	502	190	0.02	0.17	4.6	—
155	Scallops, frozen, breaded, fried, reheated.	6 scallops	90	60	175	16	8	—	—	—	9	—	—	—	—	—	—	—	—	—
156	Shad, baked with butter or margarine, bacon.	3 oz	85	64	170	20	10	—	—	—	0	20	266	0.5	320	30	0.11	0.22	7.3	—
	Shrimp:																			
157	Canned meat	3 oz	85	70	100	21	1	0.1	0.1	Tr	1	98	224	2.6	104	50	0.01	0.03	1.5	—
158	French fried[16]	3 oz	85	57	190	17	9	2.3	3.7	2.0	9	61	162	1.7	195	—	0.03	0.07	2.3	—
159	Tuna, canned in oil, drained solids.	3 oz	85	61	170	24	7	1.7	1.7	0.7	0	7	199	1.6	—	70	0.04	0.10	10.1	—
160	Tuna salad[17]	1 cup	205	70	350	30	22	4.3	6.3	6.7	7	41	291	2.7	—	590	0.08	0.23	10.3	2
	Meat and meat products:																			
161	Bacon, (20 slices per lb, raw), broiled or fried, crisp.	2 slices	15	8	85	4	8	2.5	3.7	0.7	Tr	2	34	0.5	35	0	0.08	0.05	0.8	—
	Beef,[18] cooked:																			
	Cuts braised, simmered or pot roasted:																			

TABLE A-9. (Continued)

Item No. (a)	Foods, Approximate Measures, Units, and Weight (edible part unless footnotes indicate otherwise) (b)			Water (c)	Food Energy (d)	Protein (e)	Fat (f)	Fatty Acids: Saturated (total) (g)	Fatty Acids: Unsaturated: Oleic (h)	Fatty Acids: Unsaturated: Linoleic (i)	Carbohydrate (j)	Calcium (k)	Phosphorus (l)	Iron (m)	Potassium (n)	Vitamin A Value (o)	Thiamin (p)	Riboflavin (q)	Niacin (r)	Ascorbic Acid (s)
			grams	per-cent	Cal-ories	grams	grams	grams	grams	grams	grams	milli-grams	milli-grams	milli-grams	milli-grams	inter-national units	milli-grams	milli-grams	milli-grams	milli-grams
162	Lean and fat (piece, 2 1/2 by 2 1/2 by 3/4 in.)	3 oz	85	53	245	23	16	6.8	6.5	0.4	0	10	114	2.9	184	30	0.04	0.18	3.6	—
163	Lean only from item 162	2.5 oz	72	62	140	22	5	2.1	1.8	0.2	0	10	108	2.7	176	10	0.04	0.17	3.3	—
	Ground beef, broiled:																			
164	Lean with 10% fat	3 oz or patty 3 by 5/8 in.	85	60	185	23	10	4.0	3.9	0.3	0	10	196	3.0	261	20	0.08	0.20	5.1	—
165	Lean with 21% fat	2.9 oz or patty 3 by 5/8 in.	82	54	235	20	17	7.0	6.7	0.4	0	9	159	2.6	221	30	0.07	0.17	4.4	—
	Roast, oven cooked, no liquid added:																			
	Relatively fat, such as rib:																			
166	Lean and fat (2 pieces, 4 1/8 by 2 1/4 by 1/4 in.).	3 oz	85	40	375	17	33	14.0	13.6	0.8	0	8	158	2.2	189	70	0.05	0.13	3.1	—
167	Lean only from item 166	1.8 oz	51	57	125	14	7	3.0	2.5	0.3	0	6	131	1.8	161	10	0.04	0.11	2.6	—
	Relatively lean, such as heel of round:																			
168	Lean and fat (2 pieces, 4 1/8 by 2 1/4 by 1/4 in.).	3 oz	85	62	165	25	7	2.8	2.7	0.2	0	11	208	3.2	279	10	0.06	0.19	4.5	—
169	Lean only from item 168	2.8 oz	78	65	125	24	3	1.2	1.0	0.1	0	10	199	3.0	268	Tr	0.06	0.18	4.3	—
	Steak:																			
	Relatively fat-sirloin, broiled:																			
170	Lean and fat (piece, 2 1/2 by 2 1/2 by 3/4 in.).	3 oz	85	44	330	20	27	11.3	11.1	0.6	0	9	162	2.5	220	50	0.05	0.15	4.0	—
171	Lean only from item 170	2.0 oz	56	59	115	18	4	1.8	1.6	0.2	0	7	146	2.2	202	10	0.05	0.14	3.6	—
	Relatively lean-round, braised:																			
172	Lean and fat (piece, 4 1/8 by 2 1/4 by 1/2 in.).	3 oz	85	55	220	24	13	5.5	5.2	0.4	0	10	213	3.0	272	20	0.07	0.19	4.8	—

nutrients in indicated quantity

TABLE A–9. (Continued)

Item No. (a)	Foods, Approximate Measures, Units, and Weight (edible part unless footnotes indicate otherwise) (b)			Water (c)	Food Energy (d)	Protein (e)	Fat (f)	Fatty Acids: Saturated (total) (g)	Fatty Acids: Unsaturated: Oleic (h)	Fatty Acids: Unsaturated: Linoleic (i)	Carbohydrate (j)	Calcium (k)	Phosphorus (l)	Iron (m)	Potassium (n)	Vitamin A Value (o)	Thiamin (p)	Riboflavin (q)	Niacin (r)	Ascorbic Acid (s)
			grams	per-cent	Cal-ories	grams	grams	grams	grams	grams	grams	milli-grams	milli-grams	milli-grams	milli-grams	inter-national units	milli-grams	milli-grams	milli-grams	milli-grams
211	Drumstick, fried,[23] bones removed (2 oz with bones).	1.3 oz	38	55	90	12	4	1.1	1.3	0.9	Tr	6	89	0.9	—	50	0.03	0.15	2.7	—
212	Half broiler, broiled, bones removed (10.4 oz with bones).	6.2 oz	176	71	240	42	7	2.2	2.5	1.3	0	16	355	3.0	483	160	0.09	0.34	15.5	—
213	Chicken, canned, boneless	3 oz	85	65	170	18	10	3.2	3.8	2.0	0	18	210	1.3	117	200	0.03	0.11	3.7	3
214	Chicken a la king, cooked (home recipe).	1 cup	245	68	470	27	34	12.7	14.3	3.3	12	127	358	2.5	404	1,130	0.10	0.42	5.4	12
215	Chicken and noodles, cooked (home recipe).	1 cup	240	71	365	22	18	5.9	7.1	3.5	26	26	247	2.2	149	430	0.05	0.17	4.3	Tr
	Chicken chow mein:																			
216	Canned	1 cup	250	89	95	7	Tr	—	—	—	18	45	85	1.3	418	150	0.05	0.10	1.0	13
217	From home recipe	1 cup	250	78	255	31	10	2.4	3.4	3.1	10	58	293	2.5	473	280	0.08	0.23	4.3	10
218	Chicken potpie (home recipe), baked,[19] piece (1/3 or 9-in. diam. pie).	1 piece	232	57	545	23	31	11.3	10.9	5.6	42	70	232	3.0	343	3,090	0.34	0.31	5.5	5
	Turkey, roasted, flesh without skin:																			
219	Dark meat, piece, 2 1/2 by 1 5/8 by 1/4 in.	4 pieces	85	61	175	26	7	2.1	1.5	1.5	0	—	—	2.0	338	—	0.03	0.20	3.6	—
220	Light meat, piece, 4 by 2 by 1/4 in.	2 pieces	85	62	150	28	3	0.9	0.6	0.7	0	—	—	1.0	349	—	0.04	0.12	9.4	—
	Light and dark meat:																			
221	Chopped or diced	1 cup	140	61	265	44	9	2.5	1.7	1.8	0	11	351	2.5	514	—	0.07	0.25	10.8	—
222	Pieces (1 slice white meat, 4 by 2 by 1/4 in. with 2 slices dark meat, 2 1/2 by 1 5/8 by 1/4 in.).	3 pieces	85	61	160	27	5	1.5	1.0	1.1	0	7	213	1.5	312	—	0.04	0.15	6.5	—
	fruits and fruit products																			
	Apples, raw, unpeeled, without cores:																			
223	2 3/4-in. diam. (about 3 per lb with cores).	1 apple	138	84	80	Tr	1	—	—	—	20	10	14	0.4	152	120	0.04	0.03	0.1	6

TABLE A–9. (Continued)

Item No. (a)	Foods, Approximate Measures, Units, and Weight (edible part unless footnotes indicate otherwise) (b)			Water (c)	Food Energy (d)	Protein (e)	Fat (f)	Fatty Acids: Saturated (total) (g)	Fatty Acids: Unsaturated: Oleic (h)	Fatty Acids: Unsaturated: Linoleic (i)	Carbohydrate (j)	Calcium (k)	Phosphorus (l)	Iron (m)	Potassium (n)	Vitamin A Value (o)	Thiamin (p)	Riboflavin (q)	Niacin (r)	Ascorbic Acid (s)
			grams	per-cent	Cal-ories	grams	grams	grams	grams	grams	grams	milli-grams	milli-grams	milli-grams	milli-grams	inter-national units	milli-grams	milli-grams	milli-grams	milli-grams
173	Lean only from item 172	2.4 oz	68	61	130	21	4	1.7	1.5	0.2	0	9	182	2.5	238	10	0.05	0.16	4.1	—
	Beef, canned:																			
174	Corned beef	3 oz	85	59	185	22	10	4.9	4.5	0.2	0	17	90	3.7	—	—	0.01	0.20	2.9	—
175	Corned beef hash	1 cup	220	67	400	19	25	11.9	10.9	0.5	24	29	147	4.4	440	—	0.02	0.20	4.6	—
176	Beef, dried, chipped	2 1/2-oz jar	71	48	145	24	4	2.1	2.0	0.1	0	14	287	3.6	142	—	0.05	0.23	2.7	0
177	Beef and vegetable stew	1 cup	245	82	220	16	11	4.9	4.5	0.2	15	29	184	2.9	613	2,400	0.15	0.17	4.7	17
178	Beef potpie (home recipe), baked[19] (piece, 1/3 of 9-in. diam. pie).	1 piece	210	55	515	21	30	7.9	12.8	6.7	39	29	149	3.8	334	1,720	0.30	0.30	5.5	6
179	Chili con carne with beans, canned.	1 cup	255	72	340	19	16	7.5	6.8	0.3	31	82	321	4.3	594	150	0.08	0.18	3.3	—
180	Chop suey with beef and pork (home recipe).	1 cup	250	75	300	26	17	8.5	6.2	0.7	13	60	248	4.8	425	600	0.28	0.38	5.0	33
181	Heart, beef, lean, braised	3 oz	85	61	160	27	5	1.5	1.1	0.6	1	5	154	5.0	197	20	0.21	1.04	6.5	1
	Lamb, cooked:																			
	Chop, rib (cut 3 per lb with bone), broiled:																			
182	Lean and fat	3.1 oz	89	43	360	18	32	14.8	12.1	1.2	0	8	139	1.0	200	—	0.11	0.19	4.1	—
183	Lean only from item 182	2 oz	57	60	120	16	6	2.5	2.1	0.2	0	6	121	1.1	174	—	0.09	0.15	3.4	—
	Leg, roasted:																			
184	Lean and fat (2 pieces, 4 1/8 by 2 1/4 by 1/4 in.).	3 oz	85	54	235	22	16	7.3	6.0	0.6	0	9	177	1.4	241	—	0.13	0.23	4.7	—
185	Lean only from item 184	2.5 oz	71	62	130	20	5	2.1	1.8	0.2	0	9	169	1.4	227	—	0.12	0.21	4.4	—
	Shoulder, roasted:																			
186	Lean and fat (3 pieces, 2 1/2 by 2 1/2 by 1/4 in.).	3 oz	85	50	285	18	23	10.8	8.8	0.9	0	9	146	1.0	206	—	0.11	0.20	4.0	—
187	Lean only from item 186	2.3 oz	64	61	130	17	6	3.6	2.3	0.2	0	8	140	1.0	193	—	0.10	0.18	3.7	—
188	Liver, beef, fried[20] (slice, 6 1/2 by 2 3/8 by 3/8 in.).	3 oz	85	56	195	22	9	2.5	3.5	0.9	5	9	405	7.5	323	45,390[21]	0.22	3.56	14.0	23
	Pork, cured, cooked:																			

TABLE A-9. (Continued)

nutrients in indicated quantity

Item No. (a)	Foods, Approximate Measures, Units, and Weight (edible part unless footnotes indicate otherwise) (b)			Water (c)	Food Energy (d)	Protein (e)	Fat (f)	Fatty Acids: Saturated (total) (g)	Fatty Acids: Unsaturated: Oleic (h)	Fatty Acids: Unsaturated: Linoleic (i)	Carbohydrate (j)	Calcium (k)	Phosphorus (l)	Iron (m)	Potassium (n)	Vitamin A Value (o)	Thiamin (p)	Riboflavin (q)	Niacin (r)	Ascorbic Acid (s)
			grams	per-cent	Cal-ories	grams	grams	grams	grams	grams	grams	milli-grams	milli-grams	milli-grams	milli-grams	inter-national units	milli-grams	milli-grams	milli-grams	milli-grams
189	Ham, light cure, lean and fat, roasted (2 pieces, 4 1/8 by 2 1/4 by 1/4 in.).[22]	3 oz	85	54	245	18	19	6.8	7.9	1.7	0	8	146	2.2	199	0	0.40	0.15	3.1	—
	Luncheon meat:																			
190	Boiled ham, slice (8 per 8-oz pkg.).	1 oz	28	59	65	5	5	1.7	2.0	0.4	0	3	47	0.8	—	0	0.12	0.04	0.7	—
	Canned, spiced or unspiced:																			
191	Slice, approx. 3 by 2 by 1/2 in.	1 slice	60	55	175	9	15	5.4	6.7	1.0	1	5	65	1.3	133	0	0.19	0.13	1.8	—
	Pork, fresh,[18] cooked:																			
	Chop, loin (cut 3 per lb with bone), broiled:																			
192	Lean and fat	2.7 oz	78	42	305	19	25	8.9	10.4	2.2	0	9	209	2.7	216	0	0.75	0.22	4.5	—
193	Lean only from item 192	2 oz	56	53	150	17	9	3.1	3.6	0.8	0	7	181	2.2	192	0	0.63	0.18	3.8	—
	Roast, oven cooked, no liquid added:																			
194	Lean and fat (piece, 2 1/2 by 2 1/2 by 3/4 in.).	3 oz	85	46	310	21	24	8.7	10.2	2.2	0	9	218	2.7	233	0	0.78	0.22	4.8	—
195	Lean only from item 194	2.4 oz	68	55	175	20	10	3.5	4.1	0.8	0	9	211	2.6	224	0	0.73	0.21	4.4	—
	Shoulder cut, simmered:																			
196	Lean and fat (3 pieces, 2 1/2 by 2 1/2 by 1/4 in.).	3 oz	85	46	320	20	26	9.3	10.9	2.3	0	9	118	2.6	158	0	0.46	0.21	4.1	—
197	Lean only from item 196	2.2 oz	63	60	135	18	6	2.2	2.6	0.6	0	8	111	2.3	146	0	0.42	0.19	3.7	—
	Sausages [see also Luncheon meat (items 190–191)]:																			
198	Bologna, slice (8 per 8-oz pkg.).	1 slice	28	56	85	3	8	3.0	3.4	0.5	Tr	2	36	0.5	65	—	0.05	0.06	0.7	—

TABLE A-9. (Continued)

nutrients in indicated quantity

Item No. (a)	Foods, Approximate Measures, Units, and Weight (edible part unless footnotes indicate otherwise) (b)			Water (c)	Food Energy (d)	Protein (e)	Fat (f)	Fatty Acids: Saturated (total) (g)	Fatty Acids: Unsaturated: Oleic (h)	Fatty Acids: Unsaturated: Linoleic (i)	Carbohydrate (j)	Calcium (k)	Phosphorus (l)	Iron (m)	Potassium (n)	Vitamin A Value (o)	Thiamin (p)	Riboflavin (q)	Niacin (r)	Ascorbic Acid (s)
			grams	per-cent	Cal-ories	grams	grams	grams	grams	grams	grams	milli-grams	milli-grams	milli-grams	milli-grams	inter-national units	milli-grams	milli-grams	milli-grams	milli-grams
199	Braunschweiger, slice (6 per 6-oz pkg.).	1 slice	28	53	90	4	8	2.6	3.4	0.8	1	3	69	1.7	—	1,850	0.05	0.41	2.3	—
200	Brown and serve (10–11 per 8-oz pkg.), browned.	1 link	17	40	70	3	6	2.3	2.8	0.7	Tr	—	—	—	—	—	—	—	—	—
201	Deviled ham, canned	1 tbsp	13	51	45	2	4	1.5	1.8	0.4	0	1	12	0.3	—	0	0.02	0.01	0.2	—
202	Frankfurter (8 per 1-lb pkg.), cooked (reheated).	1 frankfurter	56	57	170	7	15	5.6	6.5	1.2	1	3	57	0.8	—	—	0.08	0.11	1.4	—
203	Meat, potted (beef, chicken, turkey), canned.	1 tbsp	13	61	30	2	2	—	—	—	0	—	—	—	—	—	Tr	0.03	0.2	—
204	Pork link (16 per 1-lb pkg.), cooked.	1 link	13	35	60	2	6	2.1	2.4	0.5	Tr	1	21	0.3	35	0	0.10	0.04	0.5	—
	Salami:																			
205	Dry type, slice (12 per 4-oz pkg.).	1 slice	10	30	45	2	4	1.6	1.6	0.1	Tr	1	28	0.4	—	—	0.04	0.03	0.5	—
206	Cooked type, slice (8 per 8-oz pkg.).	1 slice	28	51	90	5	7	3.1	3.0	0.2	Tr	3	57	0.7	—	—	0.07	0.07	1.2	—
207	Vienna sausage (7 per 4-oz can).	1 sausage	16	63	40	2	3	1.2	1.4	0.2	Tr	1	24	0.3	—	—	0.01	0.02	0.4	—
	Veal, medium fat, cooked, bone removed:																			
208	Cutlet (4 1/8 by 2 1/4 by 1/2 in.), braised or broiled.	3 oz	85	60	185	23	9	4.0	3.4	0.4	0	9	196	2.7	258	—	0.06	0.21	4.6	—
209	Rib (2 pieces, 4 1/8 by 2 1/4 by 1/4 in.), roasted.	3 oz	85	55	230	23	14	6.1	5.1	0.6	0	10	211	2.9	259	—	0.11	0.26	6.6	—
	Poultry and poultry products:																			
	Chicken, cooked:																			
210	Breast, fried,[23] bones removed, 1/2 breast (3.3 oz with bones).	2.8 oz	79	58	160	26	5	1.4	1.8	1.1	1	9	218	1.3	—	70	0.04	0.17	11.6	—

TABLE A-9. (Continued)

Item No. (a)	Foods, Approximate Measures, Units, and Weight (edible part unless footnotes indicate otherwise) (b)			Water (c)	Food Energy (d)	Protein (e)	Fat (f)	Fatty Acids: Saturated (total) (g)	Fatty Acids: Unsaturated: Oleic (h)	Fatty Acids: Unsaturated: Linoleic (i)	Carbohydrate (j)	Calcium (k)	Phosphorus (l)	Iron (m)	Potassium (n)	Vitamin A Value (o)	Thiamin (p)	Riboflavin (q)	Niacin (r)	Ascorbic Acid (s)
			grams	percent	Calories	grams	grams	grams	grams	grams	grams	milligrams	milligrams	milligrams	milligrams	international units	milligrams	milligrams	milligrams	milligrams
224	3 1/4 in. diam. (about 2 per lb with cores).	1 apple	212	84	125	Tr	1	—	—	—	31	15	21	0.6	233	190	0.06	0.04	0.2	8
225	Applejuice, bottled or canned[24]	1 cup	248	88	120	Tr	Tr	—	—	—	30	15	22	1.5	250	—	0.02	0.05	0.2	2[25]
	Applesauce, canned:																			
226	Sweetened	1 cup	255	76	230	1	Tr	—	—	—	61	10	13	1.3	166	100	0.05	0.03	0.1	3[25]
227	Unsweetened	1 cup	244	89	100	Tr	Tr	—	—	—	26	10	12	1.2	190	100	0.05	0.02	0.1	2[25]
	Apricots:																			
228	Raw, without pits (about 12 per lb with pits).	3 apricots	107	85	55	1	Tr	—	—	—	14	18	25	0.5	301	2,890	0.03	0.04	0.6	11
229	Canned in heavy sirup (halves and sirup).	1 cup	258	77	220	2	Tr	—	—	—	57	28	39	0.8	604	4,490	0.05	0.05	1.0	10
	Dried:																			
230	Uncooked (28 large or 37 medium halves per cup).	1 cup	130	25	340	7	1	—	—	—	86	87	140	7.2	1,273	14,170	0.01	0.21	4.3	16
231	Cooked, unsweetened, fruit and liquid.	1 cup	250	76	215	4	1	—	—	—	54	55	88	4.5	795	7,500	0.01	0.13	2.5	8
232	Apricot nectar, canned	1 cup	251	85	145	1	Tr	—	—	—	37	23	30	0.5	379	2,380	0.03	0.03	0.5	36[26]
	Avocados, raw, whole, without skins and seeds:																			
233	California, mid- and late-winter (with skin and seed, 3 1/8-in. diam.; wt., 10 oz).	1 avocado	216	74	370	5	37	5.5	22.0	3.7	13	22	91	1.3	1,303	630	0.24	0.43	3.5	30
234	Florida, late summer and fall (with skin and seed, 3 5/8-in. diam.; wt., 1 lb).	1 avocado	304	78	390	4	33	6.7	15.7	5.3	27	30	128	1.8	1,836	880	0.33	0.61	4.9	43
235	Banana without peel (about 2.6 per lb with peel).	1 banana	119	76	100	1	Tr	—	—	—	26	10	31	0.8	440	230	0.06	0.07	0.8	12
236	Banana flakes	1 tbsp	6	3	20	Tr	Tr	—	—	—	5	2	6	0.2	92	50	0.01	0.01	0.2	Tr
237	Blackberries, raw	1 cup	144	85	85	2	1	—	—	—	19	46	27	1.3	245	290	0.04	0.06	0.6	30

nutrients in indicated quantity

TABLE A–9. (Continued)

Item No. (a)	Foods, Approximate Measures, Units, and Weight (edible part unless footnotes indicate otherwise) (b)			Water (c)	Food Energy (d)	Protein (e)	Fat (f)	Fatty Acids: Saturated (total) (g)	Fatty Acids: Unsaturated: Oleic (h)	Fatty Acids: Unsaturated: Linoleic (i)	Carbohydrate (j)	Calcium (k)	Phosphorus (l)	Iron (m)	Potassium (n)	Vitamin A Value (o)	Thiamin (p)	Riboflavin (q)	Niacin (r)	Ascorbic Acid (s)
			grams	per-cent	Cal-ories	grams	grams	grams	grams	grams	grams	milli-grams	milli-grams	milli-grams	milli-grams	inter-national units	milli-grams	milli-grams	milli-grams	milli-grams
238	Blueberries, raw	1 cup	145	83	90	1	1	—	—	—	22	22	19	1.5	117	150	0.04	0.09	0.7	20
	Cantaloup. See Muskmelons (item 271).																			
	Cherries:																			
239	Sour (tart), red, pitted, canned, water pack.	1 cup	244	88	105	2	Tr	—	—	—	26	37	32	0.7	317	1,660	0.07	0.05	0.5	12
240	Sweet, raw, without pits and stems.	10 cherries	68	80	45	1	Tr	—	—	—	12	15	13	0.3	129	70	0.03	0.04	0.3	7
241	Cranberry juice cocktail, bottled, sweetened.	1 cup	253	83	165	Tr	Tr	—	—	—	42	13	8	0.8	25	Tr	0.03	0.03	0.1	81[27]
242	Cranberry sauce, sweetened, canned, strained.	1 cup	277	62	405	Tr	1	—	—	—	104	17	11	0.6	83	60	0.03	0.03	0.1	6
	Dates:																			
243	Whole, without pits	10 dates	80	23	220	2	Tr	—	—	—	58	47	50	2.4	518	40	0.07	0.08	1.8	0
244	Chopped	1 cup	178	23	490	4	1	—	—	—	130	105	112	5.3	1,153	90	0.16	0.18	3.9	0
245	Fruit cocktail, canned, in heavy sirup.	1 cup	255	80	195	1	Tr	—	—	—	50	23	31	1.0	411	360	0.05	0.03	1.0	5
	Grapefruit:																			
	Raw, medium, 3 3/4-in. diam. (about 1 lb 1 oz):																			
246	Pink or red	1/2 grapefruit with peel[28]	241	89	50	1	Tr	—	—	—	13	20	20	0.5	166	540	0.05	0.02	0.2	44
247	White	1/2 grapefruit with peel[28]	241	89	45	1	Tr	—	—	—	12	19	19	0.5	159	10	0.05	0.02	0.2	44
248	Canned, sections with sirup	1 cup	254	81	180	2	Tr	—	—	—	45	33	36	0.8	343	30	0.08	0.05	0.5	76
	Grapefruit juice:																			
249	Raw, pink, red, or white	1 cup	246	90	95	1	Tr	—	—	—	23	22	37	0.5	399	([29])	0.10	0.05	0.5	93
	Canned, white:																			
250	Unsweetened	1 cup	247	89	100	1	Tr	—	—	—	24	20	35	1.0	400	20	0.07	0.05	0.5	84
251	Sweetened	1 cup	250	86	135	1	Tr	—	—	—	32	20	35	1.0	405	30	0.08	0.05	0.5	78
	Frozen, concentrate, unsweetened:																			
252	Undiluted, 6-fl oz can	1 can	207	62	300	4	1	—	—	—	72	70	124	0.8	1,250	60	0.29	0.12	1.4	286

TABLE A–9. (Continued)

Item No. (a)	Foods, Approximate Measures, Units, and Weight (edible part unless footnotes indicate otherwise) (b)			Water (c)	Food Energy (d)	Protein (e)	Fat (f)	Fatty Acids: Saturated (total) (g)	Fatty Acids: Unsaturated: Oleic (h)	Fatty Acids: Unsaturated: Linoleic (i)	Carbohydrate (j)	Calcium (k)	Phosphorus (l)	Iron (m)	Potassium (n)	Vitamin A Value (o)	Thiamin (p)	Riboflavin (q)	Niacin (r)	Ascorbic Acid (s)
			grams	percent	Calories	grams	grams	grams	grams	grams	grams	milligrams	milligrams	milligrams	milligrams	international units	milligrams	milligrams	milligrams	milligrams
253	Diluted with 3 parts water by volume.	1 cup	247	89	100	1	Tr	—	—	—	24	25	42	0.2	420	20	0.10	0.04	0.5	96
254	Dehydrated crystals, prepared with water (1 lb yields about 1 gal).	1 cup	247	90	100	1	Tr	—	—	—	24	22	40	0.2	412	20	0.10	0.05	0.5	91
	Grapes, European type (adherent skin), raw:																			
255	Thompson Seedless	10 grapes	50	81	35	Tr	Tr	—	—	—	9	6	10	0.2	87	50	0.03	0.02	0.2	2
256	Tokay and Emperor, seeded types	10 grapes[30]	60	81	40	Tr	Tr	—	—	—	10	7	11	0.2	99	60	0.03	0.02	0.2	2
	Grapejuice:																			
257	Canned or bottled	1 cup	253	83	165	1	Tr	—	—	—	42	28	30	0.8	293	—	0.10	0.05	0.5	Tr[25]
	Frozen concentrate, sweetened:																			
258	Undiluted, 6-fl oz can	1 can	216	53	395	1	Tr	—	—	—	100	22	32	0.9	255	40	0.13	0.22	1.5	32[31]
259	Diluted with 3 parts water by volume.	1 cup	250	86	135	1	Tr	—	—	—	33	8	10	0.3	85	10	0.05	0.08	0.5	10[31]
260	Grape drink, canned	1 cup	250	86	135	Tr	Tr	—	—	—	35	8	10	0.3	88	—	0.03[32]	0.03[32]	0.3	([32])
261	Lemon, raw, size 165, without peel and seeds (about 4 per lb with peels and seeds).	1 lemon	74	90	20	1	Tr	—	—	—	6	19	12	0.4	102	10	0.03	0.01	0.1	39
	Lemon juice:																			
262	Raw	1 cup	244	91	60	1	Tr	—	—	—	20	17	24	0.5	344	50	0.07	0.02	0.2	112
263	Canned, or bottled, unsweetened	1 cup	244	92	55	1	Tr	—	—	—	19	17	24	0.5	344	50	0.07	0.02	0.2	102
264	Frozen, single strength, unsweetened, 6-fl oz can.	1 can	183	92	40	1	Tr	—	—	—	13	13	16	0.5	258	40	0.05	0.02	0.2	81
	Lemonade concentrate, frozen:																			
265	Undiluted, 6-fl oz can	1 can	219	49	425	Tr	Tr	—	—	—	112	9	13	0.4	153	40	0.05	0.06	0.7	66

nutrients in indicated quantity

TABLE A–9. (Continued)

Item No. (a)	Foods, Approximate Measures, Units, and Weight (edible part unless footnotes indicate otherwise) (b)		Weight	Water (c)	Food Energy (d)	Protein (e)	Fat (f)	Fatty Acids: Saturated (total) (g)	Fatty Acids: Unsaturated: Oleic (h)	Fatty Acids: Unsaturated: Linoleic (i)	Carbohydrate (j)	Calcium (k)	Phosphorus (l)	Iron (m)	Potassium (n)	Vitamin A Value (o)	Thiamin (p)	Riboflavin (q)	Niacin (r)	Ascorbic Acid (s)
			grams	per-cent	Cal-ories	grams	grams	grams	grams	grams	grams	milli-grams	milli-grams	milli-grams	milli-grams	inter-national units	milli-grams	milli-grams	milli-grams	milli-grams
266	Diluted with 4 1/3 parts water by volume.	1 cup	248	89	105	Tr	Tr	—	—	—	28	2	3	0.1	40	10	0.01	0.02	0.2	17
	Limeade concentrate, frozen:																			
267	Undiluted, 6-fl oz can	1 can	218	50	410	Tr	Tr	—	—	—	108	11	13	0.2	129	Tr	0.02	0.02	0.2	26
268	Diluted with 4 1/3 parts water by volume.	1 cup	247	89	100	Tr	Tr	—	—	—	27	3	3	Tr	32	Tr	Tr	Tr	Tr	6
	Limejuice:																			
269	Raw	1 cup	246	90	65	1	Tr	—	—	—	22	22	27	0.5	256	20	0.05	0.02	0.2	79
270	Canned, unsweetened	1 cup	246	90	65	1	Tr	—	—	—	22	22	27	0.5	256	20	0.05	0.02	0.2	52
	Muskmelons, raw, with rind, without seed cavity:																			
271	Cantaloup, orange-fleshed (with rind and seed cavity, 5-in. diam., 2 1/3 lb).	1/2 melon with rind[33]	477	91	80	2	Tr	—	—	—	20	38	44	1.1	682	9,240	0.11	0.08	1.6	90
272	Honeydew (with rind and seed cavity, 6 1/2-in. diam., 5 1/4 lb).	1/10 melon with rind[33]	226	91	50	1	Tr	—	—	—	11	21	24	0.6	374	60	0.06	0.04	0.9	34
	Oranges,all commercial varieties, raw:																			
273	Whole, 2 5/8-in. diam., without peel and seeds (about 2 1/2 per lb with peel and seeds).	1 orange	131	86	65	1	Tr	—	—	—	16	54	26	0.5	263	260	0.13	0.05	0.5	66
274	Sections without membranes	1 cup	180	86	90	2	Tr	—	—	—	22	74	36	0.7	360	360	0.18	0.07	0.7	90
	Orange juice:																			
275	Raw, all varieties	1 cup	248	88	110	2	Tr	—	—	—	26	27	42	0.5	496	500	0.22	0.07	1.0	124
276	Canned, unsweetened	1 cup	249	87	120	2	Tr	—	—	—	28	25	45	1.0	496	500	0.17	0.05	0.7	100
	Frozen concentrate:																			
277	Undiluted, 6-fl oz can	1 can	213	55	360	5	Tr	—	—	—	87	75	126	0.9	1,500	1,620	0.68	0.11	2.8	360

nutrients in indicated quantity

TABLE A-9. (Continued)

Item No. (a)	Foods, Approximate Measures, Units, and Weight (edible part unless footnotes indicate otherwise) (b)			Water (c)	Food Energy (d)	Protein (e)	Fat (f)	Fatty Acids: Saturated (total) (g)	Fatty Acids: Unsaturated: Oleic (h)	Fatty Acids: Unsaturated: Linoleic (i)	Carbohydrate (j)	Calcium (k)	Phosphorus (l)	Iron (m)	Potassium (n)	Vitamin A Value (o)	Thiamin (p)	Riboflavin (q)	Niacin (r)	Ascorbic Acid (s)
			grams	per-cent	Cal-ories	grams	grams	grams	grams	grams	grams	milli-grams	milli-grams	milli-grams	milli-grams	inter-national units	milli-grams	milli-grams	milli-grams	milli-grams
278	Diluted with 3 parts water by volume	1 cup	249	87	120	2	Tr	—	—	—	29	25	42	0.2	503	540	0.23	0.03	0.9	120
279	Dehydrated crystals, prepared with water (1 lb yields about 1 gal).	1 cup	248	88	115	1	Tr	—	—	—	27	25	40	0.5	518	500	0.20	0.07	1.0	109
	Orange and grapefruit juice:																			
	Frozen concentrate:																			
280	Undiluted, 6-fl oz can	1 cup	210	59	330	4	1	—	—	—	78	61	99	0.8	1,308	800	0.48	0.06	2.3	302
281	Diluted with 3 parts water by volume.	1 cup	248	88	110	1	Tr	—	—	—	26	20	32	0.2	439	270	0.15	0.02	0.7	102
282	Papayas, raw, 1/2-in cubes	1 cup	140	89	55	1	Tr	—	—	—	14	28	22	0.4	328	2,450	0.06	0.06	0.4	78
	Peaches:																			
	Raw:																			
283	Whole, 2 1/2-in. diam., peeled, pitted (about 4 per lb with peels and pits).	1 peach	100	89	40	1	Tr	—	—	—	10	9	19	0.5	202	1,330[34]	0.02	0.05	1.0	7
284	Sliced	1 cup	170	89	65	1	Tr	—	—	—	16	15	32	0.9	343	2,260[34]	0.03	0.09	1.7	12
	Canned, yellow-fleshed, solids and liquid (halves or slices):																			
285	Sirup pack	1 cup	256	79	200	1	Tr	—	—	—	51	10	31	0.8	333	1,100	0.03	0.05	1.5	8
286	Water pack	1 cup	244	91	75	1	Tr	—	—	—	20	10	32	0.7	334	1,100	0.02	0.07	1.5	7
	Dried:																			
287	Uncooked	1 cup	160	25	420	5	1	—	—	—	109	77	187	9.6	1,520	6,240	0.02	0.30	8.5	29
288	Cooked, unsweetened, halves and juice	1 cup	250	77	205	3	1	—	—	—	54	38	93	4.8	743	3,050	0.01	0.15	3.8	5
	Frozen, sliced, sweetened:																			
289	10-oz container	1 container	284	77	250	1	Tr	—	—	—	64	11	37	1.4	352	1,850	0.03	0.11	2.0	116[35]
290	Cup	1 cup	250	77	220	1	Tr	—	—	—	57	10	33	1.3	310	1,630	0.03	0.10	1.8	103[35]

TABLE A-9. (Continued)

Item No. (a)	Foods, Approximate Measures, Units, and Weight (edible part unless footnotes indicate otherwise) (b)			Water (c)	Food Energy (d)	Protein (e)	Fat (f)	Fatty Acids: Saturated (total) (g)	Fatty Acids: Unsaturated: Oleic (h)	Fatty Acids: Unsaturated: Linoleic (i)	Carbohydrate (j)	Calcium (k)	Phosphorus (l)	Iron (m)	Potassium (n)	Vitamin A Value (o)	Thiamin (p)	Riboflavin (q)	Niacin (r)	Ascorbic Acid (s)
			grams	per-cent	Cal-ories	grams	grams	grams	grams	grams	grams	milli-grams	milli-grams	milli-grams	milli-grams	inter-national units	milli-grams	milli-grams	milli-grams	milli-grams
	Pears:																			
	Raw, with skin, cored:																			
291	Bartlett, 2 1/2-in. diam. (about 2 1/2 per lb with cores and stems).	1 pear	164	83	100	1	1	—	—	—	25	13	18	0.5	213	30	0.03	0.07	0.2	7
292	Bosc, 2 1/2-in. diam. (about 3 per lb with cores and stems).	1 pear	141	83	85	1	1	—	—	—	22	11	16	0.4	83	30	0.03	0.06	0.1	6
293	D'Anjou, 3-in. diam. (about 2 per lb with cores and stems).	1 pear	200	83	120	1	1	—	—	—	31	16	22	0.6	260	40	0.04	0.08	0.2	8
294	Canned, solids and liquid, sirup pack, heavy (halves or slices).	1 cup	255	80	195	1	1	—	—	—	50	13	18	0.5	214	10	0.03	0.05	0.3	3
	Pineapple:																			
295	Raw, diced	1 cup	155	85	80	1	Tr	—	—	—	21	26	12	0.8	226	110	0.14	0.05	0.3	26
	Canned, heavy sirup pack, solids and liquid:																			
296	Crushed, chunks, tidbits	1 cup	255	80	190	1	Tr	—	—	—	49	28	13	0.8	245	130	0.20	0.05	0.5	18
	Slices and liquid:																			
297	Large	1 slice: 2 1/4 tbsp liquid.	105	80	80	Tr	Tr	—	—	—	20	12	5	0.3	101	50	0.08	0.02	0.2	7
298	Medium	1 slice; 1 1/4 tbsp liquid.	58	80	45	Tr	Tr	—	—	—	11	6	3	0.2	56	30	0.05	0.01	0.1	4
299	Pineapple juice, unsweetened, canned.	1 cup	250	86	140	1	Tr	—	—	—	34	38	23	0.8	373	130	0.13	0.05	0.5	80[27]
	Plums:																			
	Raw, without pits:																			
300	Japanese and hybrid (2 1/8-in. diam., about 6 1/2 lb with pits).	1 plum	66	87	30	Tr	Tr	—	—	—	8	8	12	0.3	112	160	0.02	0.02	0.3	4

TABLE A–9. (Continued)

Item No. (a)	Foods, Approximate Measures, Units, and Weight (edible part unless footnotes indicate otherwise) (b)		Weight (grams)	Water (c) (per-cent)	Food Energy (d) (Cal-ories)	Pro-tein (e) (grams)	Fat (f) (grams)	Fatty Acids: Satu-rated (total) (g) (grams)	Fatty Acids: Unsatu-rated: Oleic (h) (grams)	Fatty Acids: Unsatu-rated: Lino-leic (i) (grams)	Carbo-hydrate (j) (grams)	Calcium (k) (milli-grams)	Phos-phorus (l) (milli-grams)	Iron (m) (milli-grams)	Potas-sium (n) (milli-grams)	Vitamin A Value (o) (inter-national units)	Thiamin (p) (milli-grams)	Ribo-flavin (q) (milli-grams)	Niacin (r) (milli-grams)	Ascorbic Acid (s) (milli-grams)
											nutrients in indicated quantity									
301	Prune-type (1 1/2-in. diam., about 15 per lb with pits).	1 plum	28	79	20	Tr	Tr	—	—	—	6	3	5	0.1	48	80	0.01	0.01	0.1	1
	Canned, heavy sirup pack (Italian prunes), with pits and liquid:																			
302	Cup	1 cup[36]	272	77	215	1	Tr	—	—	—	56	23	26	2.3	367	3,130	0.05	0.05	1.0	5
303	Portion	3 plums; 2 3/4 tbsp liquid.[36]	140	77	110	1	Tr	—	—	—	29	12	13	1.2	189	1,610	0.03	0.03	0.5	3
	Prunes, dried, "softenized," with pits:																			
304	Uncooked	4 extra large or 5 large prunes.[36]	49	28	110	1	Tr	—	—	—	29	22	34	1.7	298	690	0.04	0.07	0.7	1
305	Cooked, unsweetened, all sizes, fruit and liquid.	1 cup[36]	250	66	255	2	1	—	—	—	67	51	79	3.8	695	1,590	0.07	0.15	1.5	2
306	Prune juice, canned or bottled	1 cup	256	80	195	1	Tr	—	—	—	49	36	51	1.8	602	—	0.03	0.03	1.0	5
	Raisins, seedless:																			
307	Cup, not pressed down	1 cup	145	18	420	4	Tr	—	—	—	112	90	146	5.1	1,106	30	0.16	0.12	0.7	1
308	Packet, 1/2 oz (1 1/2 tbsp)	1 packet	14	18	40	Tr	Tr	—	—	—	11	9	14	0.5	107	Tr	0.02	0.01	0.1	Tr
	Raspberries, red:																			
309	Raw, capped, whole	1 cup	123	84	70	1	1	—	—	—	17	27	27	1.1	207	160	0.04	0.11	1.1	31
310	Frozen, sweetened, 10-oz container	1 container	284	74	280	2	1	—	—	—	70	37	48	1.7	284	200	0.06	0.17	1.7	60
	Rhubarb, cooked, added sugar:																			
311	From raw	1 cup	270	63	380	1	Tr	—	—	—	97	211	41	1.6	548	220	0.05	0.14	0.8	16
312	From frozen, sweetened	1 cup	270	63	385	1	1	—	—	—	98	211	32	1.9	475	190	0.05	0.11	0.5	16
	Strawberries:																			
313	Raw, whole berries, capped	1 cup	149	90	55	1	1	—	—	—	13	31	31	1.5	244	90	0.04	0.10	0.9	88
	Frozen, sweetened:																			
314	Sliced, 10-oz container	1 container	284	71	310	1	1	—	—	—	79	40	48	2.0	318	90	0.06	0.17	1.4	151

TABLE A–9. (Continued)

Item No. (a)	Foods, Approximate Measures, Units, and Weight (edible part unless footnotes indicate otherwise) (b)			Water (c)	Food Energy (d)	Protein (e)	Fat (f)	Fatty Acids: Saturated (total) (g)	Fatty Acids: Unsaturated: Oleic (h)	Fatty Acids: Unsaturated: Linoleic (i)	Carbohydrate (j)	Calcium (k)	Phosphorus (l)	Iron (m)	Potassium (n)	Vitamin A Value (o)	Thiamin (p)	Riboflavin (q)	Niacin (r)	Ascorbic Acid (s)
			grams	per-cent	Cal-ories	grams	grams	grams	grams	grams	grams	milli-grams	milli-grams	milli-grams	milli-grams	inter-national units	milli-grams	milli-grams	milli-grams	milli-grams
315	Whole, 1-lb container (about 1 3/4 cups).	1 container	454	76	415	2	1	—	—	—	107	59	73	2.7	472	140	0.09	0.27	2.3	249
316	Tangerine, raw, 2 3/8-in. diam., size 176, without peel (about 4 per lb with peels and seeds).	1 tangerine	86	87	40	1	Tr	—	—	—	10	34	15	0.3	108	360	0.05	0.02	0.1	27
317	Tangerine juice, canned, sweetened.	1 cup	249	87	125	1	Tr	—	—	—	30	44	35	0.5	440	1,040	0.15	0.05	0.2	54
318	Watermelon, raw, 4 by 8 in. wedge with rind and seeds (1/16 of 32 2/3-lb melon, 10 by 16 in.).	1 wedge with rind and seeds[37]	926	93	110	2	1	—	—	—	27	30	43	2.1	426	2,510	0.13	0.13	0.9	30
	grain products																			
	Bagel, 3-in. diam.:																			
319	Egg	1 bagel	55	32	165	6	2	0.5	0.9	0.8	28	9	43	1.2	41	30	0.14	0.10	1.2	0
320	Water	1 bagel	55	29	165	6	1	0.2	0.4	0.6	30	8	41	1.2	42	0	0.15	0.11	1.4	0
321	Barley, pearled, light, uncooked	1 cup	200	11	700	16	2	0.3	0.2	0.8	158	32	378	4.0	320	0	0.24	0.10	6.2	0
	Biscuits, baking powder, 2-in. diam. (enriched flour, vegetable shortening):																			
322	From home recipe	1 biscuit	28	27	105	2	5	1.2	2.0	1.2	13	34	49	0.4	33	Tr	0.08	0.08	0.7	Tr
323	From mix	1 biscuit	28	29	90	2	3	0.6	1.1	0.7	15	19	65	0.6	32	Tr	0.09	0.08	0.8	Tr
	Breadcrumbs (enriched):[38]																			
324	Dry, grated	1 cup	100	7	390	13	5	1.0	1.6	1.4	73	122	141	3.6	152	Tr	0.35	0.35	4.8	Tr
	Soft. See White bread (items 349–350).																			
	Breads:																			
325	Boston brown bread, canned, slice, 3 1/4 by 1/2 in.[38]	1 slice	45	45	95	2	1	0.1	0.2	0.2	21	41	72	0.9	131	0[39]	0.06	0.04	0.7	0

TABLE A-9. (Continued)

Item No. (a)	Foods, Approximate Measures, Units, and Weight (edible part unless footnotes indicate otherwise) (b)			Water (c)	Food Energy (d)	Protein (e)	Fat (f)	Fatty Acids: Saturated (total) (g)	Fatty Acids: Unsaturated: Oleic (h)	Fatty Acids: Unsaturated: Linoleic (i)	Carbohydrate (j)	Calcium (k)	Phosphorus (l)	Iron (m)	Potassium (n)	Vitamin A Value (o)	Thiamin (p)	Riboflavin (q)	Niacin (r)	Ascorbic Acid (s)
			grams	per-cent	Cal-ories	grams	grams	grams	grams	grams	grams	milli-grams	milli-grams	milli-grams	milli-grams	inter-national units	milli-grams	milli-grams	milli-grams	milli-grams
	Cracked-wheat bread (3/4 enriched wheat flour, 1/4 cracked wheat):[38]																			
326	Loaf, 1 lb	1 loaf	454	35	1,195	39	10	2.2	3.0	3.9	236	399	581	9.5	608	Tr	1.52	1.13	14.4	Tr
327	Slice (18 per loaf)	1 slice	25	35	65	2	1	0.1	0.2	0.2	13	22	32	0.5	34	Tr	0.08	0.06	0.8	Tr
	French or vienna bread, enriched:[38]																			
328	Loaf, 1 lb	1 loaf	454	31	1,315	41	14	3.2	4.7	4.6	251	195	386	10.0	408	Tr	1.80	1.10	15.0	Tr
	Slice:																			
329	French (5 by 2 1/2 by 1 in.)	1 slice	35	31	100	3	1	0.2	0.4	0.4	19	15	30	0.8	32	Tr	0.14	0.08	1.2	Tr
330	Vienna (4 3/4 by 4 by 1/2 in.).	1 slice	25	31	75	2	1	0.2	0.3	0.3	14	11	21	0.6	23	Tr	0.10	0.06	0.8	Tr
	Italian bread, enriched:																			
331	Loaf, 1 lb	1 loaf	454	32	1,250	41	4	0.6	0.3	1.5	256	77	349	10.0	336	0	1.80	1.10	15.0	0
332	Slice, 4 1/2 by 3 1/4 by 3/4 in.	1 slice	30	32	85	3	Tr	Tr	Tr	0.1	17	5	23	0.7	22	0	0.12	0.07	1.0	0
	Raisin bread, enriched[38]																			
333	Loaf, 1 lb	1 loaf	454	35	1,190	30	13	3.0	4.7	3.9	243	322	395	10.0	1,057	Tr	1.70	1.07	10.7	Tr
334	Slice (18 per loaf)	1 slice	25	35	65	2	1	0.2	0.3	0.2	13	18	22	0.6	58	Tr	0.09	0.06	0.6	Tr
	Rye Bread:																			
	American, light (2/3 enriched wheat flour, 1/3 rye flour):																			
335	Loaf, 1 lb	1 loaf	454	36	1,100	41	5	0.7	0.5	2.2	236	340	667	9.1	658	0	1.35	0.98	12.9	0
336	Slice (4 3/4 by 3 3/4 by 7/16 in.).	1 slice	25	36	60	2	Tr	Tr	Tr	0.1	13	19	37	0.5	36	0	0.07	0.05	0.7	0
	Pumpernickel (2/3 rye flour, 1/3 enriched wheat flour):																			
337	Loaf, 1 lb	1 loaf	454	34	1,115	41	5	0.7	0.5	2.4	241	381	1,039	11.8	2,059	0	1.30	0.93	8.5	0

Nutrients in indicated quantity: columns (c) through (s).

TABLE A-9. (Continued)

Item No. (a)	Foods, Approximate Measures, Units, and Weight (edible part unless footnotes indicate otherwise) (b)			Water (c)	Food Energy (d)	Protein (e)	Fat (f)	Fatty Acids: Saturated (total) (g)	Fatty Acids: Unsaturated: Oleic (h)	Fatty Acids: Unsaturated: Linoleic (i)	Carbohydrate (j)	Calcium (k)	Phosphorus (l)	Iron (m)	Potassium (n)	Vitamin A Value (o)	Thiamin (p)	Riboflavin (q)	Niacin (r)	Ascorbic Acid (s)
								nutrients in indicated quantity												
			grams	percent	Calories	grams	grams	grams	grams	grams	grams	milligrams	milligrams	milligrams	milligrams	international units	milligrams	milligrams	milligrams	milligrams
338	Slice (5 by 4 by 3/8 in.)	1 slice	32	34	80	3	Tr	0.1	Tr	0.2	17	27	73	0.8	145	0	0.09	0.07	0.6	0
	White bread, enriched:[38]																			
	Soft-crumb type:																			
339	Loaf, 1 lb	1 loaf	454	36	1,225	39	15	3.4	5.3	4.6	229	381	440	11.3	476	Tr	1.80	1.10	15.0	Tr
340	Slice (18 per loaf)	1 slice	25	36	70	2	1	0.2	0.3	0.3	13	21	24	0.6	26	Tr	0.10	0.06	0.8	Tr
341	Slice, toasted	1 slice	22	25	70	2	1	0.2	0.3	0.3	13	21	24	0.6	26	Tr	0.08	0.06	0.8	Tr
342	Slice (22 per loaf)	1 slice	20	36	55	2	1	0.2	0.2	0.2	10	17	19	0.5	21	Tr	0.08	0.05	0.7	Tr
343	Slice, toasted	1 slice	17	25	55	2	1	0.2	0.2	0.2	10	17	19	0.5	21	Tr	0.06	0.05	0.7	Tr
344	Loaf, 1 1/2 lb	1 loaf	680	36	1,835	59	22	5.2	7.9	6.9	343	571	660	17.0	714	Tr	2.70	1.65	22.5	Tr
345	Slice (24 per loaf)	1 slice	28	36	75	2	1	0.2	0.3	0.3	14	24	27	0.7	29	Tr	0.11	0.07	0.9	Tr
346	Slice, toasted	1 slice	24	25	75	2	1	0.2	0.3	0.3	14	24	27	0.7	29	Tr	0.09	0.07	0.9	Tr
347	Slice (28 per loaf)	1 slice	24	36	65	2	1	0.2	0.3	0.2	12	20	23	0.6	25	Tr	0.10	0.06	0.8	Tr
348	Slice, toasted	1 slice	21	25	65	2	1	0.2	0.3	0.2	12	20	23	0.6	25	Tr	0.08	0.06	0.8	Tr
349	Cubes	1 cup	30	36	80	3	1	0.2	0.3	0.3	15	25	29	0.8	32	Tr	0.12	0.07	1.0	Tr
350	Crumbs	1 cup	45	36	120	4	1	0.3	0.5	0.5	23	38	44	1.1	47	Tr	0.18	0.11	1.5	Tr
	Firm-crumb type:																			
351	Loaf, 1 lb	1 loaf	454	35	1,245	41	17	3.9	5.9	5.2	228	435	463	11.3	549	Tr	1.80	1.10	15.0	Tr
352	Slice (20 per loaf)	1 slice	23	35	65	2	1	0.2	0.3	0.3	12	22	23	0.6	28	Tr	0.09	0.06	0.8	Tr
353	Slice, toasted	1 slice	20	24	65	2	1	0.2	0.3	0.3	12	22	23	0.6	28	Tr	0.07	0.06	0.8	Tr
354	Loaf, 2 lb	1 loaf	907	35	2,495	82	34	7.7	11.8	10.4	455	871	925	22.7	1,097	Tr	3.60	2.20	30.0	Tr
355	Slice (34 per loaf)	1 slice	27	35	75	2	1	0.2	0.3	0.3	14	26	28	0.7	33	Tr	0.11	0.06	0.9	Tr
356	Slice, toasted	1 slice	23	24	75	2	1	0.2	0.3	0.3	14	26	28	0.7	33	Tr	0.09	0.06	0.9	Tr
	Whole-wheat bread:																			
	Soft-crumb type:[38]																			
357	Loaf, 1 lb	1 loaf	454	36	1,095	41	12	2.2	2.9	4.2	224	381	1,152	13.6	1,161	Tr	1.37	0.45	12.7	Tr
358	Slice (16 per loaf)	1 slice	28	36	65	3	1	0.1	0.2	0.2	14	24	71	0.8	72	Tr	0.09	0.03	0.8	Tr
359	Slice, toasted	1 slice	24	24	65	3	1	0.1	0.2	0.2	14	24	71	0.8	72	Tr	0.07	0.03	0.8	Tr
	Firm-crumb type:[38]																			
360	Loaf, 1 lb	1 loaf	454	36	1,100	48	14	2.5	3.3	4.9	216	449	1,034	13.6	1,238	Tr	1.17	0.54	12.7	Tr
361	Slice (18 per loaf)	1 slice	25	36	60	3	1	0.1	0.2	0.3	12	25	57	0.8	68	Tr	0.06	0.03	0.7	Tr
362	Slice, toasted	1 slice	21	24	60	3	1	0.1	0.2	0.3	12	25	57	0.8	68	Tr	0.05	0.03	0.7	Tr

TABLE A-9. (Continued)

Item No. (a)	Foods, Approximate Measures, Units, and Weight (edible part unless footnotes indicate otherwise) (b)			Water (c)	Food Energy (d)	Protein (e)	Fat (f)	Fatty Acids: Saturated (total) (g)	Fatty Acids: Unsaturated: Oleic (h)	Fatty Acids: Unsaturated: Linoleic (i)	Carbohydrate (j)	Calcium (k)	Phosphorus (l)	Iron (m)	Potassium (n)	Vitamin A Value (o)	Thiamin (p)	Riboflavin (q)	Niacin (r)	Ascorbic Acid (s)
			grams	per-cent	Cal-ories	grams	grams	grams	grams	grams	grams	milli-grams	milli-grams	milli-grams	milli-grams	inter-national units	milli-grams	milli-grams	milli-grams	milli-grams
	Breakfast cereals:																			
	Hot type, cooked:																			
	Corn (hominy) grits, degermed:																			
363	Enriched	1 cup	245	87	125	3	Tr	Tr	Tr	0.1	27	2	25	0.7	27	Tr[40]	0.10	0.07	1.0	0
364	Unenriched	1 cup	245	87	125	3	Tr	Tr	Tr	0.1	27	2	25	0.2	27	Tr[40]	0.05	0.02	0.5	0
365	Farina, quick-cooking, enriched.	1 cup	245	89	105	3	Tr	Tr	Tr	0.1	22	147	113[41]	([42])	25	0	0.12	0.07	1.0	0
366	Oatmeal or rolled oats	1 cup	240	87	130	5	2	0.4	0.8	0.9	23	22	137	1.4	146	0	0.19	0.05	0.2	0
367	Wheat, rolled	1 cup	240	80	180	5	1	—	—	—	41	19	182	1.7	202	0	0.17	0.07	2.2	0
368	Wheat, whole-meal	1 cup	245	88	110	4	1	—	—	—	23	17	127	1.2	118	0	0.15	0.05	1.5	0
	Ready-to-eat:																			
369	Bran flakes (40% bran), added sugar, salt, iron, vitamins.	1 cup	35	3	105	4	1	—	—	—	28	19	125	12.4	137	1,650	0.41	0.49	4.1	12
370	Bran flakes with raisins, added sugar, salt, iron, vitamins.	1 cup	50	7	145	4	1	—	—	—	40	28	146	17.7	154	2,350	0.58	0.71	5.8	18
	Corn flakes:																			
371	Plain, added sugar, salt, iron, vitamins.	1 cup	25	4	95	2	Tr	—	—	—	21	([43])	9	0.6	30	1,180	0.29	0.35	2.9	9
372	Sugar-coated, added salt, iron, vitamins.	1 cup	40	2	155	2	Tr	—	—	—	37	1	10	1.0	27	1,880	0.46	0.56	4.6	14
373	Corn, puffed, plain, added sugar, salt, iron, vitamins.	1 cup	20	4	80	2	1	—	—	—	16	4	18	2.3	—	940	0.23	0.28	2.3	7
374	Corn, shredded, added sugar, salt, iron, thiamin, niacin.	1 cup	25	3	95	2	Tr	—	—	—	22	1	10	0.6	—	0	0.11	0.05	0.5	0
375	Oats, puffed, added sugar, salt, minerals, vitamins.	1 cup	25	3	100	3	1	—	—	—	19	44	102	2.9	—	1,180	0.29	0.35	2.9	9
	Rice, puffed:																			

TABLE A-9. (Continued)

Item No. (a)	Foods, Approximate Measures, Units, and Weight (edible part unless footnotes indicate otherwise) (b)			Water (c)	Food Energy (d)	Protein (e)	Fat (f)	Fatty Acids: Saturated (total) (g)	Fatty Acids: Unsaturated: Oleic (h)	Fatty Acids: Unsaturated: Linoleic (i)	Carbohydrate (j)	Calcium (k)	Phosphorus (l)	Iron (m)	Potassium (n)	Vitamin A Value (o)	Thiamin (p)	Riboflavin (q)	Niacin (r)	Ascorbic Acid (s)
											nutrients in indicated quantity									
			grams	percent	Calories	grams	grams	grams	grams	grams	grams	milligrams	milligrams	milligrams	milligrams	international units	milligrams	milligrams	milligrams	milligrams
376	Plain, added iron, thiamin, niacin.	1 cup	15	4	60	1	Tr	—	—	—	13	3	14	0.3	15	0	0.07	0.01	0.7	0
377	Presweetened, added salt, iron, vitamins.	1 cup	28	3	115	1	0	—	—	—	26	3	14	1.1[44]	43	1,250	0.38	0.43	5.0	15[45]
378	Wheat flakes, added sugar, salt, iron, vitamins.	1 cup	30	4	105	3	Tr	—	—	—	24	12	83	([43])	81	1,410	0.35	0.42	3.5	11
	Wheat, puffed:																			
379	Plain, added iron, thiamin, niacin.	1 cup	15	3	55	2	Tr	—	—	—	12	4	48	0.6	51	0	0.08	0.03	1.2	0
380	Presweetened, added salt, iron, vitamins.	1 cup	38	3	140	3	Tr	—	—	—	33	7	52	1.6[44]	63	1,680	0.50	0.57	6.7	20[45]
381	Wheat, shredded, plain	1 oblong biscuit or 1/2 cup spoon-size biscuits.	25	7	90	2	1	—	—	—	20	11	97	0.9	87	0	0.06	0.03	1.1	0
382	Wheat germ, without salt and sugar, toasted.	1 tbsp	6	4	25	2	1	—	—	—	3	3	70	0.5	57	10	0.11	0.05	0.3	1
383	Buckwheat flour, light, sifted	1 cup	98	12	340	6	1	0.2	0.4	0.4	78	11	86	1.0	314	0	0.08	0.04	0.4	0
384	Bulgur, canned, seasoned	1 cup	135	56	245	8	4	—	—	—	44	27	263	1.9	151	0	0.08	0.05	4.1	0
	Cake icings. See Sugars and Sweets (items 532–536).																			
	Cakes made from cake mixes with enriched flour:[46]																			
	Angelfood:																			
385	Whole cake (9 3/4-in. diam. tube cake).	1 cake	635	34	1,645	36	1	—	—	—	377	603	756	2.5	381	0	0.37	0.95	3.6	0
386	Piece, 1/12 of cake	1 piece	53	34	135	3	Tr	—	—	—	32	50	63	0.2	32	0	0.03	0.08	0.3	0
	Coffeecake:																			
387	Whole cake (7 3/4 by 5 5/8 by 1 1/4 in.).	1 cake	430	30	1,385	27	41	11.7	16.3	8.8	225	262	748	6.9	469	690	0.82	0.91	7.7	1
388	Piece, 1/6 of cake	1 piece	72	30	230	5	7	2.0	2.7	1.5	38	44	125	1.2	78	120	0.14	0.15	1.3	Tr
	Cupcakes, made with egg, milk, 2 1/2-in. diam.:																			

TABLE A-9. (Continued)

Item No. (a)	Foods, Approximate Measures, Units, and Weight (edible part unless footnotes indicate otherwise) (b)			Water (c)	Food Energy (d)	Protein (e)	Fat (f)	Fatty Acids: Saturated (total) (g)	Fatty Acids: Unsaturated: Oleic (h)	Fatty Acids: Unsaturated: Linoleic (i)	Carbohydrate (j)	Calcium (k)	Phosphorus (l)	Iron (m)	Potassium (n)	Vitamin A Value (o)	Thiamin (p)	Riboflavin (q)	Niacin (r)	Ascorbic Acid (s)
			grams	per-cent	Cal-ories	grams	grams	grams	grams	grams	grams	milli-grams	milli-grams	milli-grams	milli-grams	inter-national units	milli-grams	milli-grams	milli-grams	milli-grams
389	Without icing	1 cupcake	25	26	90	1	3	0.8	1.2	0.7	14	40	59	0.3	21	40	0.05	0.05	0.4	Tr
390	With chocolate icing	1 cupcake	36	22	130	2	5	2.0	1.6	0.6	21	47	71	0.4	42	60	0.05	0.06	0.4	Tr
	Devil's food with chocolate icing:																			
391	Whole, 2 layer cake (8- or 9-in. diam.).	1 cake	1,107	24	3,755	49	136	50.0	44.9	17.0	645	653	1,162	16.6	1,439	1,660	1.06	1.65	10.1	1
392	Piece, 1/16 of cake	1 piece	69	24	235	3	8	3.1	2.8	1.1	40	41	72	1.0	90	100	0.07	0.10	0.6	Tr
393	Cupcake, 2 1/2-in. diam	1 cupcake	35	24	120	2	4	1.6	1.4	0.5	20	21	37	0.5	46	50	0.03	0.05	0.3	Tr
	Gingerbread:																			
394	Whole cake (8-in. square)	1 cake	570	37	1,575	18	39	9.7	16.6	10.0	291	513	570	8.6	1,562	Tr	0.84	1.00	7.4	Tr
395	Piece, 1/9 of cake	1 piece	63	37	175	2	4	1.1	1.8	1.1	32	57	63	0.9	173	Tr	0.09	0.11	0.8	Tr
	White, 2 layer with chocolate icing:																			
396	Whole cake (8- or 9-in. diam.)	1 cake	1,140	21	4,000	44	122	48.2	46.4	20.0	716	1,129	2,041	11.4	1,322	680	1.50	1.77	12.5	2
397	Piece, 1/16 of cake	1 piece	71	21	250	3	8	3.0	2.9	1.2	45	70	127	0.7	82	40	0.09	0.11	0.8	Tr
	Yellow, 2 layer with chocolate icing:																			
398	Whole cake (8- or 9-in. diam.)	1 cake	1,108	26	3,735	45	125	47.8	47.8	20.3	638	1,008	2,017	12.2	1,208	1,550	1.24	1.57	10.6	2
399	Piece, 1/16 of cake	1 piece	69	26	235	3	8	3.0	3.0	1.3	40	63	126	0.8	75	100	0.08	0.10	0.7	Tr
	Cakes made from home recipes using enriched flour:[47]																			
	Boston cream pie with custard filling:																			
400	Whole cake (8-in. diam.)	1 cake	825	35	2,490	41	78	23.0	30.1	15.2	412	553	833	8.2	734[48]	1,730	1.04	1.27	9.6	2
401	Piece, 1/12 of cake	1 piece	69	35	210	3	6	1.9	2.5	1.3	34	46	70	0.7	61[48]	140	0.09	0.11	0.8	Tr
	Fruitcake, dark:																			
402	Loaf, 1-lb (7 1/2 by 2 by 1 1/2 in.).	1 loaf	454	18	1,720	22	69	14.4	33.5	14.8	271	327	513	11.8	2,250	540	0.72	0.73	4.9	2

TABLE A-9. (Continued)

Item No. (a)	Foods, Approximate Measures, Units, and Weight (edible part unless footnotes indicate otherwise) (b)			Water (c)	Food Energy (d)	Protein (e)	Fat (f)	Fatty Acids: Saturated (total) (g)	Fatty Acids: Unsaturated: Oleic (h)	Fatty Acids: Unsaturated: Linoleic (i)	Carbohydrate (j)	Calcium (k)	Phosphorus (l)	Iron (m)	Potassium (n)	Vitamin A Value (o)	Thiamin (p)	Riboflavin (q)	Niacin (r)	Ascorbic Acid (s)
			grams	per-cent	Cal-ories	grams	grams	grams	grams	grams	grams	milli-grams	milli-grams	milli-grams	milli-grams	inter-national units	milli-grams	milli-grams	milli-grams	milli-grams
403	Slice, 1/30 of loaf	1 slice	15	18	55	1	2	0.5	1.1	0.5	9	11	17	0.4	74	20	0.02	0.02	0.2	Tr
	Plain, sheet cake:																			
	Without icing:																			
404	Whole cake (9-in. square)	1 cake	777	25	2,830	35	108	29.5	44.4	23.9	434	497	793	8.5	614[48]	1,320	1.21	1.40	10.2	2
405	Piece, 1/9 of cake	1 piece	86	25	315	4	12	3.3	4.9	2.6	48	55	88	0.9	68[48]	150	0.13	0.15	1.1	Tr
	With uncooked white icing:																			
406	Whole cake (9-in. square)	1 cake	1,096	21	4,020	37	129	42.2	49.5	24.4	694	548	822	8.2	669[48]	2,190	1.22	1.47	10.2	2
407	Piece, 1/9 of cake	1 piece	121	21	445	4	14	4.7	5.5	2.7	77	61	91	0.8	74[48]	240	0.14	0.16	1.1	Tr
	Pound:[49]																			
408	Loaf, 8 1/2 by 3 1/2 by 3 1/4 in.	1 loaf	565	16	2,725	31	170	42.9	73.1	39.6	273	107	418	7.9	345	1,410	0.90	0.99	7.3	0
409	Slice, 1/17 of loaf	1 slice	33	16	160	2	10	2.5	4.3	2.3	16	6	24	0.5	20	80	0.05	0.06	0.4	0
	Spongecake:																			
410	Whole cake (9 3/4-in. diam. tube cake).	1 cake	790	32	2,345	60	45	13.1	15.8	5.7	427	237	885	13.4	687	3,560	1.10	1.64	7.4	Tr
411	Piece, 1/12 of cake	1 piece	66	32	195	5	4	1.1	1.3	0.5	36	20	74	1.1	57	300	0.09	0.14	0.6	Tr
	Cookies made with enriched flour:[50, 51]																			
	Brownies with nuts:																			
	Home-prepared, 1 3/4 by 1 3/4 by 7.8 in.:																			
412	From home recipe	1 brownie	20	10	95	1	6	1.5	3.0	1.2	10	8	30	0.4	38	40	0.04	0.03	0.2	Tr
413	From commercial recipe	1 brownie	20	11	85	1	4	0.9	1.4	1.3	13	9	27	0.4	34	20	0.03	0.02	0.2	Tr
414	Frozen, with chocolate icing,[52] 1 1/2 by 1 3/4 by 7/8 in.	1 brownie	25	13	105	1	5	2.0	2.2	0.7	15	10	31	0.4	44	50	0.03	0.03	0.2	Tr
	Chocolate chip:																			
415	Commercial, 2 1/4-in. diam., 3/8 in. thick.	4 cookies	42	3	200	2	9	2.8	2.9	2.2	29	16	48	1.0	56	50	0.10	0.17	0.9	Tr
416	From home recipe, 2 1/3-in. diam.	4 cookies	40	3	205	2	12	3.5	4.5	2.9	24	14	40	0.8	47	40	0.06	0.06	0.5	Tr

nutrients in indicated quantity

TABLE A-9. (Continued)

Item No. (a)	Foods, Approximate Measures, Units, and Weight (edible part unless footnotes indicate otherwise) (b)			Water (c)	Food Energy (d)	Protein (e)	Fat (f)	Fatty Acids: Saturated (total) (g)	Fatty Acids: Unsaturated: Oleic (h)	Fatty Acids: Unsaturated: Linoleic (i)	Carbohydrate (j)	Calcium (k)	Phosphorus (l)	Iron (m)	Potassium (n)	Vitamin A Value (o)	Thiamin (p)	Riboflavin (q)	Niacin (r)	Ascorbic Acid (s)
			grams	per-cent	Cal-ories	grams	grams	grams	grams	grams	grams	milli-grams	milli-grams	milli-grams	milli-grams	inter-national units	milli-grams	milli-grams	milli-grams	milli-grams
417	Fig bars, square (1 5/8 by 1 5/8 by 3/8 in.) or rectangular (1 1/2 by 1 3/4 by 1/2 in.).	4 cookies	56	14	200	2	3	0.8	1.2	0.7	42	44	34	1.0	111	60	0.04	0.14	0.9	Tr
418	Gingersnaps, 2-in. diam., 1/4 in. thick.	4 cookies	28	3	90	2	2	0.7	1.0	0.6	22	20	13	0.7	129	20	0.08	0.06	0.7	0
419	Macaroons, 2 3/4-in diam., 1/4 in. thick.	2 cookies	38	4	180	2	9	—	—	—	25	10	32	0.3	176	0	0.02	0.06	0.2	0
420	Oatmeal with raisins, 2 5/8-in. diam., 1/4 in. thick.	4 cookies	52	3	235	3	8	2.0	3.3	2.0	38	11	53	1.4	192	30	0.15	0.10	1.0	Tr
421	Plain, prepared from commercial chilled dough, 2 1/2-in. diam., 1/4 in. thick.	4 cookies	48	5	240	2	12	3.0	5.2	2.9	31	17	35	0.6	23	30	0.10	0.08	0.9	0
422	Sandwich type (chocolate or vanilla), 1 3/4-in. diam., 3/8 in. thick.	4 cookies	40	2	200	2	9	2.2	3.9	2.2	28	10	96	0.7	15	0	0.06	0.10	0.7	0
423	Vanilla wafers, 1 3/4-in. diam., 1/4 in. thick.	10 cookies	40	3	185	2	6	—	—	—	30	16	25	0.6	29	50	0.10	0.09	0.8	0
	Cornmeal:																			
424	Whole-ground, unbolted, dry form.	1 cup	122	12	435	11	5	0.5	1.0	2.5	90	24	312	2.9	346	620[53]	0.46	0.13	2.4	0
425	Bolted (nearly whole-grain), dry form.	1 cup	122	12	440	11	4	0.5	0.9	2.1	91	21	272	2.2	303	590[53]	0.37	0.10	2.3	0
	Degermed, enriched:																			
426	Dry form	1 cup	138	12	500	11	2	0.2	0.4	0.9	108	8	137	4.0	166	610[53]	0.61	0.36	4.8	0
427	Cooked	1 cup	240	88	120	3	Tr	Tr	0.1	0.2	26	2	34	1.0	38	140[53]	0.14	0.10	1.2	0
	Degermed, unenriched:																			
428	Dry form	1 cup	138	12	500	11	2	0.2	0.4	0.9	108	8	137	1.5	166	610[53]	0.19	0.07	1.4	0
429	Cooked	1 cup	240	88	120	3	Tr	Tr	0.1	0.2	26	2	34	0.5	38	140[53]	0.05	0.02	0.2	0
	Crackers:[38]																			

nutrients in indicated quantity

TABLE A–9. (Continued)

Item No. (a)	Foods, Approximate Measures, Units, and Weight (edible part unless footnotes indicate otherwise) (b)			Water (c)	Food Energy (d)	Protein (e)	Fat (f)	Fatty Acids: Saturated (total) (g)	Fatty Acids: Unsaturated Oleic (h)	Fatty Acids: Unsaturated Linoleic (i)	Carbohydrate (j)	Calcium (k)	Phosphorus (l)	Iron (m)	Potassium (n)	Vitamin A Value (o)	Thiamin (p)	Riboflavin (q)	Niacin (r)	Ascorbic Acid (s)
			grams	per-cent	Cal-ories	grams	grams	grams	grams	grams	grams	milli-grams	milli-grams	milli-grams	milli-grams	inter-national units	milli-grams	milli-grams	milli-grams	milli-grams
430	Graham, plain, 2 1/2-in. square	2 crackers	14	6	55	1	1	0.3	0.5	0.3	10	6	21	0.5	55	0	0.02	0.08	0.5	0
431	Rye wafers, whole-grain, 1 7/8 by 3 1/2 in.	2 wafers	13	6	45	2	Tr	—	—	—	10	7	50	0.5	78	0	0.04	0.03	0.2	0
432	Saltines, made with enriched flour.	4 crackers or 1 packet	11	4	50	1	1	0.3	0.5	0.4	8	2	10	0.5	13	0	0.05	0.05	0.4	0
	Danish pastry (enriched flour), plain without fruit or nuts:[54]																			
433	Packaged ring, 12 oz	1 ring	340	22	1,435	25	80	24.3	31.7	16.5	155	170	371	6.1	381	1,050	0.97	1.01	8.6	Tr
434	Round piece, about 4 1/4-in. diam. by 1 in.	1 pastry	65	22	275	5	15	4.7	6.1	3.2	30	33	71	1.2	73	200	0.18	0.19	1.7	Tr
435	Ounce	1 oz	28	22	120	2	7	2.0	2.7	1.4	13	14	31	0.5	32	90	0.08	0.08	0.7	Tr
	Doughnuts, made with enriched flour:[38]																			
436	Cake type, plain, 2 1/2-in. diam., 1 in. high.	1 doughnut	25	24	100	1	5	1.2	2.0	1.1	13	10	48	0.4	23	20	0.05	0.05	0.4	Tr
437	Yeast-leavened, glazed, 3 3/4-in. diam., 1 1/4 in. high.	1 doughnut	50	26	205	3	11	3.3	5.8	3.3	22	16	33	0.6	34	25	0.10	0.10	0.8	0
	Macaroni, enriched, cooked (cut lengths, elbows, shells):																			
438	Firm stage (hot)	1 cup	130	64	190	7	1	—	—	—	39	14	85	1.4	103	0	0.23	0.13	1.8	0
	Tender stage:																			
439	Cold macaroni	1 cup	105	73	115	4	Tr	—	—	—	24	8	53	0.9	64	0	0.15	0.08	1.2	0
440	Hot macaroni	1 cup	140	73	155	5	1	—	—	—	32	11	70	1.3	85	0	0.20	0.11	1.5	0
	Macaroni (enriched) and cheese:																			
441	Canned[55]	1 cup	240	80	230	9	10	4.2	3.1	1.4	26	199	182	1.0	139	260	0.12	0.24	1.0	Tr
442	From home recipe (served hot)[56]	1 cup	200	58	430	17	22	8.9	8.8	2.9	40	362	322	1.8	240	860	0.20	0.40	1.8	Tr

nutrients in indicated quantity

TABLE A-9. (Continued)

Item No. (a)	Foods, Approximate Measures, Units, and Weight (edible part unless footnotes indicate otherwise) (b)			Water (c)	Food Energy (d)	Protein (e)	Fat (f)	Fatty Acids: Saturated (total) (g)	Fatty Acids: Unsaturated: Oleic (h)	Fatty Acids: Unsaturated: Linoleic (i)	Carbohydrate (j)	Calcium (k)	Phosphorus (l)	Iron (m)	Potassium (n)	Vitamin A Value (o)	Thiamin (p)	Riboflavin (q)	Niacin (r)	Ascorbic Acid (s)
			grams	percent	Calories	grams	grams	grams	grams	grams	grams	milligrams	milligrams	milligrams	milligrams	international units	milligrams	milligrams	milligrams	milligrams
	Muffins made with enriched flour:[38]																			
	From home recipe:																			
443	Blueberry, 2 3/8-in. diam., 1 1/2 in. high.	1 muffin	40	39	110	3	4	1.1	1.4	0.7	17	34	53	0.6	46	90	0.09	0.10	0.7	Tr
444	Bran	1 muffin	40	35	105	3	4	1.2	1.4	0.8	17	57	162	1.5	172	90	0.07	0.10	1.7	Tr
	Muffins made with enriched flour[38] (cont'd)																			
	From home recipe (cont'd)																			
445	Corn (enriched degermed cornmeal and flour), 2 3/8-in. diam., 1 1/2 in. high.	1 muffin	40	33	125	3	4	1.2	1.6	0.9	19	42	68	0.7	54	120[57]	0.10	0.10	0.7	Tr
446	Plain, 3-in. diam., 1 1/2 in. high.	1 muffin	40	38	120	3	4	1.0	1.7	1.0	17	42	60	0.6	50	40	0.09	0.12	0.9	Tr
	From mix, egg, milk:																			
447	Corn, 2 3/8-in. diam., 1 1/2 in. high.[58]	1 muffin	40	30	130	3	4	1.2	1.7	0.9	20	96	152	0.6	44	100[57]	0.08	0.09	0.7	Tr
448	Noodles (egg noodles), enriched, cooked.	1 cup	160	71	200	7	2	—	—	—	37	16	94	1.4	70	110	0.22	0.13	1.9	0
449	Noodles, chow mein, canned	1 cup	45	1	220	6	11	—	—	—	26	—	—	—	—	—	—	—	—	—
	Pancakes, (4-in. diam.):[38]																			
450	Buckwheat, made from mix (with buckwheat and enriched flours), egg and milk added.	1 cake	27	58	55	2	2	0.8	0.9	0.4	6	59	91	0.4	66	60	0.04	0.05	0.2	Tr
	Plain:																			
451	Made from home recipe using enriched flour.	1 cake	27	50	60	2	2	0.5	0.8	0.5	9	27	38	0.4	33	30	0.06	0.07	0.5	Tr
452	Made from mix with enriched flour, egg and milk added.	1 cake	27	51	60	2	2	0.7	0.7	0.3	9	58	70	0.3	42	70	0.04	0.06	0.2	Tr

Nutrients in indicated quantity (columns c–s).

TABLE A-9. (Continued)

Item No. (a)	Foods, Approximate Measures, Units, and Weight (edible part unless footnotes indicate otherwise) (b)			Water (c)	Food Energy (d)	Protein (e)	Fat (f)	Fatty Acids: Saturated (total) (g)	Fatty Acids: Unsaturated: Oleic (h)	Fatty Acids: Unsaturated: Linoleic (i)	Carbohydrate (j)	Calcium (k)	Phosphorus (l)	Iron (m)	Potassium (n)	Vitamin A Value (o)	Thiamin (p)	Riboflavin (q)	Niacin (r)	Ascorbic Acid (s)
			grams	per-cent	Cal-ories	grams	grams	grams	grams	grams	grams	milli-grams	milli-grams	milli-grams	milli-grams	inter-national units	milli-grams	milli-grams	milli-grams	milli-grams
	Pies, piecrust made with enriched flour, vegetable shortening (9-in. diam.):																			
	Apple:																			
453	Whole	1 pie	945	48	2,420	21	105	27.0	44.5	25.2	360	76	208	6.6	756	280	1.06	0.79	9.3	9
454	Sector, 1/7 of pie	1 sector	135	48	345	3	15	3.9	6.4	3.6	51	11	30	0.9	108	40	0.15	0.11	1.3	2
	Banana cream:																			
455	Whole	1 pie	910	54	2,010	41	85	26.7	33.2	16.2	279	601	746	7.3	1,847	2,280	0.77	1.51	7.0	9
456	Sector, 1/7 of pie	1 sector	130	54	285	6	12	3.8	4.7	2.3	40	86	107	1.0	264	330	0.11	0.22	1.0	1
	Blueberry:																			
457	Whole	1 pie	945	51	2,285	23	102	24.8	43.7	25.1	330	104	217	9.5	614	280	1.03	0.80	10.0	28
458	Sector, 1/7 of pie	1 sector	135	51	325	3	15	3.5	6.2	3.6	47	15	31	1.4	88	40	0.15	0.11	1.4	4
	Cherry:																			
459	Whole	1 pie	945	47	2,465	25	107	28.2	45.0	25.3	363	132	236	6.6	992	4,160	1.09	0.84	9.8	Tr
460	Sector, 1/7 of pie	1 sector	135	47	350	4	15	4.0	6.4	3.6	52	19	34	0.9	142	590	0.16	0.12	1.4	Tr
	Custard:																			
461	Whole	1 pie	910	58	1,985	56	101	33.9	38.5	17.5	213	874	1,028	8.2	1,247	2,090	0.79	1.92	5.6	0
462	Sector, 1/7 of pie	1 sector	130	58	285	8	14	4.8	5.5	2.5	30	125	147	1.2	178	300	0.11	0.27	0.8	0
	Lemon meringue:																			
463	Whole	1 pie	840	47	2,140	31	86	26.1	33.8	16.4	317	118	412	6.7	420	1,430	0.61	0.84	5.2	25
464	Sector, 1/7 of pie	1 sector	120	47	305	4	12	3.7	4.8	2.3	45	17	59	1.0	60	200	0.09	0.12	0.7	4
	Mince:																			
465	Whole	1 pie	945	43	2,560	24	109	28.0	45.9	25.2	389	265	359	13.3	1,682	20	0.96	0.86	9.8	9
466	Sector, 1/7 of pie	1 sector	135	43	365	3	16	4.0	6.6	3.6	56	38	51	1.9	240	Tr	0.14	0.12	1.4	1
	Peach:																			
467	Whole	1 pie	945	48	2,410	24	101	24.8	43.7	25.1	361	95	274	8.5	1,408	6,900	1.04	0.97	14.0	28
468	Sector, 1/7 of pie	1 sector	135	48	345	3	14	3.5	6.2	3.6	52	14	39	1.2	201	990	0.15	0.14	2.0	4
	Pecan:																			
469	Whole	1 pie	825	20	3,450	42	189	27.8	101.0	44.2	423	388	850	25.6	1,015	1,320	1.80	0.95	6.9	Tr
470	Sector, 1/7 of pie	1 sector	118	20	495	6	27	4.0	14.4	6.3	61	55	122	3.7	145	190	0.26	0.14	1.0	Tr
	Pumpkin:																			
471	Whole	1 pie	910	59	1,920	36	102	37.4	37.5	16.6	223	464	628	7.3	1,456	22,480	0.78	1.27	7.0	Tr

nutrients in indicated quantity

TABLE A–9. (Continued)

Item No. (a)	Foods, Approximate Measures, Units, and Weight (edible part unless footnotes indicate otherwise) (b)			Water (c)	Food Energy (d)	Protein (e)	Fat (f)	Fatty Acids: Saturated (total) (g)	Fatty Acids: Unsaturated: Oleic (h)	Fatty Acids: Unsaturated: Linoleic (i)	Carbohydrate (j)	Calcium (k)	Phosphorus (l)	Iron (m)	Potassium (n)	Vitamin A Value (o)	Thiamin (p)	Riboflavin (q)	Niacin (r)	Ascorbic Acid (s)
			grams	per-cent	Cal-ories	grams	grams	grams	grams	grams	grams	milli-grams	milli-grams	milli-grams	milli-grams	inter-national units	milli-grams	milli-grams	milli-grams	milli-grams
472	Sector, 1/7 of pie	1 sector	130	59	275	5	15	5.4	5.4	2.4	32	66	90	1.0	208	3,210	0.11	0.18	1.0	Tr
473	Piecrust (home recipe) made with enriched flour and vegetable shortening, baked.	1 pie shell, 9-in.	180	15	900	11	60	14.8	26.1	14.9	79	25	90	3.1	89	0	0.47	0.40	5.0	0
474	Piecrust mix with enriched flour and vegetable shortening, 10-oz pkg. prepared and baked.	Piecrust for 2-crust pie, 9-in. diam.	320	19	1,485	20	93	22.7	39.7	23.4	141	131	272	6.1	179	0	1.07	0.79	9.9	0
475	Pizza (cheese) baked, 4 3/4-in. sector; 1/8 of 12-in. diam. pie.[19]	1 sector	60	45	145	6	4	1.7	1.5	0.6	22	86	89	1.1	67	230	0.16	0.18	1.6	4
	Popcorn, popped:																			
476	Plain, large kernel	1 cup	6	4	25	1	Tr	Tr	0.1	0.2	5	1	17	0.2	—	—	—	0.01	0.1	0
477	With oil (coconut) and salt added, large kernel.	1 cup	9	3	40	1	2	1.5	0.2	0.2	5	1	19	0.2	—	—	—	0.01	0.2	0
478	Sugar coated	1 cup	35	4	135	2	1	0.5	0.2	0.4	30	2	47	0.5	—	—	—	0.02	0.4	0
	Pretzels, made with enriched flour:																			
479	Dutch, twisted, 2 3/4 by 2 5/8 in.	1 pretzel	16	5	60	2	1	—	—	—	12	4	21	0.2	21	0	0.05	0.04	0.7	0
480	Thin, twisted, 3 1/4 by 2 1/4 by 1/4 in.	10 pretzels	60	5	235	6	3	—	—	—	46	13	79	0.9	78	0	0.20	0.15	2.5	0
481	Stick, 2 1/4 in long	10 pretzels	3	5	10	Tr	Tr	—	—	—	2	1	4	Tr	4	0	0.01	0.01	0.1	0
	Rice, white, enriched:																			
482	Instant, ready-to-serve, hot	1 cup	165	73	180	4	Tr	Tr	Tr	Tr	40	5	31	1.3	—	0	0.21	([59])	1.7	0
	Long grain:																			
483	Raw	1 cup	185	12	670	12	1	0.2	0.2	0.2	149	44	174	5.4	170	0	0.81	0.06	6.5	0
484	Cooked, served hot	1 cup	205	73	225	4	Tr	0.1	0.1	0.1	50	21	57	1.8	57	0	0.23	0.02	2.1	0
	Parboiled:																			
485	Raw	1 cup	185	10	685	14	1	0.2	0.1	0.2	150	111	370	5.4	278	0	0.81	0.07	6.5	0
486	Cooked, served hot	1 cup	175	73	185	4	Tr	0.1	0.1	0.1	41	33	100	1.4	75	0	0.19	0.02	2.1	0

TABLE A-9. (Continued)

Item No. (a)	Foods, Approximate Measures, Units, and Weight (edible part unless footnotes indicate otherwise) (b)			Water (c)	Food Energy (d)	Protein (e)	Fat (f)	Fatty Acids: Saturated (total) (g)	Fatty Acids: Unsaturated: Oleic (h)	Fatty Acids: Unsaturated: Linoleic (i)	Carbohydrate (j)	Calcium (k)	Phosphorus (l)	Iron (m)	Potassium (n)	Vitamin A Value (o)	Thiamin (p)	Riboflavin (q)	Niacin (r)	Ascorbic Acid (s)
			grams	per-cent	Cal-ories	grams	grams	grams	grams	grams	grams	milli-grams	milli-grams	milli-grams	milli-grams	inter-national units	milli-grams	milli-grams	milli-grams	milli-grams
	Rolls, enriched:[38]																			
	Commercial:																			
487	Brown-and-serve (12 per 12-oz pkg.), browned.	1 roll	26	27	85	2	2	0.4	0.7	0.5	14	20	23	0.5	25	Tr	0.10	0.06	0.9	Tr
488	Cloverleaf or pan, 2 1/2-in. diam., 2 in. high.	1 roll	28	31	85	2	2	0.4	0.6	0.4	15	21	24	0.5	27	Tr	0.11	0.07	0.9	Tr
489	Frankfurter and hamburger (8 per 11 1/2-oz pkg.).	1 roll	40	31	120	3	2	0.5	0.8	0.6	21	30	34	0.8	38	Tr	0.16	0.10	1.3	Tr
490	Hard, 3 3/4-in. diam., 2 in. high.	1 roll	50	25	155	5	2	0.4	0.6	0.5	30	24	46	1.2	49	Tr	0.20	0.12	1.7	Tr
491	Hoagie or submarine, 11 1/2 by 3 by 2 1/2 in.	1 roll	135	31	390	12	4	0.9	1.4	1.4	75	58	115	3.0	122	Tr	0.54	0.32	4.5	Tr
	From home recipe:																			
492	Cloverleaf, 2 1/2-in. diam., 2 in. high.	1 roll	35	26	120	3	3	0.8	1.1	0.7	20	16	36	0.7	41	30	0.12	0.12	1.2	Tr
	Spaghetti, enriched, cooked:																			
493	Firm stage, "al dente," served hot.	1 cup	130	64	190	7	1	—	—	—	39	14	85	1.4	103	0	0.23	0.13	1.8	0
494	Tender stage, served hot	1 cup	140	73	155	5	1	—	—	—	32	11	70	1.3	85	0	0.20	0.11	1.5	0
	Spaghetti (enriched) in tomato sauce with cheese:																			
495	From home recipe	1 cup	250	77	260	9	9	2.0	5.4	0.7	37	80	135	2.3	408	1,080	0.25	0.18	2.3	13
496	Canned	1 cup	250	80	190	6	2	0.5	0.3	0.4	39	40	88	2.8	303	930	0.35	0.28	4.5	10
	Spaghetti (enriched) with meat balls and tomato sauce:																			
497	From home recipe	1 cup	248	70	330	19	12	3.3	6.3	0.9	39	124	236	3.7	665	1,590	0.25	0.30	4.0	22
498	Canned	1 cup	250	78	260	12	10	2.2	3.3	3.9	29	53	113	3.3	245	1,000	0.15	0.18	2.3	6
499	Toaster pastries	1 pastry	50	12	200	3	6	—	—	—	36	54[60]	67[60]	1.9	74[60]	500	0.16	0.17	2.1	([60])
	Waffles, made with enriched flour, 7-in. diam.:[38]																			

TABLE A-9. (Continued)

Item No. (a)	Foods, Approximate Measures, Units, and Weight (edible part unless footnotes indicate otherwise) (b)			Water (c)	Food Energy (d)	Protein (e)	Fat (f)	Fatty Acids: Saturated (total) (g)	Fatty Acids: Unsaturated: Oleic (h)	Fatty Acids: Unsaturated: Linoleic (i)	Carbohydrate (j)	Calcium (k)	Phosphorus (l)	Iron (m)	Potassium (n)	Vitamin A Value (o)	Thiamin (p)	Riboflavin (q)	Niacin (r)	Ascorbic Acid (s)
			grams	per-cent	Cal-ories	grams	grams	grams	grams	grams	grams	milli-grams	milli-grams	milli-grams	milli-grams	inter-national units	milli-grams	milli-grams	milli-grams	milli-grams
500	From home recipe	1 waffle	75	41	210	7	7	2.3	2.8	1.4	28	85	130	1.3	109	250	0.17	0.23	1.4	Tr
501	From mix, egg and milk added	1 waffle	75	42	205	7	8	2.8	2.9	1.2	27	179	257	1.0	146	170	0.14	0.22	0.9	Tr
	Wheat flours:																			
	All-purpose or family flour, enriched:																			
502	Sifted, spooned	1 cup	115	12	420	12	1	0.2	0.1	0.5	88	18	100	3.3	109	0	0.74	0.46	6.1	0
503	Unsifted, spooned	1 cup	125	12	455	13	1	0.2	0.1	0.5	95	20	109	3.6	119	0	0.80	0.50	6.6	0
504	Cake or pastry flour, enriched, sifted, spooned.	1 cup	96	12	350	7	1	0.1	0.1	0.3	76	16	70	2.8	91	0	0.61	0.38	5.1	0
505	Self-rising, enriched, unsifted, spooned.	1 cup	125	12	440	12	1	0.2	0.1	0.5	93	331	583	3.6	—	0	0.80	0.50	6.6	0
506	Whole-wheat, from hard wheats, stirred.	1 cup	120	12	400	16	2	0.4	0.2	1.0	85	49	446	4.0	444	0	0.66	0.14	5.2	0
	legumes (dry), nuts, seeds; related products																			
	Almonds, shelled:																			
507	Chopped (about 130 almonds)	1 cup	130	5	775	24	70	5.6	47.7	12.8	25	304	655	6.1	1,005	0	0.31	1.20	4.6	Tr
508	Slivered, not pressed down (about 115 almonds).	1 cup	115	5	690	21	62	5.0	42.2	11.3	22	269	580	5.4	889	0	0.28	1.06	4.0	Tr
	Beans, dry:																			
	Common varieties as Great Northern, navy, and others:																			
	Cooked, drained:																			
509	Great Northern	1 cup	180	69	210	14	1	—	—	—	38	90	266	4.9	749	0	0.25	0.13	1.3	0
510	Pea (navy)	1 cup	190	69	225	15	1	—	—	—	40	95	281	5.1	790	0	0.27	0.13	1.3	0
	Canned, solids and liquid:																			
	White with—																			
511	Frankfurters (sliced)	1 cup	255	71	365	19	18	—	—	—	32	94	303	4.8	668	330	0.18	0.15	3.3	Tr
512	Pork and tomato sauce	1 cup	255	71	310	16	7	2.4	2.8	0.6	48	138	235	4.6	536	330	0.20	0.08	1.5	5

TABLE A–9. (Continued)

Item No. (a)	Foods, Approximate Measures, Units, and Weight (edible part unless footnotes indicate otherwise) (b)			Water (c)	Food Energy (d)	Protein (e)	Fat (f)	Fatty Acids: Saturated (total) (g)	Fatty Acids: Unsaturated: Oleic (h)	Fatty Acids: Unsaturated: Linoleic (i)	Carbohydrate (j)	Calcium (k)	Phosphorus (l)	Iron (m)	Potassium (n)	Vitamin A Value (o)	Thiamin (p)	Riboflavin (q)	Niacin (r)	Ascorbic Acid (s)
			grams	per-cent	Cal-ories	grams	grams	grams	grams	grams	grams	milli-grams	milli-grams	milli-grams	milli-grams	inter-national units	milli-grams	milli-grams	milli-grams	milli-grams
513	Pork and sweet sauce	1 cup	255	66	385	16	12	4.3	5.0	1.1	54	161	291	5.9	—	—	0.15	0.10	1.3	—
514	Red kidney	1 cup	255	76	230	15	1	—	—	—	42	74	278	4.6	673	10	0.13	0.10	1.5	—
515	Lima, cooked, drained	1 cup	190	64	260	16	1	—	—	—	49	55	293	5.9	1,163	—	0.25	0.11	1.3	—
516	Blackeye peas, dry, cooked (with residual cooking liquid).	1 cup	250	80	190	13	1	—	—	—	35	43	238	3.3	573	30	0.40	0.10	1.0	—
517	Brazil nuts, shelled (6–8 large kernels).	1 oz	28	5	185	4	19	4.8	6.2	7.1	3	53	196	1.0	203	Tr	0.27	0.03	0.5	—
518	Cashew nuts, roasted in oil	1 cup	140	5	785	24	64	12.9	36.8	10.2	41	53	522	5.3	650	140	0.60	0.35	2.5	—
	Coconut meat, fresh:																			
519	Piece, about 2 by 2 by 1/2 in.	1 piece	45	51	155	2	16	14.0	0.9	0.3	4	6	43	0.8	115	0	0.02	0.01	0.2	1
520	Shredded or grated, not pressed down.	1 cup	80	51	275	3	28	24.8	1.6	0.5	8	10	76	1.4	205	0	0.04	0.02	0.4	2
521	Filberts (hazelnuts), chopped (about 80 kernels).	1 cup	115	6	730	14	72	5.1	55.2	7.3	19	240	388	3.9	810	—	0.53	—	1.0	Tr
522	Lentils, whole, cooked	1 cup	200	72	210	16	Tr	—	—	—	39	50	238	4.2	498	40	0.14	0.12	1.2	0
523	Peanuts, roasted in oil, salted (whole, halves, chopped).	1 cup	144	2	840	37	72	13.7	33.0	20.7	27	107	577	3.0	971	—	0.46	0.19	24.8	0
524	Peanut butter	1 tbsp	16	2	95	4	8	1.5	3.7	2.3	3	9	61	0.3	100	—	0.02	0.02	2.4	0
525	Peas, split, dry, cooked	1 cup	200	70	230	16	1	—	—	—	42	22	178	3.4	592	80	0.30	0.18	1.8	—
526	Pecans, chopped or pieces (about 120 large halves).	1 cup	118	3	810	11	84	7.2	50.5	20.0	17	86	341	2.8	712	150	1.01	0.15	1.1	2
527	Pumpkin and squash kernels, dry, hulled.	1 cup	140	4	775	41	65	11.8	23.5	27.5	21	71	1,602	15.7	1,386	100	0.34	0.27	3.4	—
528	Sunflower seeds, dry, hulled	1 cup	145	5	810	35	69	8.2	13.7	43.2	29	174	1,214	10.3	1,334	70	2.84	0.33	7.8	—
	Walnuts:																			
	Black:																			
529	Chopped or broken kernels	1 cup	125	3	785	26	74	6.3	13.3	45.7	19	Tr	713	7.5	575	380	0.28	0.14	0.9	—
530	Ground (finely)	1 cup	80	3	500	16	47	4.0	8.5	29.2	12	Tr	456	4.8	368	240	0.18	0.09	0.6	—

Columns (c)–(s): nutrients in indicated quantity

TABLE A–9. (Continued)

Item No. (a)	Foods, Approximate Measures, Units, and Weight (edible part unless footnotes indicate otherwise) (b)			Water (c)	Food Energy (d)	Protein (e)	Fat (f)	Fatty Acids: Saturated (total) (g)	Fatty Acids: Unsaturated: Oleic (h)	Fatty Acids: Unsaturated: Linoleic (i)	Carbohydrate (j)	Calcium (k)	Phosphorus (l)	Iron (m)	Potassium (n)	Vitamin A Value (o)	Thiamin (p)	Riboflavin (q)	Niacin (r)	Ascorbic Acid (s)
			grams	per-cent	Cal-ories	grams	grams	grams	grams	grams	grams	milli-grams	milli-grams	milli-grams	milli-grams	inter-national units	milli-grams	milli-grams	milli-grams	milli-grams
531	Persian or English, chopped (about 60 halves).	1 cup	120	4	780	18	77	8.4	11.8	42.2	19	119	456	3.7	540	40	0.40	0.16	1.1	2
	sugars and sweets																			
	Cake icings:																			
	Boiled, white:																			
532	Plain	1 cup	94	18	295	1	0	0	0	0	75	2	2	Tr	17	0	Tr	0.03	Tr	0
533	With coconut	1 cup	166	15	605	3	13	11.0	0.9	Tr	124	10	50	0.8	277	0	0.02	0.07	0.3	0
	Uncooked:																			
534	Chocolate made with milk and butter.	1 cup	275	14	1,035	9	38	23.4	11.7	1.0	185	165	305	3.3	536	580	0.06	0.28	0.6	1
535	Creamy fudge from mix and water.	1 cup	245	15	830	7	16	5.1	6.7	3.1	183	96	218	2.7	238	Tr	0.05	0.20	0.7	Tr
536	White	1 cup	319	11	1,200	2	21	12.7	5.1	0.5	260	48	38	Tr	57	860	Tr	0.06	Tr	Tr
	Candy:																			
537	Caramels, plain or chocolate	1 oz	28	8	115	1	3	1.6	1.1	0.1	22	42	35	0.4	54	Tr	0.01	0.05	0.1	Tr
	Chocolate:																			
538	Milk, plain	1 oz	28	1	145	2	9	5.5	3.0	0.3	16	65	65	0.3	109	80	0.02	0.10	0.1	Tr
539	Semisweet, small pieces (60 per oz).	1 cup or 6-oz pkg	170	1	860	7	61	36.2	19.8	1.7	97	51	255	4.4	553	30	0.02	0.14	0.9	0
540	Chocolate-coated peanuts	1 oz	28	1	160	5	12	4.0	4.7	2.1	11	33	84	0.4	143	Tr	0.10	0.05	2.1	Tr
541	Fondant, uncoated (mints, candy corn, other).	1 oz	28	8	105	Tr	1	0.1	0.3	0.1	25	4	2	0.3	1	0	Tr	Tr	Tr	0
542	Fudge, chocolate, plain	1 oz	28	8	115	1	3	1.3	1.4	0.6	21	22	24	0.3	42	Tr	0.01	0.03	0.1	Tr
543	Gum drops	1 oz	28	12	100	Tr	Tr	—	—	—	25	2	Tr	0.1	1	0	0	Tr	Tr	0
544	Hard	1 oz	28	1	110	0	Tr	—	—	—	28	6	2	0.5	1	0	0	0	0	0
545	Marshmallows	1 oz	28	17	90	1	Tr	—	—	—	23	5	2	0.5	2	0	0	Tr	Tr	0
	Chocolate-flavored beverage powders (about 4 heaping tsp per oz):																			

nutrients in indicated quantity

TABLE A–9. (Continued)

Item No. (a)	Foods, Approximate Measures, Units, and Weight (edible part unless footnotes indicate otherwise) (b)			Water (c)	Food Energy (d)	Protein (e)	Fat (f)	Fatty Acids: Saturated (total) (g)	Fatty Acids: Unsaturated: Oleic (h)	Fatty Acids: Unsaturated: Linoleic (i)	Carbohydrate (j)	Calcium (k)	Phosphorus (l)	Iron (m)	Potassium (n)	Vitamin A Value (o)	Thiamin (p)	Riboflavin (q)	Niacin (r)	Ascorbic Acid (s)
			grams	per-cent	Cal-ories	grams	grams	grams	grams	grams	grams	milli-grams	milli-grams	milli-grams	milli-grams	inter-national units	milli-grams	milli-grams	milli-grams	milli-grams
546	With nonfat dry milk	1 oz	28	2	100	5	1	0.5	0.3	Tr	20	167	155	0.5	227	10	0.04	0.21	0.2	1
547	Without milk	1 oz	28	1	100	1	1	0.4	0.2	Tr	25	9	48	0.6	142	—	0.01	0.03	0.1	0
548	Honey, strained or extracted	1 tbsp	21	17	65	Tr	0	0	0	0	17	1	1	0.1	11	0	Tr	0.01	0.1	Tr
549	Jams and preserves	1 tbsp	20	29	55	Tr	Tr	—	—	—	14	4	2	0.2	18	Tr	Tr	0.01	Tr	Tr
550		1 packet	14	29	40	Tr	Tr	—	—	—	10	3	1	0.1	12	Tr	Tr	Tr	Tr	Tr
551	Jellies	1 tbsp	18	29	50	Tr	Tr	—	—	—	13	4	1	0.3	14	Tr	Tr	0.01	Tr	1
552		1 packet	14	29	40	Tr	Tr	—	—	—	10	3	1	0.2	11	Tr	Tr	Tr	Tr	1
	Sirups:																			
	Chocolate-flavored sirup or topping:																			
553	Thin type	1 fl oz or 2 tbsp	38	32	90	1	1	0.5	0.3	Tr	24	6	35	0.6	106	Tr	0.01	0.03	0.2	0
554	Fudge type	1 fl oz or 2 tbsp	38	25	125	2	5	3.1	1.6	0.1	20	48	60	0.5	107	60	0.02	0.08	0.2	Tr
	Molasses, cane:																			
555	Light (first extraction)	1 tbsp	20	24	50	—	—	—	—	—	13	33	9	0.9	183	—	0.01	0.01	Tr	—
556	Blackstrap (third extraction)	1 tbsp	20	24	45	—	—	—	—	—	11	137	17	3.2	585	—	0.02	0.04	0.4	—
557	Sorghum	1 tbsp	21	23	55	—	—	—	—	—	14	35	5	2.6	—	—	—	0.02	Tr	—
558	Table blends, chiefly corn, light and dark.	1 tbsp	21	24	60	0	0	0	0	0	15	9	3	0.8	1	0	0	0	0	0
	Sugars:																			
559	Brown, pressed down	1 cup	220	2	820	0	0	0	0	0	212	187	42	7.5	757	0	0.02	0.07	0.4	0
	White:																			
560	Granulated	1 cup	200	1	770	0	0	0	0	0	199	0	0	0.2	6	0	0	0	0	0
561		1 tbsp	12	1	45	0	0	0	0	0	12	0	0	Tr	Tr	0	0	0	0	0
562		1 packet	6	1	23	0	0	0	0	0	6	0	0	Tr	Tr	0	0	0	0	0
563	Powdered, sifted, spooned into cup.	1 cup	100	1	385	0	0	0	0	0	100	0	0	0.1	3	0	0	0	0	0

vegetable and vegetable products

Asparagus, green:

Cooked, drained:

TABLE A-9. (Continued)

Item No. (a)	Foods, Approximate Measures, Units, and Weight (edible part unless footnotes indicate otherwise) (b)			Water (c)	Food Energy (d)	Protein (e)	Fat (f)	Fatty Acids: Saturated (total) (g)	Fatty Acids: Unsaturated: Oleic (h)	Fatty Acids: Unsaturated: Linoleic (i)	Carbohydrate (j)	Calcium (k)	Phosphorus (l)	Iron (m)	Potassium (n)	Vitamin A Value (o)	Thiamin (p)	Riboflavin (q)	Niacin (r)	Ascorbic Acid (s)
			grams	per-cent	Cal-ories	grams	grams	grams	grams	grams	grams	milli-grams	milli-grams	milli-grams	milli-grams	inter-national units	milli-grams	milli-grams	milli-grams	milli-grams
	Cuts and tips, 1 1/2- to 2-in. lengths:																			
564	From raw	1 cup	145	94	30	3	Tr	—	—	—	5	30	73	0.9	265	1,310	0.23	0.26	2.0	38
565	From frozen	1 cup	180	93	40	6	Tr	—	—	—	6	40	115	2.2	396	1,530	0.25	0.23	1.8	41
	Spears, 1/2-in. diam. at base:																			
566	From raw	4 spears	60	94	10	1	Tr	—	—	—	2	13	30	0.4	110	540	0.10	0.11	0.8	16
567	From frozen	4 spears	60	92	15	2	Tr	—	—	—	2	13	40	0.7	143	470	0.10	0.08	0.7	16
568	Canned, spears, 1/2-in. diam. at base.	4 spears	80	93	15	2	Tr	—	—	—	3	15	42	1.5	133	640	0.05	0.08	0.6	12
	Beans:																			
	Lima, immature seeds, frozen, cooked, drained:																			
569	Thick-seeded types (Ford-hooks)	1 cup	170	74	170	10	Tr	—	—	—	32	34	153	2.9	724	390	0.12	0.09	1.7	29
570	Thin-seeded types (baby limas)	1 cup	180	69	210	13	Tr	—	—	—	40	63	227	4.7	709	400	0.16	0.09	2.2	22
	Snap:																			
	Green:																			
	Cooked, drained:																			
571	From raw (cuts and French style).	1 cup	125	92	30	2	Tr	—	—	—	7	63	46	0.8	189	680	0.09	0.11	0.6	15
	From frozen:																			
572	Cuts	1 cup	135	92	35	2	Tr	—	—	—	8	54	43	0.9	205	780	0.09	0.12	0.5	7
573	French style	1 cup	130	92	35	2	Tr	—	—	—	8	49	39	1.2	177	690	0.08	0.10	0.4	9
574	Canned, drained solids (cuts).	1 cup	135	92	30	2	Tr	—	—	—	7	61	34	2.0	128	630	0.04	0.07	0.4	5
	Yellow or wax:																			
	Cooked, drained:																			
575	From raw (cuts and French style).	1 cup	125	93	30	2	Tr	—	—	—	6	63	46	0.8	189	290	0.09	0.11	0.6	16

Nutrients in indicated quantity: columns (c) through (s).

TABLE A-9. (Continued)

Item No. (a)	Foods, Approximate Measures, Units, and Weight (edible part unless footnotes indicate otherwise) (b)			Water (c)	Food Energy (d)	Protein (e)	Fat (f)	Fatty Acids: Saturated (total) (g)	Fatty Acids: Unsaturated: Oleic (h)	Fatty Acids: Unsaturated: Linoleic (i)	Carbohydrate (j)	Calcium (k)	Phosphorus (l)	Iron (m)	Potassium (n)	Vitamin A Value (o)	Thiamin (p)	Riboflavin (q)	Niacin (r)	Ascorbic Acid (s)
			grams	percent	Calories	grams	grams	grams	grams	grams	grams	milligrams	milligrams	milligrams	milligrams	international units	milligrams	milligrams	milligrams	milligrams
576	From frozen (cuts)	1 cup	135	92	35	2	Tr	—	—	—	8	47	42	0.9	221	140	0.09	0.11	0.5	8
577	Canned, drained solids (cuts).	1 cup	135	92	30	2	Tr	—	—	—	7	61	34	2.0	128	140	0.04	0.07	0.4	7
	Beans, mature. See Beans, dry (items 509–515) and Blackeye peas, dry (item 516).																			
	Bean sprouts (mung):																			
578	Raw	1 cup	105	89	35	4	Tr	—	—	—	7	20	67	1.4	234	20	0.14	0.14	0.8	20
579	Cooked, drained	1 cup	125	91	35	4	Tr	—	—	—	7	21	60	1.1	195	30	0.11	0.13	0.9	8
	Beets:																			
	Cooked, drained, peeled:																			
580	Whole beets, 2-in. diam.	2 beets	100	91	30	1	Tr	—	—	—	7	14	23	0.5	208	20	0.03	0.04	0.3	6
581	Diced or sliced	1 cup	170	91	55	2	Tr	—	—	—	12	24	39	0.9	354	30	0.05	0.07	0.5	10
	Canned, drained solids:																			
582	Whole beets, small	1 cup	160	89	60	2	Tr	—	—	—	14	30	29	1.1	267	30	0.02	0.05	0.2	5
583	Diced or sliced	1 cup	170	89	65	2	Tr	—	—	—	15	32	31	1.2	284	30	0.02	0.05	0.2	5
584	Beet greens, leaves and stems, cooked, drained.	1 cup	145	94	25	2	Tr	—	—	—	5	144	36	2.8	481	7,400	0.10	0.22	0.4	22
	Blackeye peas, immature seeds, cooked and drained:																			
585	From raw	1 cup	165	72	180	13	1	—	—	—	30	40	241	3.5	625	580	0.50	0.18	2.3	28
586	From frozen	1 cup	170	66	220	15	1	—	—	—	40	43	286	4.8	573	290	0.68	0.19	2.4	15
	Broccoli, cooked, drained:																			
	From raw:																			
587	Stalk, medium size	1 stalk	180	91	45	6	1	—	—	—	8	158	112	1.4	481	4,500	0.16	0.36	1.4	162
588	Stalks cut into 1/2-in. pieces	1 cup	155	91	40	5	Tr	—	—	—	7	136	96	1.2	414	3,880	0.14	0.31	1.2	140
	From frozen:																			
589	Stalk, 4 1/2 to 5 in. long	1 stalk	30	91	10	1	Tr	—	—	—	1	12	17	0.2	66	570	0.02	0.03	0.2	22
590	Chopped	1 cup	185	92	50	5	1	—	—	—	9	100	104	1.3	392	4,810	0.11	0.22	0.9	105

nutrients in indicated quantity

TABLE A-9. (Continued)

Item No. (a)	Foods, Approximate Measures, Units, and Weight (edible part unless footnotes indicate otherwise) (b)			Water (c)	Food Energy (d)	Protein (e)	Fat (f)	Fatty Acids: Saturated (total) (g)	Fatty Acids: Unsaturated: Oleic (h)	Fatty Acids: Unsaturated: Linoleic (i)	Carbohydrate (j)	Calcium (k)	Phosphorus (l)	Iron (m)	Potassium (n)	Vitamin A Value (o)	Thiamin (p)	Riboflavin (q)	Niacin (r)	Ascorbic Acid (s)
			grams	per-cent	Cal-ories	grams	grams	grams	grams	grams	grams	milli-grams	milli-grams	milli-grams	milli-grams	inter-national units	milli-grams	milli-grams	milli-grams	milli-grams
	Brussels sprouts, cooked, drained:																			
591	From raw, 7–8 sprouts (1 1/4- to 1 1/2-in. diam.).	1 cup	155	88	55	7	1	—	—	—	10	50	112	1.7	423	810	0.12	0.22	1.2	135
592	From frozen	1 cup	155	89	50	5	Tr	—	—	—	10	33	95	1.2	457	880	0.12	0.16	0.9	126
	Cabbage:																			
	Common varieties:																			
	Raw:																			
593	Coarsely shredded or sliced	1 cup	70	91	15	1	Tr	—	—	—	4	34	20	0.3	163	90	0.04	0.04	0.2	33
594	Finely shredded or chopped	1 cup	90	92	20	1	Tr	—	—	—	5	44	26	0.4	210	120	0.05	0.05	0.3	42
595	Cooked, drained	1 cup	145	94	30	2	Tr	—	—	—	6	64	29	0.4	236	190	0.06	0.06	0.4	48
	Common varieties (cont'd):																			
596	Red, raw, coarsely shredded or sliced.	1 cup	70	90	20	1	Tr	—	—	—	5	29	25	0.6	188	30	0.06	0.04	0.3	43
597	Savoy, raw, coarsely shredded or sliced.	1 cup	70	92	15	2	Tr	—	—	—	3	47	38	0.6	188	140	0.04	0.06	0.2	39
598	Cabbage, celery (also called pe-tsai or wongbok), raw, 1-in. pieces.	1 cup	75	95	10	1	Tr	—	—	—	2	32	30	0.5	190	110	0.04	0.03	0.5	19
599	Cabbage, white mustard (also called bokchoy or pakchoy), cooked drained.	1 cup	170	95	25	2	Tr	—	—	—	4	252	56	1.0	364	5,270	0.07	0.14	1.2	26
	Carrots:																			
	Raw, without crowns and tips, scraped:																			
600	Whole, 7 1/2 by 1 1/8 in. or strips, 2 1/2 to 3 in. long.	1 carrot or 18 strips	72	88	30	1	Tr	—	—	—	7	27	26	0.5	246	7,930	0.04	0.04	0.4	6
601	Grated	1 cup	110	88	45	1	Tr	—	—	—	11	41	40	0.8	375	12,100	0.07	0.06	0.7	9

nutrients in indicated quantity

TABLE A–9. (Continued)

Item No. (a)	Foods, Approximate Measures, Units, and Weight (edible part unless footnotes indicate otherwise) (b)			Water (c)	Food Energy (d)	Protein (e)	Fat (f)	Fatty Acids: Saturated (total) (g)	Fatty Acids: Unsaturated: Oleic (h)	Fatty Acids: Unsaturated: Linoleic (i)	Carbohydrate (j)	Calcium (k)	Phosphorus (l)	Iron (m)	Potassium (n)	Vitamin A Value (o)	Thiamin (p)	Riboflavin (q)	Niacin (r)	Ascorbic Acid (s)
			grams	per-cent	Cal-ories	grams	grams	grams	grams	grams	grams	milli-grams	milli-grams	milli-grams	milli-grams	inter-national units	milli-grams	milli-grams	milli-grams	milli-grams
602	Cooked (crosswise cuts), drained	1 cup	155	91	50	1	Tr	—	—	—	11	51	48	0.9	344	16,280	0.08	0.08	0.8	9
	Canned:																			
603	Sliced, drained solids	1 cup	155	91	45	1	Tr	—	—	—	10	47	34	1.1	186	23,250	0.03	0.05	0.6	3
604	Strained or junior (baby food)	1 oz (1 3/4 to 2 tbsp)	28	92	10	Tr	Tr	—	—	—	2	7	6	0.1	51	3,690	0.01	0.01	0.1	1
	Cauliflower:																			
605	Raw, chopped	1 cup	115	91	31	3	Tr	—	—	—	6	29	64	1.3	339	70	0.13	0.12	0.8	90
	Cooked, drained:																			
606	From raw (flower buds)	1 cup	125	93	30	3	Tr	—	—	—	5	26	53	0.9	258	80	0.11	0.10	0.8	69
607	From frozen (flowerets)	1 cup	180	94	30	3	Tr	—	—	—	6	31	68	0.9	373	50	0.07	0.09	0.7	74
	Celery, Pascal type, raw:																			
608	Stalk, large outer, 8 by 1 1/2 in., at root end.	1 stalk	40	94	5	Tr	Tr	—	—	—	2	16	11	0.1	136	110	0.01	0.01	0.1	4
609	Pieces, diced	1 cup	120	94	20	1	Tr	—	—	—	5	47	34	0.4	409	320	0.04	0.04	0.4	11
	Collards, cooked, drained:																			
610	From raw (leaves without stems)	1 cup	190	90	65	7	1	—	—	—	10	357	99	1.5	498	14,820	0.21	0.38	2.3	144
611	From frozen (chopped)	1 cup	170	90	50	5	1	—	—	—	10	299	87	1.7	401	11,560	0.10	0.24	1.0	56
	Corn, sweet:																			
	Cooked, drained:																			
612	From raw, ear 5 by 1 3/4 in.	1 ear[61]	140	74	70	2	1	—	—	—	16	2	69	0.5	151	310[62]	0.09	0.08	1.1	7
	From frozen:																			
613	Ear, 5 in. long	1 ear[61]	229	73	120	4	1	—	—	—	27	4	121	1.0	291	440[62]	0.18	0.10	2.1	9
614	Kernels	1 cup	165	77	130	5	1	—	—	—	31	5	120	1.3	304	580[62]	0.15	0.10	2.5	8
	Canned:																			
615	Cream style	1 cup	256	76	210	5	2	—	—	—	51	8	143	1.5	248	840[62]	0.08	0.13	2.6	13
	Whole Kernel:																			
616	Vacuum pack	1 cup	210	76	175	5	1	—	—	—	43	6	153	1.1	204	740[62]	0.06	0.13	2.3	11
617	Wet pack, drained solids	1 cup	165	76	140	4	1	—	—	—	33	8	81	0.8	160	580[62]	0.05	0.08	1.5	7

TABLE A-9. (Continued)

Item No. (a)	Foods, Approximate Measures, Units, and Weight (edible part unless footnotes indicate otherwise) (b)			Water (c)	Food Energy (d)	Protein (e)	Fat (f)	Fatty Acids: Saturated (total) (g)	Fatty Acids: Unsaturated: Oleic (h)	Fatty Acids: Unsaturated: Linoleic (i)	Carbohydrate (j)	Calcium (k)	Phosphorus (l)	Iron (m)	Potassium (n)	Vitamin A Value (o)	Thiamin (p)	Riboflavin (q)	Niacin (r)	Ascorbic Acid (s)
			grams	percent	Calories	grams	grams	grams	grams	grams	grams	milligrams	milligrams	milligrams	milligrams	international units	milligrams	milligrams	milligrams	milligrams
	Cowpeas. See Blackeye peas, (items 585–586).																			
	Cucumber slices, 1/8 in. thick, (large, 2 1/8-in. diam.; small, 1 3/4-in. diam.):																			
618	With peel	6 large or 8 small slices	28	95	5	Tr	Tr	—	—	—	1	7	8	0.3	45	70	0.01	0.01	0.1	3
619	Without peel	6 1/2 large or 9 small pieces	28	96	5	Tr	Tr	—	—	—	1	5	5	0.1	45	Tr	0.01	0.01	0.1	3
620	Dandelion greens, cooked, drained	1 cup	105	90	35	2	1	—	—	—	7	147	44	1.9	244	12,290	0.14	0.17	—	19
621	Endive, curly (including escarole), raw, small pieces.	1 cup	50	93	10	1	Tr	—	—	—	2	41	27	0.9	147	1,650	0.04	0.07	0.3	5
	Kale, cooked, drained:																			
622	From raw (leaves without stems and midribs).	1 cup	110	88	45	5	1	—	—	—	7	206	64	1.8	243	9,130	0.11	0.20	1.8	102
623	From frozen (leaf style)	1 cup	130	91	40	4	1	—	—	—	7	157	62	1.3	251	10,660	0.08	0.20	0.9	49
	Lettuce, raw:																			
	Butterhead, as Boston types:																			
624	Head, 5-in. diam	1 head[63]	220	95	25	2	Tr	—	—	—	4	57	42	3.3	430	1,580	0.10	0.10	0.5	13
625	Leaves	1 outer or 2 inner or 3 heart leaves.	15	95	Tr	Tr	Tr	—	—	—	Tr	5	4	0.3	40	150	0.01	0.01	Tr	1
	Crisphead, as Iceberg:																			
626	Head, 6-in. diam.	1 head[64]	567	96	70	5	1	—	—	—	16	108	118	2.7	943	1,780	0.32	0.32	1.6	32
627	Wedge, 1/4 of head	1 wedge	135	96	20	1	Tr	—	—	—	4	27	30	0.7	236	450	0.08	0.08	0.4	8
628	Pieces, chopped or shredded	1 cup	55	96	5	Tr	Tr	—	—	—	2	11	12	0.3	96	180	0.03	0.03	0.2	3
629	Looseleaf (bunching varieties including romaine or cos), chopped or shredded pieces.	1 cup	55	94	10	1	Tr	—	—	—	2	37	14	0.8	145	1,050	0.03	0.04	0.2	10

nutrients in indicated quantity

TABLE A-9. (Continued)

Item No. (a)	Foods, Approximate Measures, Units, and Weight (edible part unless footnotes indicate otherwise) (b)			Water (c)	Food Energy (d)	Protein (e)	Fat (f)	Fatty Acids: Saturated (total) (g)	Fatty Acids: Unsaturated: Oleic (h)	Fatty Acids: Unsaturated: Linoleic (i)	Carbohydrate (j)	Calcium (k)	Phosphorus (l)	Iron (m)	Potassium (n)	Vitamin A Value (o)	Thiamin (p)	Riboflavin (q)	Niacin (r)	Ascorbic Acid (s)
					nutrients in indicated quantity															
			grams	percent	Calories	grams	grams	grams	grams	grams	grams	milligrams	milligrams	milligrams	milligrams	international units	milligrams	milligrams	milligrams	milligrams
630	Mushrooms, raw, sliced or chopped	1 cup	70	90	20	2	Tr	—	—	—	3	4	81	0.6	290	Tr	0.07	0.32	2.9	2
631	Mustard greens, without stems and midribs, cooked, drained.	1 cup	140	93	30	3	1	—	—	—	6	193	45	2.5	308	8,120	0.11	0.20	0.8	67
632	Okra pods, 3 by 5/8 in., cooked	10 pods	106	91	30	2	Tr	—	—	—	6	98	43	0.5	184	520	0.14	0.19	1.0	21
	Onions:																			
	Mature:																			
	Raw:																			
633	Chopped	1 cup	170	89	65	3	Tr	—	—	—	15	46	61	0.9	267	Tr[65]	0.05	0.07	0.3	17
634	Sliced	1 cup	115	89	45	2	Tr	—	—	—	10	31	41	0.6	181	Tr[65]	0.03	0.05	0.2	12
635	Cooked (whole or sliced), drained.	1 cup	210	92	60	3	Tr	—	—	—	14	50	61	0.8	231	Tr[65]	0.06	0.06	0.4	15
636	Young green, bulb (3/8 in. diam.) and white portion of top.	6 onions	30	88	15	Tr	Tr	—	—	—	3	12	12	0.2	69	Tr	0.02	0.01	0.1	8
637	Parsley, raw, chopped	1 tbsp	4	85	Tr	Tr	Tr	—	—	—	Tr	7	2	0.2	25	300	Tr	0.01	Tr	6
638	Parsnips, cooked (diced or 2-in. lengths).	1 cup	155	82	100	2	1	—	—	—	23	70	96	0.9	587	50	0.11	0.12	0.2	16
	Peas, green:																			
	Canned:																			
639	Whole, drained solids	1 cup	170	77	150	8	1	—	—	—	29	44	129	3.2	163	1,170	0.15	0.10	1.4	14
640	Strained (baby food)	1 oz (1 3/4 to 2 tbsp)	28	86	15	1	Tr	—	—	—	3	3	18	0.3	28	140	0.02	0.03	0.3	3
641	Frozen, cooked, drained	1 cup	160	82	110	8	Tr	—	—	—	19	30	138	3.0	216	960	0.43	0.14	2.7	21
642	Peppers, hot, red, without seeds, dried (ground chili powder, added seasonings).	1 tsp	2	9	5	Tr	Tr	—	—	—	1	5	4	0.3	20	1,300	Tr	0.02	0.2	Tr
	Peppers, sweet (about 5 per lb, whole), stem and seeds removed:																			

TABLE A–9. (Continued)

Item No. (a)	Foods, Approximate Measures, Units, and Weight (edible part unless footnotes indicate otherwise) (b)			Water (c)	Food Energy (d)	Protein (e)	Fat (f)	Fatty Acids: Saturated (total) (g)	Fatty Acids: Unsaturated Oleic (h)	Fatty Acids: Unsaturated Linoleic (i)	Carbohydrate (j)	Calcium (k)	Phosphorus (l)	Iron (m)	Potassium (n)	Vitamin A Value (o)	Thiamin (p)	Riboflavin (q)	Niacin (r)	Ascorbic Acid (s)
			grams	per-cent	Cal-ories	grams	grams	grams	grams	grams	grams	milli-grams	milli-grams	milli-grams	milli-grams	inter-national units	milli-grams	milli-grams	milli-grams	milli-grams
643	Raw	1 pod	74	93	15	1	Tr	—	—	—	4	7	16	0.5	157	310	0.06	0.06	0.4	94
644	Cooked, boiled, drained	1 pod	73	95	15	1	Tr	—	—	—	3	7	12	0.4	109	310	0.05	0.05	0.4	70
	Potatoes, cooked:																			
645	Baked, peeled after baking (about 2 per lb, raw).	1 potato	156	75	145	4	Tr	—	—	—	33	14	101	1.1	782	Tr	0.15	0.07	2.7	31
	Boiled (about 3 per lb, raw):																			
646	Peeled after boiling	1 potato	137	80	105	3	Tr	—	—	—	23	10	72	0.8	556	Tr	0.12	0.05	2.0	22
647	Peeled before boiling	1 potato	135	83	90	3	Tr	—	—	—	20	8	57	0.7	385	Tr	0.12	0.05	1.6	22
	French-fried, strip, 2 to 3 1/2 in. long:																			
648	Prepared from raw	10 strips	50	45	135	2	7	1.7	1.2	3.3	18	8	56	0.7	427	Tr	0.07	0.04	1.6	11
649	Frozen, oven heated	10 strips	50	53	110	2	4	1.1	0.8	2.1	17	5	43	0.9	326	Tr	0.07	0.01	1.3	11
650	Hashed brown, prepared from frozen.	1 cup	155	56	345	3	18	4.6	3.2	9.0	45	28	78	1.9	439	Tr	0.11	0.03	1.6	12
	Mashed, prepared from Raw:																			
651	Milk added	1 cup	210	83	135	4	2	0.7	0.4	Tr	27	50	103	0.8	548	40	0.17	0.11	2.1	21
652	Milk and butter added	1 cup	210	80	195	4	9	5.6	2.3	0.2	26	50	101	0.8	525	360	0.17	0.11	2.1	19
653	Dehydrated flakes (without milk), water, milk, butter, and salt added.	1 cup	210	79	195	4	7	3.6	2.1	0.2	30	65	99	0.6	601	270	0.08	0.08	1.9	11
654	Potato chips, 1 3/4 by 2 1/2 in. oval cross section.	10 chips	20	2	115	1	8	2.1	1.4	4.0	10	8	28	0.4	226	Tr	0.04	0.01	1.0	3
655	Potato salad, made with cooked salad dressing.	1 cup	250	76	250	7	7	2.0	2.7	1.3	41	80	160	1.5	798	350	0.20	0.18	2.8	28
656	Pumpkin, canned	1 cup	245	90	80	2	1	—	—	—	19	61	64	1.0	588	15,680	0.07	0.12	1.5	12
657	Radishes, raw (prepackaged) stem ends, rootlets cut off.	4 radishes	18	95	5	Tr	Tr	—	—	—	1	5	6	0.2	58	Tr	0.01	0.01	0.1	5
658	Sauerkraut, canned, solids and liquid.	1 cup	235	93	40	2	Tr	—	—	—	9	85	42	1.2	329	120	0.07	0.09	0.5	33
	Southern peas. See Blackeye peas (items 585–586).																			

Columns (c)–(s): nutrients in indicated quantity.

TABLE A-9. (Continued)

Item No. (a)	Foods, Approximate Measures, Units, and Weight (edible part unless footnotes indicate otherwise) (b)			Water (c)	Food Energy (d)	Protein (e)	Fat (f)	Fatty Acids: Saturated (total) (g)	Fatty Acids: Unsaturated: Oleic (h)	Fatty Acids: Unsaturated: Linoleic (i)	Carbohydrate (j)	Calcium (k)	Phosphorus (l)	Iron (m)	Potassium (n)	Vitamin A Value (o)	Thiamin (p)	Riboflavin (q)	Niacin (r)	Ascorbic Acid (s)
								nutrients in indicated quantity												
			grams	per-cent	Cal-ories	grams	grams	grams	grams	grams	grams	milli-grams	milli-grams	milli-grams	milli-grams	inter-national units	milli-grams	milli-grams	milli-grams	milli-grams
	Spinach:																			
659	Raw, chopped	1 cup	55	91	15	2	Tr	—	—	—	2	51	28	1.7	259	4,460	0.06	0.11	0.3	28
	Cooked, drained:																			
660	From raw	1 cup	180	92	40	5	1	—	—	—	6	167	68	4.0	583	14,580	0.13	0.25	0.9	50
	From frozen:																			
661	Chopped	1 cup	205	92	45	6	1	—	—	—	8	232	90	4.3	683	16,200	0.14	0.31	0.8	39
662	Leaf	1 cup	190	92	45	6	1	—	—	—	7	200	84	4.8	688	15,390	0.15	0.27	1.0	53
663	Canned, drained solids	1 cup	205	91	50	6	1	—	—	—	7	242	53	5.3	513	16,400	0.04	0.25	0.6	29
	Squash, cooked:																			
664	Summer (all varieties), diced, drained.	1 cup	210	96	30	2	Tr	—	—	—	7	53	53	0.8	296	820	0.11	0.17	1.7	21
665	Winter (all varieties), baked, mashed.	1 cup	205	81	130	4	1	—	—	—	32	57	98	1.6	945	8,610	0.10	0.27	1.4	27
	Sweetpotatoes:																			
	Cooked (raw, 5 by 2 in.; about 2 1/2 per lb):																			
666	Baked in skin, peeled	1 potato	114	64	160	2	1	—	—	—	37	46	66	1.0	342	9,230	0.10	0.08	0.8	25
667	Boiled in skin, peeled	1 potato	151	71	170	3	1	—	—	—	40	48	71	1.1	367	11,940	0.14	0.09	0.9	26
668	Candied, 2 1/2 by 2-in. piece	1 piece	105	60	175	1	3	2.0	0.8	0.1	36	39	45	0.9	200	6,620	0.06	0.04	0.4	11
	Canned:																			
669	Solid pack (mashed)	1 cup	255	72	275	5	1	—	—	—	63	64	105	2.0	510	19,890	0.13	0.10	1.5	36
670	Vacuum pack, piece 2 3/4 by 1 in.	1 piece	40	72	45	1	Tr	—	—	—	10	10	16	0.3	80	3,120	0.02	0.02	0.2	6
	Tomatoes:																			
671	Raw, 2 3/5-in. diam. (3 per 12 oz pkg.).	1 tomato[66]	135	94	25	1	Tr	—	—	—	6	16	33	0.6	300	1,110	0.07	0.05	0.9	28[6]
672	Canned, solids and liquid	1 cup	241	94	50	2	Tr	—	—	—	10	14[68]	46	1.2	523	2,170	0.12	0.07	1.7	41
673	Tomato catsup	1 cup	273	69	290	5	1	—	—	—	69	60	137	2.2	991	3,820	0.25	0.19	4.4	41
674		1 tbsp	15	69	15	Tr	Tr	—	—	—	4	3	8	0.1	54	210	0.01	0.01	0.2	2
	Tomato juice, canned:																			
675	Cup	1 cup	243	94	45	2	Tr	—	—	—	10	17	44	2.2	552	1,940	0.12	0.07	1.9	39
676	Glass (6 fl oz)	1 glass	182	94	35	2	Tr	—	—	—	8	13	33	1.6	413	1,460	0.09	0.05	1.5	29

TABLE A-9. (Continued)

Item No. (a)	Foods, Approximate Measures, Units, and Weight (edible part unless footnotes indicate otherwise) (b)			Water (c)	Food Energy (d)	Protein (e)	Fat (f)	Fatty Acids: Saturated (total) (g)	Fatty Acids: Unsaturated: Oleic (h)	Fatty Acids: Unsaturated: Linoleic (i)	Carbohydrate (j)	Calcium (k)	Phosphorus (l)	Iron (m)	Potassium (n)	Vitamin A Value (o)	Thiamin (p)	Riboflavin (q)	Niacin (r)	Ascorbic Acid (s)
			grams	per-cent	Cal-ories	grams	grams	grams	grams	grams	grams	milli-grams	milli-grams	milli-grams	milli-grams	inter-national units	milli-grams	milli-grams	milli-grams	milli-grams
677	Turnips, cooked, diced	1 cup	155	94	35	1	Tr	—	—	—	8	54	37	0.6	291	Tr	0.06	0.08	0.5	34
	Turnip greens, cooked, drained:																			
678	From raw (leaves and stems)	1 cup	145	94	30	3	Tr	—	—	—	5	252	49	1.5	—	8,270	0.15	0.33	0.7	68
679	From frozen (chopped)	1 cup	165	93	40	4	Tr	—	—	—	6	195	64	2.6	246	11,390	0.08	0.15	0.7	31
680	Vegetables, mixed, frozen, cooked	1 cup	182	83	115	6	1	—	—	—	24	46	115	2.4	348	9,010	0.22	0.13	2.0	15
	miscellaneous items																			
	Baking powders for home use:																			
	Sodium aluminum sulfate:																			
681	With monocalcium phosphate monohydrate.	1 tsp	3.0	2	5	Tr	Tr	0	0	0	1	58	87	—	5	0	0	0	0	0
682	With monocalcium phosphate monohydrate, calcium sulfate.	1 tsp	2.9	1	5	Tr	Tr	0	0	0	1	183	45	—	—	0	0	0	0	0
683	Straight phosphate	1 tsp	3.8	2	5	Tr	Tr	0	0	0	1	239	359	—	6	0	0	0	0	0
684	Low sodium	1 tsp	4.3	2	5	Tr	Tr	0	0	0	2	207	314	—	471	0	0	0	0	0
685	Barbecue sauce	1 cup	250	81	230	4	17	2.2	4.3	10.0	20	53	50	2.0	435	900	0.03	0.03	0.8	13
	Beverages, alcoholic:																			
686	Beer	12 fl oz	360	92	150	1	0	0	0	0	14	18	108	Tr	90	—	0.01	0.11	2.2	—
	Gin, rum, vodka, whisky:																			
687	80-proof	1 1/2-fl oz jigger	42	67	95	—	—	0	0	0	Tr	—	—	—	1	—	—	—	—	—
688	86-proof	1 1/2-fl oz jigger	42	64	105	—	—	0	0	0	Tr	—	—	—	1	—	—	—	—	—
689	90-proof	1 1/2-fl oz jigger	42	62	110	—	—	0	0	0	Tr	—	—	—	1	—	—	—	—	—
	Wines:																			
690	Dessert	3 1/2-fl oz glass	103	77	140	Tr	0	0	0	0	8	8	—	—	77	—	0.01	0.02	0.2	—
691	Table	3 1/2-fl oz glass	102	86	85	Tr	0	0	0	0	4	9	10	0.4	94	—	Tr	0.01	0.1	—
	Beverages, carbonated, sweetened, nonalcoholic:																			
692	Carbonated water	12 fl oz	366	92	115	0	0	0	0	0	29	—	—	—	—	0	0	0	0	0
693	Cola type	12 fl oz	369	90	145	0	0	0	0	0	37	—	—	—	—	0	0	0	0	0

TABLE A-9. (Continued)

Item No. (a)	Foods, Approximate Measures, Units, and Weight (edible part unless footnotes indicate otherwise) (b)			Water (c)	Food Energy (d)	Protein (e)	Fat (f)	Fatty Acids: Saturated (total) (g)	Fatty Acids: Unsaturated: Oleic (h)	Fatty Acids: Unsaturated: Linoleic (i)	Carbohydrate (j)	Calcium (k)	Phosphorus (l)	Iron (m)	Potassium (n)	Vitamin A Value (o)	Thiamin (p)	Riboflavin (q)	Niacin (r)	Ascorbic Acid (s)
								nutrients in indicated quantity												
			grams	percent	Calories	grams	grams	grams	grams	grams	grams	milligrams	milligrams	milligrams	milligrams	international units	milligrams	milligrams	milligrams	milligrams
694	Fruit-flavored sodas and Tom Collins mixer.	12 fl oz	372	88	170	0	0	0	0	0	45	—	—	—	—	0	0	0	0	0
695	Ginger ale	12 fl oz	366	92	115	0	0	0	0	0	29	—	—	—	0	0	0	0	0	0
696	Root beer	12 fl oz	370	90	150	0	0	0	0	0	39	—	—	—	0	0	0	0	0	0
	Chili powder. See Peppers, hot, red (item 642).																			
	Chocolate:																			
697	Bitter or baking	1 oz	28	2	145	3	15	8.9	4.9	0.4	8	22	109	1.9	235	20	0.01	0.07	0.4	0
	Semisweet, see Candy, chocolate (item 539).																			
698	Gelatin, dry	1, 7-g envelope	7	13	25	6	Tr	0	0	0	0	—	—	—	—	—	—	—	—	—
699	Geletin dessert prepared with gelatin dessert powder and water.	1 cup	240	84	140	4	0	0	0	0	34	—	—	—	—	—	—	—	—	—
700	Mustard, prepared, yellow	1 tsp or individual serving pouch or cup.	5	80	5	Tr	Tr	—	—	—	Tr	4	4	0.1	7	—	—	—	—	—
	Olives, pickled, canned:																			
701	Green	4 medium or 3 extra large or 2 giant.[69]	16	78	15	Tr	2	0.2	1.2	0.1	Tr	8	1	0.2	7	40	—	—	—	—
702	Ripe, Mission	3 small or 2 large[69]	10	73	15	Tr	2	0.2	1.2	0.1	Tr	9	2	0.1	2	10	Tr	Tr	—	—
	Pickles, cucumber:																			
703	Dill, medium, whole, 3 3/4 in. long, 1 1/4-in. diam.	1 pickle	65	93	5	Tr	Tr	—	—	—	1	17	14	0.7	130	70	Tr	0.01	Tr	4
704	Fresh-pack, slices 1 1/2-in. diam., 1/4 in. thick.	2 slices	15	79	10	Tr	Tr	—	—	—	3	5	4	0.3	—	20	Tr	Tr	Tr	1
705	Sweet, gherkin, small, whole, about 2 1/2 in. long, 3/4-in. diam.	1 pickle	15	61	20	Tr	Tr	—	—	—	5	2	2	0.2	—	10	Tr	Tr	Tr	1
706	Relish, finely chopped, sweet	1 tbsp	15	63	20	Tr	Tr	—	—	—	5	3	2	0.1	—	—	—	—	—	—
	Popcorn. See items 476–478.																			

TABLE A-9. (Continued)

Item No. (a)	Foods, Approximate Measures, Units, and Weight (edible part unless footnotes indicate otherwise) (b)			Water (c)	Food Energy (d)	Protein (e)	Fat (f)	Fatty Acids: Saturated (total) (g)	Fatty Acids: Unsaturated: Oleic (h)	Fatty Acids: Unsaturated: Linoleic (i)	Carbohydrate (j)	Calcium (k)	Phosphorus (l)	Iron (m)	Potassium (n)	Vitamin A Value (o)	Thiamin (p)	Riboflavin (q)	Niacin (r)	Ascorbic Acid (s)
			grams	per-cent	Cal-ories	grams	grams	grams	grams	grams	grams	milli-grams	milli-grams	milli-grams	milli-grams	inter-national units	milli-grams	milli-grams	milli-grams	milli-grams
														nutrients in indicated quantity						
707	Popsicle, 3-fl oz size	1 popsicle	95	80	70	0	0	0	0	0	18	0	—	Tr	—	0	0	0	0	0
	Soups:																			
	Canned, condensed:																			
	Prepared with equal volume of milk:																			
708	Cream of chicken	1 cup	245	85	180	7	10	4.2	3.6	1.3	15	172	152	0.5	260	610	0.05	0.27	0.7	2
709	Cream of mushroom	1 cup	245	83	215	7	14	5.4	2.9	4.6	16	191	169	0.5	279	250	0.05	0.34	0.7	1
710	Tomato	1 cup	250	84	175	7	7	3.4	1.7	1.0	23	168	155	0.8	418	1,200	0.10	0.25	1.3	15
	Prepared with equal volume of water:																			
711	Bean with pork	1 cup	250	84	170	8	6	1.2	1.8	2.4	22	63	128	2.3	395	650	0.13	0.08	1.0	3
712	Beef broth, bouillon, consomme.	1 cup	240	96	30	5	0	0	0	0	3	Tr	31	0.5	130	Tr	Tr	0.02	1.2	—
713	Beef noodle	1 cup	240	93	65	4	3	0.6	0.7	0.8	7	7	48	1.0	77	50	0.05	0.07	1.0	Tr
714	Clam chowder, Manhattan type (with tomatoes, without milk).	1 cup	245	92	80	2	3	0.5	0.4	1.3	12	34	47	1.0	184	880	0.02	0.02	1.0	—
715	Cream of chicken	1 cup	240	92	95	3	6	1.6	2.3	1.1	8	24	34	0.5	79	410	0.02	0.05	0.5	Tr
716	Cream of mushroom	1 cup	240	90	135	2	10	2.6	1.7	4.5	10	41	50	0.5	98	70	0.02	0.12	0.7	Tr
717	Minestrone	1 cup	245	90	105	5	3	0.7	0.9	1.3	14	37	59	1.0	314	2,350	0.07	0.05	1.0	—
718	Split pea	1 cup	245	85	145	9	3	1.1	1.2	0.4	21	29	149	1.5	270	440	0.25	0.15	1.5	1
719	Tomato	1 cup	245	91	90	2	3	0.5	0.5	1.0	16	15	34	0.7	230	1,000	0.05	0.05	1.2	12
720	Vegetable beef	1 cup	245	92	80	5	2	—	—	—	10	12	49	0.7	162	2,700	0.05	0.05	1.0	—
721	Vegetarian	1 cup	245	92	80	2	2	—	—	—	13	20	39	1.0	172	2,940	0.05	0.05	1.0	—
	Dehydrated:																			
722	Bouillon cube, 1/2 in.	1 cube	4	4	5	1	Tr	—	—	—	Tr	—	—	—	4	—	—	—	—	—
	Mixes:																			
	Unprepared:																			
723	Onion	1 1/2-oz pkg	43	3	150	6	5	1.1	2.3	1.0	23	42	49	0.6	238	30	0.05	0.03	0.3	6
	Prepared with water:																			
724	Chicken noodle	1 cup	240	95	55	2	1	—	—	—	8	7	19	0.2	19	50	0.07	0.05	0.5	Tr
725	Onion	1 cup	240	96	35	1	1	—	—	—	6	10	12	0.2	58	Tr	Tr	Tr	Tr	2

TABLE A–9. (Continued)

Item No. (a)	Foods, Approximate Measures, Units, and Weight (edible part unless footnotes indicate otherwise) (b)			Water (c)	Food Energy (d)	Protein (e)	Fat (f)	Fatty Acids: Saturated (total) (g)	Fatty Acids: Unsaturated: Oleic (h)	Fatty Acids: Unsaturated: Linoleic (i)	Carbohydrate (j)	Calcium (k)	Phosphorus (l)	Iron (m)	Potassium (n)	Vitamin A Value (o)	Thiamin (p)	Riboflavin (q)	Niacin (r)	Ascorbic Acid (s)
			grams	percent	Calories	grams	grams	grams	grams	grams	grams	milligrams	milligrams	milligrams	milligrams	international units	milligrams	milligrams	milligrams	milligrams
726	Tomato vegetable with noodles.	1 cup	240	93	65	1	1	—	—	—	12	7	19	0.2	29	480	0.05	0.02	0.5	5
727	Vinegar, cider	1 tbsp	15	94	Tr	Tr	0	0	0	0	1	1	1	0.1	15	—	—	—	—	—
728	White sauce, medium, with enriched flour.	1 cup	250	73	405	10	31	19.3	7.8	0.8	22	288	233	0.5	348	1,150	0.12	0.43	0.7	2
	Yeast:																			
729	Baker's, dry, active	1 pkg	7	5	20	3	Tr	—	—	—	3	3	90	1.1	140	Tr	0.16	0.38	2.6	Tr
730	Brewer's, dry	1 tbsp	8	5	25	3	Tr	—	—	—	3	17[70]	140	1.4	152	Tr	1.25	0.34	3.0	Tr

NOTE: Dashes (—) denote lack of reliable data for a constituent believed to be present in measurable amount.

1 Vitamin A value is largely from beta-carotene used for coloring. Riboflavin value for items 40–41 apply to products with added riboflavin.
2 Applies to product without added vitamin A. With added vitamin A, value is 500 International Units (I.U.).
3 Applies to product without vitamin A added.
4 Applies to product with added vitamin A. Without added vitamin A, value is 20 International Units (I.U.).
5 Yields 1 qt of fluid milk when reconstituted according to package directions.
6 Applies to product with added vitamin A.
7 Weight applies to product with label claim of 1 1/3 cups equal 3.2 oz.
8 Applies to products made from thick shake mixes and that do not contain added ice cream. Products made from milk shake mixes are higher in fat and usually contain added ice cream.
9 Content of fat, vitamin A, and carbohydrate varies. Consult the label when precise values are needed for special diets.
10 Applies to product made with milk containing no added vitamin A.
11 Based on year-round average.
12 Based on average vitamin A content of fortified margarine. Federal specifications for fortified margarine require a minimum of 15,000 International Units (I.U.) of vitamin A per pound.
13 Fatty acid values apply to product made with regular-type margarine.
14 Dipped in egg, milk or water, and breadcrumbs; fried in vegetable shortening.
15 If bones are discarded, value for calcium will be greatly reduced.
16 Dipped in egg, breadcrumbs, and flour or batter.
17 Prepared with tuna, celery, salad dressing (mayonnaise type), pickle, onion, and egg.
18 Outer layer of fat on the cut was removed to within approximately 1/2 in. of the lean. Deposits of fat within the cut were not removed.
19 Crust made with vegetable shortening and enriched flour.
20 Regular-type margarine used.
21 Value varies widely.
22 About one-fourth of the outer layer of fat on the cut was removed. Deposits of fat within the cut were not removed.
23 Vegetable shortening used.
24 Also applies to pasteurized apple cider.

TABLE A-9. (Continued)

[25] Applies to product without added ascorbic acid. For value of product with added ascorbic acid, refer to label.
[26] Based on product with label claim of 45% of U.S. RDA in 6 fl oz.
[27] Based on product with label claim of 100% of U.S. RDA in 6 fl oz.
[28] Weight includes peel and membranes between sections. Without these parts, the weight of the edible portion is 123 g for item 246 and 118 g for item 247.
[29] For white-fleshed varieties, value is about 20 International Units (I.U.) per cup; for red-fleshed varieties, 1,080 I.U.
[30] Weight includes seeds. Without seeds, weight of the edible portion is 57 g.
[31] Applies to product without added ascorbic acid. With added ascorbic acid, based on claim that 6 fl oz of reconstituted juice contain 45% or 50% of the U.S. RDA, value in milligrams is 108 or 120 for a 6-fl oz can (item 258), 36 or 40 for 1 cup of diluted juice (item 259).
[32] For products with added thiamin and riboflavin but without added ascorbic acid, values in milligrams would be 0.60 for thiamin, 0.80 for riboflavin, and trace for ascorbic acid. For products with only ascorbic acid added, value varies with the brand. Consult the label.
[33] Weight includes rind. Without rind, the weight of the edible portion is 272 g for item 271 and 149 g for item 272.
[34] Represents yellow-fleshed varieties. For white-fleshed varieties, value is 50 International Units (I.U.) for 1 peach, 90 I.U. for 1 cup of slices.
[35] Value represents products with added ascorbic acid. For products without added ascorbic acid, value in milligrams is 116 for a 10-oz container, 103 for 1 cup.
[36] Weight includes pits. After removal of the pits, the weight of the edible portion is 258 g for item 302, 133 g for item 303, 43 g for item 304, and 213 g for item 305.
[37] Weight includes rind and seeds. Without rind and seeds, weight of the edible portion is 426 g.
[38] Made with vegetable shortening.
[39] Applies to product made with white cornmeal. With yellow cornmeal, value is 30 International Units (I.U.).
[40] Applies to white varieties. For yellow varieties, value is 150 International Units (I.U.).
[41] Applies to products that do not contain di-sodium phosphate. If di-sodium phosphate is an ingredient, value is 162 mg.
[42] Value may range from less than 1 mg to about 8 mg depending on the brand. Consult the label.
[43] Value varies with the brand. Consult the label.
[44] Value varies with the brand. Consult the label.
[45] Applies to product with added ascorbic acid. Without added ascorbic acid, value is trace.
[46] Excepting angelfood cake, cakes were made from mixes containing vegetable shortening; icings, with butter
[47] Excepting spongecake, vegetable shortening used for cake portion; butter, for icing. If butter or margarine used for cake portion, vitamin A values would be higher.
[48] Applies to product made with a sodium aluminum-sulfate type baking powder. With a low-sodium type baking powder containing potassium, value would be about twice the amount shown.
[49] Equal weights of flour, sugar, eggs, and vegetable shortening.
[50] Products are commercial unless otherwise specified.
[51] Made with enriched flour and vegetable shortening except for macaroons which do not contain flour or shortening.
[52] Icing made with butter.
[53] Applies to yellow varieties; white varieties contain only a trace.
[54] Contains vegetable shortening and butter.
[55] Made with corn oil.
[56] Made with regular margarine.
[57] Applies to product made with yellow cornmeal.
[58] Made with enriched degermed cornmeal and enriched flour.
[59] Product may or may not be enriched with riboflavin. Consult the label.
[60] Value varies with the brand. Consult the label.
[61] Weight includes cob. Without cob, weight is 77 g for item 612, 126 g for item 613.
[62] Based on yellow varieties. For white varieties, value is trace.
[63] Weight includes refuse of outer leaves and core. Without these parts, weight is 163 g.
[64] Weight includes core. Without core, weight is 539 g.
[65] Value based on white-fleshed varieties. For yellow-fleshed varieties, value in International Units (I.U.) is 70 for item 633, 50 for item 634, and 80 for item 635.
[66] Weight includes cores and stem ends. Without these parts, weight is 123 g.
[67] Based on year-round average. For tomatoes marketed from November through May, value is about 12 mg; from June through October, 32 mg.
[68] Applies to product without calcium salts added. Value for products with calcium salts added may be as much as 63 mg for whole tomatoes, 241 mg for cut forms.
[69] Weight includes pits. Without pits, weight is 13 g for item 701, 9 g for item 702.
[70] Value may vary from 6 to 60 mg.

index